MW01254051

Statistical Methods for Modeling Human Dynamics

An Interdisciplinary Dialogue

The Notre Dame Series on Quantitative Methodology

Building on the strength of Notre Dame as a center for training in quantitative psychology, the Notre Dame Series on Quantitative Methodology (NDSQM) offers advanced training in quantitative methods for social and behavioral research. Leading experts in data analytic techniques provide instruction in state--of--the--art methods designed to enhance quantitative skills in a selected substantive domain.

Each volume is the outcome from an annual conference that brings together expert methodologists and a workshop audience of substantive researchers. The substantive researchers are challenged with innovative techniques and the methodologists are challenged by innovative applications. The goal of each conference is to stimulate an emergent substantive and methodological synthesis, enabling the solution of existing problems and bringing forth the realization of new questions that need to be asked. The resulting volumes are targeted towards researchers in a specific substantive area, but also contain innovative techniques of interest to pure methodologists.

The books in the series are:

Methodological issues in aging research, co--edited by Cindy S. Bergeman and Steven M. Boker (2006)

Data Analytic Techniques for Dynamical Systems, co--edited by Steven M. Boker and Michael J. Wenger (2007)

Statistical and Process Models for Cognitive Neuroscience and Aging, co--edited by Michael J. Wenger and Christof Schuster (2007)

Statistical Methods for Modeling Human Dynamics: An Interdisciplinary Dialogue, co--edited by Sy-Miin Chow, Emilio Ferrer and Fushing Hsieh (2010)

Statistical Methods for Modeling Human Dynamics

An Interdisciplinary Dialogue

Edited by

Sy-Miin Chow
University of North Carolina at Chapel Hill

Emilio Ferrer
University of California, Davis

Fushing Hsieh
University of California, Davis

Routledge
Taylor & Francis Group
New York London

Routledge
Taylor & Francis Group
270 Madison Avenue
New York, NY 10016

Routledge
Taylor & Francis Group
27 Church Road
Hove, East Sussex BN3 2FA

Printed in the United States of America on acid-free paper
10 9 8 7 6 5 4 3 2 1

International Standard Book Number: 978-1-84872-825-7 (Hardback)

Visit the Taylor & Francis Web site at
http://www.taylorandfrancis.com

and the Psychology Press Web site at
http://www.psypress.com

Contents

PART III: Modeling Interindividual Differences in Change and Interpersonal Dynamics

Preface

We are pleased to present *Statistical Methods for Modeling Human Dynamics: An Interdisciplinary Dialogue*, the fourth volume of the *Notre Dame Series on Quantitative Methodology*. As its title indicates, the focus of this volume is on methodological techniques for examining complex time-related processes from an interdisciplinary perspective. In particular, our purpose for putting this volume together was to integrate approaches to human dynamics from several scientific disciplines.

Human dynamics are complex and comprise multiple processes that unfold over different time scales. The need to consider complex ways of representing change is unavoidable and requires the use of increasingly sophisticated methodology. Two significant changes relevant to quantitative methodology have taken place in areas related to the study of human dynamics. First, traditional behavioral and physiological methods have been expanded by information from neuroscience, particularly in the area of brain imaging, and these methods have revealed a set of important challenges for statistical analysis and mathematical modeling. Second, the theoretical language for investigating human dynamics has been augmented by the inclusion of formal models (mathematical, algorithmic, and computational) of the dynamic processes under study. These advantages present important challenges to both quantitative methodologists and substantive researchers.

While studies of human dynamics have been pursued from a variety of complementary perspectives—neuroscience, computational and mathematical modeling, and traditional biobehavioral assessment—much research is still conducted within disciplinary boundaries. For instance, although researchers in the physical and life sciences have developed methodologies for evaluating more complex patterns of change, some of these techniques remain relatively unfamiliar to behavioral and social scientists.

This volume was developed to address this need for further interdisciplinary exchanges. We have brought together researchers from the fields of psychology, physics, statistics, computer science, engineering, and neuroscience, who can provide different perspectives on ways to study human dynamics. Our goal was to promote the use of state-of-the-art dynamic techniques for analyzing data in the behavioral and social sciences through such interdisciplinary exchanges. With such goals in mind, we have compiled a number of chapters that combine technical advances in statistical methodology with applications in various research areas, including emotion, cognitive psychology, and electrophysiology.

The same need for interdisciplinary exchanges that motivated us to bring researchers from various disciplines is the goal we had in mind when we thought about the interested audience. This volume is addressed to social science researchers with a methodological emphasis, as well as statisticians, computer scientists, engineers, neuroscientists, and researchers in general who believe their questions can only be addressed by an interdisciplinary team and sophisticated methodology.

Because of the different nature of the various contributions, with emphasis from different disciplines and research questions, we have grouped the chapters into three thematic sections: *Parametric and Exploratory Approaches for Extracting Within-Person Nonstationarities*, *Representing and Extracting Intraindividual Change*, and *Modeling Interindividual Differences in Change and Interpersonal Dynamics*. We have chosen these as important topics that define current research in human dynamics. Although each chapter can stand alone and be read separately, the chapters within each section complement each other, providing a broader perspective on the particular theme.

Advances in quantitative methodology typically go hand in hand with improvements in computer programming. The authors of each chapter have generously provided the syntax necessary to run each of the analyses presented in the volume. Most of the computer programs are in R, the ever-expanding language of the statistical and methodological community. Some other codes are written in general programs such as MATLAB®, SAS, and WinBUGS. Yet others are specific to particular types of analysis, such as DyFA. Interested readers can access these computer programs at www.psypress.com/chow and apply the statistical techniques to their own data sets.

In sum, as we believe our initial goals for this volume were worthy, we hope such goals are met so that this volume can serve as a template for ideas on how to model human processes in dynamic terms.

MATLAB is a registered trademark of The MathWorks, Inc. For product information, please contact:

Sy-Miin Chow
Emilio Ferrer
Fushing Hsieh

Acknowledgments

Editing a book is a joint undertaking that needs input and help from many people. We would like to acknowledge such extensive help here. First, we would like to express our appreciation to Steven Boker, the series editor. Dr. Boker developed the idea of the *Notre Dame Series on Quantitative Methodologies* and initiated the meetings at Notre Dame. Since the first conference meeting in 2003, the Notre Dame Series have helped facilitate numerous exchanges of ideas and the pursuit of new research endeavors in many areas of quantitative methodologies. We are indebted to the faculty of the University of Notre Dame and the conference attendants for the many intellectual discourses that helped shape the contents of this volume. We would especially like to thank other previous NDSQM editors and conference organizers for their help and support over the years. They include, again, Steven Boker, Guangjian Zhang, Scott Maxwell, Cindy Bergeman, Michael Wenger, Christof Schuster, Ke-Hai Yuan, and Gitta Lubke. Of course, the Notre Dame Series would not have continued for so long without the kind help and support of the graduate students at Notre Dame. We would like to thank Jiyun Zu, Manshu Yang, Robert Perera, Jeff Spies, Eric Covey, Stacey Tiberio, Stephen Tueller, Tim Brick, and many others for their help in making the past conference a success. We are privileged to contribute with this year's volume.

We would like to thank each of the authors for their major effort in contributing their best work to this volume. Any value of this volume is, clearly, theirs. We tried simply to give coherence to the progression of chapters. We would also like to thank a number of colleagues and friends who generously donated time and expertise to review manuscripts, raise critical questions, provide helpful advice, and, in sum, enhance the quality of each chapter. They are, in alphabetical order, Alexander Aue (University of California, Davis), Daniel Bauer (UNC-Chapel Hill), Ryan Bowles (Michigan State University), Li Cai (UCLA), Patrick Curran (UNC-Chapel Hill), Pascal Deboeck (University of Kansas), Conor Dolan (University of Amsterdam), Stephen Du Toit (Scientific Software International), Michael

Edwards (Ohio State University), Konstantinos Fokianos (University of Cyprus), Stefanos Georgiadis (University of Kuopio), Kevin Grimm (University of California, Davis), Fumiaki Hamagami (University of Virginia), Ellen Hamaker (Utrecht University), David MacKinnon (Arizona State University), Peter Molenaar (Penn State University), James Roberts (Georgia Institute of Technology), Mika Tarvainen (University of Kuopio), Lijuan Wang (Notre Dame University), and Zhiyong Zhang (Notre Dame University). Their help is much appreciated.

In addition, several graduate students at the University of California, Davis, proofread each chapter and provided important editorial comments. These are Laura Castro-Schilo, Jonathan Helm, Hairong Song, and Joel Steele. We appreciate their meticulous and invaluable help.

Our work as coeditors of this volume has been generously supported by the National Science Foundation (grants BCS-0527766, BCS-0826844, and BCS-0827021) and the National Institutes of Health-NINDS (grant R01 NS057146-01). We would also like to thank the National Institute on Aging, the Institute for Scholarship in Liberal Arts (ISLA), and the Office of Research at the University of Notre Dame for funding the series in previous years.

Finally, this volume could in no way have been completed as scheduled without the support and unconditional patience of Debra Riegert at Taylor & Francis. And speaking of patience and support, wholehearted thanks go to our respective families.

1

Introduction and Section Overview

Sy-Miin Chow, Emilio Ferrer, and Fushing Hsieh

1.1 PART I: PARAMETRIC AND EXPLORATORY APPROACHES FOR EXTRACTING WITHIN-PERSON NONSTATIONARITIES

1.1.1 Nonstationarity

Stationarity is a mathematical property that allows a dynamic system to repeat itself indefinitely according to some prescribed laws. Most models of intraindividual change—including longitudinal panel models, time series models, dynamical systems models, and state-space models—assume some level of stationarity. Strict stationarity refers to the invariance of all distributional characteristics of a set of data over time. Weak stationarity, namely invariance of the mean and covariance structures of a data set, is routinely assumed in many modeling contexts.

Stationarity comprises at its core the notion of invariance. This very concept is of fundamental importance to many scientific disciplines, including the field of psychometrics. In particular, much of the research on psychometrics in the past four decades has been motivated in part by the need to search for invariant principles of dynamics or measurement (Harris, 1963; Horn, McArdle, & Mason, 1983; Lord & Novick, 1968; Meredith, 1993; Stevens, 1946). It is fair to say that the quest for invariance has been, and will remain in decades to come, one of the key driving forces behind many scientific endeavors.

In spite of the need to establish invariance principles, nonstationarity may be the norm, as opposed to a source of statistical artifacts, in the study of complex human dynamics (Molenaar, 2004). For instance, evidence for nonstationarities has been reported in studies of psychomotor dynamics (Haken, Kelso, & Bunz, 1985; Molenaar & Newell, 2003), human perceptual rhythms (Lavie, 1977), biomedical and physiological changes (Tarvainen, Georgiadis, Ranta-aho, & Karjalainen, 2006; Weber, Molenaar & Van der Molen, 1992), interpersonal dynamics (Boker & Rotondo, 2003; Newtson, 1993), and emotions (Chow, Hamaker, Fujita, & Boker, in press). Decades of research on change and invariance have led to a renewed perspective, however, on ways to reconcile issues pertaining to nonstationary processes. In particular, contemporary researchers have come to recognize the importance of finding invariance amid nonstationarity and instability.

Nonstationarity has no specific "form." Different dynamic systems can manifest a variety of unknown and yet characteristically distinct forms of nonstationarity. This section of the book includes four chapters focussing on different dynamic techniques for identifying and representing different kinds of nonstationarities in time series data. Central to the four chapters are empirical applications illustrating instances of nonstationarities in intensive repeated measurement data over time. Often, the questions of interest to substantive researchers are not whether we can find evidence for nonstationarities, but rather ways of deducing meaningful, theoretically relevant information while taking such nonstationarities into account. The four chapters provide several practical examples along these lines. The programming codes in the supplementary CD serve as a starting point for readers interested in implementing the algorithms discussed in the chapters.

1.1.2 Section Outline

The chapter by Molenaar and Ram discusses the concept of ergodicity and its relevance in ensuring that the results based on intraindividual variations can be compared with the results derived from interindividual differences. Heterogeneity (across subjects) and nonstationarity are cited as two important causes for nonergodicity. Their discussion is followed by two methods for tracking the ebbs and flows of nonstationary dynamic processes. The first technique, termed extended Kalman filtering with iteration and smoothing (EKFIS), is one possible nonlinear counterpart of the linear Kalman filtering and smoothing techniques considered in a later chapter by Tarvainen (this volume). The EKFIS can be used to estimate linear and nonlinear time-varying processes and parameters over time. Compared with the linear modeling framework adopted by Tarvainen, relaxing the constraints of linearity allows multivariate processes and multiple indicators to be incorporated more readily into the modeling process. The second technique features an approach based on control theory for determining the optimal (and possibly time-varying) external input needed to maintain some desired level of a dynamic process.

Tarvainen considers two empirical examples that utilize classic state-space estimation techniques such as the Kalman filter and the Kalman smoother to handle nonstationarities inherent in electroencephalogram (EEG) and heart rate variability data. In particular, the author demonstrates how autoregressive moving average (ARMA) models with time-varying parameters can be formulated in the frequency domain. Tarvainen illustrates the practical importance of this approach in the analysis of biomedical data.

Gao, Ombao, and Ho present an approach for clustering time series data. They accompany their presentation with an empirical example involving clustering EEG data into normal versus epileptic seizure signals. Wavelet packet analysis is used to extract the time-varying spectral properties of the data on which subsequent clustering is based. The discussion on model fit and selection issues (e.g., to guide the selection of wavelet packet basis and its associated features, and to assess the optimal number of clusters in the sample) is of direct relevance to the work of many behavioral and social scientists.

The chapter by Prado provides a concise introductory account on the basic properties of time-varying autoregressive (TVAR) models, namely autoregressive (AR) models with time-varying AR coefficients, formulated within a dynamic linear modeling framework (West & Harrison, 1997). A simple classifier is built using estimates from a TVAR model to differentiate between the normal and the fatigue state. Guidelines on ways of handling prior information and other pertinent estimation issues within a Bayesian framework are provided.

In sum, the four chapters cover different approaches to handling models with time-varying parameters, either in the time or in the frequency domain. The chapters by Prado as well as Molenaar and Zhu place more emphasis on the former, whereas the chapters by Gao et al. and Tarvainen provide more detailed descriptions from the latter perspective (see also the joint discussion chapter by Ombao and Prado, pp. 155–157). All the empirical examples presented in this section are based on biomedical and physiological data, more notably, EEG data. Such convergence is, of course, no coincidence because EEG data are known to have directly interpretable meaning when divided into different frequency bands (e.g., the delta, theta, alpha, and beta bands). Whether frequency domain analytic techniques can gain wider appeal in the analysis of behavioral data remains an open question. Likewise, the utility of dynamic models with time-varying parameters has not been popularized in the social and behavioral sciences. In our view, such techniques are underutilized in part because many social and behavioral scientists are unfamiliar with the potential of these methods for addressing issues pertaining to change. By presenting the readers with an array of working examples gleaned from other disciplines, we hope to inspire more researchers to explore the many benefits of these techniques.

1.2 PART II: REPRESENTING AND EXTRACTING INTRAINDIVIDUAL CHANGE

1.2.1 Intraindividual Variability and Trends

Part of the complexities of studying human dynamics resides in the myriad intra- and interperson change processes that exist in our daily lives. An important distinction among such change processes was brought up by Nesselroade (1991). Specifically, Nesselroade distinguished between two kinds of intraindividual change processes, namely systematic trends that unfold at a more gradual rate (e.g., over years and decades), and transient fluctuations (occurring, e.g., over days, minutes, and seconds) that are reversible. The latter, generally referred to as intraindividual variability, has received increased recognition as an important source of individual differences (Eid & Diener, 1999; Eizenman, Nesselroade, Featherman, & Rowe, 1997; Hultsch & MacDonald, 2005). However, tools for representing these kinds of less structured, relatively transient change processes are clearly lacking in the literature.

The dividing line between trends and intraindividual variability is not always a salient one. The increased prevalence of intensive repeated measures designs in studies involving neurophysiological and biomedical makers (Cacioppo, Petty, Losch, & Kim, 1986), daily dairy or experience sampling designs (Bolger, Davis, & Rafaeli, 2003; Ong, Bergeman, & Bisconti, 2004), dyadic interaction studies (Ferrer & Nesselroade, 2003; Gottman, Murray, Swanson, Tyson, & Swanson, 2002), and studies of cognitive and sensorimotor performance (Li, Huxhold, & Schmiedek, 2004) has further eroded the traditional gap between trends and intraindividual variability. Systematic trends may very well exist in data that span close intervals (e.g., weeks) and models used to capture trends in one study may serve as an appropriate platform for capturing intraindividual variability in other studies. Researchers thus have to exercise increased sophistication in determining their study designs and modeling strategies of choice. We refer to methods described in this section more generally as methods for representing and extracting *intraindividual change*, and we hope that these approaches would offer the reader even more options for examining human dynamics—trends and intraindividual variability included.

1.2.2 Section Outline

Intraindividual change is a recurring theme that threads through the different chapters in this section. Differential equation models are one possible modeling tool for such change processes. Two chapters in this section (Boker, Deboeck, Edler & Keel; Deboeck & Boker) deal with two related estimation techniques for fitting differential equation models, both based on a cyclic oscillatory model. One technique consists of a single-indicator approach, whereas the other method allows the incorporation of multiple indicators. Particularly worth noting is both approaches' strengths and ease of use in handling irregularly spaced longitudinal data. Stochastic variations of this model have been considered in exact discrete time formulation elsewhere (e.g., Oud & Jansen, 2000; Singer, 1993). The interested reader may refer to the first volume of the Notre Dame Series on Quantitative Methodology (NDSQM) series (Boker & Wenger, 2007) for such modeling alternatives.

The chapter by Craigmille and Peruggia uses cognitive reaction time data to illustrate several methods for detrending data. Detrending—or the removal of trends—is a standard data preprocessing step routinely taken in time series analysis prior to any model fitting. Craigmille and Peruggia propose combining standard detrending techniques such as spline smoothing with an additional normalization step to aid the extraction of trends. Rationales for detrending and practical guidelines for choosing the appropriate detrending technique are also discussed.

Zhang and Browne present a structural equation-based approach for fitting dynamic factor analysis models to ordinal data. Considered to be an extension of Cattell's (Cattell, Cattell, & Rhymer, 1947) *P*-technique model, dynamic factor models combine a factor analytic model with a user's choice of a time series model at the factor level. The ARMA models are one common choice of such time series models and they include many other dynamic models as special cases. The general flexibility afforded by the dynamic factor models makes them especially suited for representing intraindividual variability processes (e.g., Hamilton, 1994; Harvey, 1993). An overview of the key properties of dynamic factor models and a description of the steps involved in fitting these models to ordinal data are provided by the authors.

Finally, Bowles takes on an item response modeling approach to representing intraindividual variability. By presenting a novel approach to capturing within-person, intratask variability, this chapter offers a unique perspective on the conceptualization of change. Using empirical data involving a working memory task, Bowles illustrates how this approach can be used to answer questions concerning age-related differences in intraindividual variability.

1.3 PART III: MODELING INTERINDIVIDUAL DIFFERENCES IN CHANGE AND INTERPERSONAL DYNAMICS

1.3.1 Interpersonal Differences and Dynamics

Much of the contemporary modeling work in the social and behavioral sciences involves making inferences concerning a group of individuals. A goal that typically goes hand in hand with the analysis of systematic change is the study of individual differences in such a change. That is, researchers are interested not only in obtaining characteristics of change that represent population estimates, but also in identifying differences in such estimates across individuals, as well as in relating those differences to other attributes of interest.

Several statistical models are now available that can be used to pursue these goals. Among some of the more commonly adopted techniques are random coefficients models (also known as mixed-effects models, and in certain special cases, multilevel and latent growth models). With such models, researchers can generate estimates that apply to the entire sample—thus, representing the population—as well as unique estimates for each individual. Random coefficients are a central feature of two of the chapters in this section. The remaining chapters address slightly different aspects, namely intergroup dynamics and interpersonal dynamics.

1.3.2 Section Outline

In this section of the book, four chapters address various issues related to the theme of interindividual differences in change and interpersonal dynamics. Cudeck and Harring's chapter deals directly with all the described questions by exploring the possibilities of a random coefficient model for nonlinear repeated measures data. Modeling nonlinear longitudinal data is an important topic, especially in many areas of social and behavioral research where most theories predict nonlinear trajectories over time and the data typically show nonlinear patterns. In spite of this, not many models are commonly used that can capture the nonlinearity of the data, let alone models that attempt to map onto theoretical nonlinear mechanisms. Cudeck et al. attempt all this in their chapter. In particular, they describe a number of alternative models for nonlinear data that are then applied to repeated measures data from one subject. After this, random effects are incorporated for determining the average change pattern for an entire sample as well as individual differences in such changes. One of the strengths of Cudeck et al.'s chapter is the authors' emphasis on different criteria for selecting an appropriate model—or response function—including fit, appropriateness, and interpretability. This balance between the fit of a selected functional form and the substantive utility of the various model parameters is much needed in the application of models to empirical data.

Hamagami, Zhang, and McArdle present in their chapter a mixed effects latent difference score (LDS) model in the context of Bayesian estimation. They compare the use of LDS models for fitting univariate and bivariate repeated measures data under Bayesian estimation and the more standard maximum likelihood via structural equation modeling. The authors use simulations as well as empirical data, and extend their innovative approach for modeling dynamic systems that involve the interrelations of two processes, as they unfold over time. The chapter gives a concise and informative summary of some key distinctions between the Bayesian and structural equation modeling (SEM) frameworks as well as important recommendations about future uses of Bayesian approaches in the social and behavioral sciences.

Wang, Zhang, and Estabrook's chapter includes a model to assess longitudinal mediation of training intervention effects. The authors extend Cole and Maxwell's mediation model (2003) into a multiple group longitudinal AR mediation model that they use to evaluate the effect of training across groups. As the previous chapters do, this chapter addresses issues related to systematic change—in this case, longitudinal changes presumably elicited by training intervention—with interindividual differences—here, differences between groups.

The final chapter by Hsieh, Chen, Chow, and Ferrer presents nonparametric methods and graphical approaches for extracting multivariate dynamics in dyadic interaction. The first nonparametric technique uses the Lempell–Ziv measure of complexity to quantify intervariable differences. The second technique, termed hierarchical segmentation (HS), is used to extract patterns of nonstationarity and identify possible regime changes from multivariate time series data. The graphical approach consists of transition networks. In addition to its use as a data visualization tool, this approach is used to derive statistics for evaluating potential linkages between variables within-person and between individuals. With appropriate adaptations, nonparametric tools such as the ones described in this chapter can be used to explore the tenability of the parametric assumptions imposed in confirmatory models of change, some examples of which have been given throughout this volume.

REFERENCES

Boker, S. M., & Rotondo, J. L. (2003). Symmetry building and symmetry breaking in synchronized movement. In M. Stamenov & V. Gallese (Eds.), *Mirror neurons and the evolution of brain and language* (pp. 163–171). Amsterdam: John Benjamins.

Boker, S. M., & Wenger, M. J. (Eds.). (2007). *Notre dame series on quantitative methodology: data analytic techniques for dynamical systems* (Vol. 1). Mahwah, NJ: Psychology Press.

Bolger, N., Davis, A., & Rafaeli, E. (2003). Dairy methods: Capturing life as it is lived. *Annual Review of Psychology, 54*, 579–616.
Cacioppo, J. T., Petty, R. E., Losch, M. E., & Kim, H. S. (1986). Electromyographic activity over facial muscle regions can differentiate the valence and intensity of affective reactions. *Journal of Personality and Social Psychology, 50*(2), 260–268.
Cattell, R. B., Cattell, A. K. S., & Rhymer, R. M. (1947). P-technique demonstrated in determining psychophysical source traits in a normal individual. *Psychometrika, 12*, 267–288.
Chow, S.-M., Hamaker, E. J., Fujita, F., & Boker, S. M. (in press). Representing time-varying cyclic dynamics using multiple-subject state-space models.
Eid, M. & Diener, E. (1999). Intraindividual variability in affect: Reliability, validity and personality correlates. *Journal of Personality and Social Psychology, 76*(4), 662–676.
Eizenman, D. R., Nesselroade, J. R., Featherman, D. L., & Rowe, J. W. (1997). Intra-individual variability in perceived control in an elderly sample: The MacArthur successful aging studies. *Psychology and Aging, 12*, 489–502.
Ferrer, E. & Nesselroade, J. R. (2003). Modeling affective processes in dyadic relations via dynamic factor analysis. *Emotion, 3*(4), 344–360.
Gottman, J. M., Murray, J. D., Swanson, C. C., Tyson, R., & Swanson, K. R. (Eds.). (2002). *The mathematics of marriage: Dynamic nonlinear models*. Cambridge, MA: MIT Press.
Haken, H., Kelso, J. A. S., & Bunz, H. (1985). A theoretical model of phase transitions in human hand movements. *Biological Cybernetics, 51*, 347–356.
Hamilton, J. D. (1994). *Time series analysis*. Princeton, NJ: Princeton University Press.
Harris, C. W. (Ed.). (1963). *Problems in measuring change*. Madison, WI: University of Wisconsin Press.
Harvey, A. C. (1993). *Time series models* (2nd ed.). Cambridge, MA: MIT Press.
Horn, J., McArdle, J. J., & Mason, R. (1983). When invariance is not invariant: A practical scientist's view of the ethereal concept of factorial invariance. *The Southern Psychologist, 1*, 179–188.
Hultsch, D. F., & MacDonald, S. W. S. (2005). Intraindividual variability in performance as a theoretical window onto cognitive aging. In R. A. Dixon, L. Bachman, & L.-G. Nilsson (Eds.), *New frontiers in cognitive aging* (pp. 65–89). New York: Oxford University Press.
Lavie, P. (1977). Nonstationarity in human perceptual ultradian rhythms. *Chronobiologia, 4*(1), 38–48.
Li, S.-C., Huxhold, O., & Schmiedek, F. (2004). Aging and attenuated processing robustness: Evidence from cognitive and sensorimotor functioning. *Gerontology, 50*(1), 28–34.
Lord, F. M., & Novick, M. R. (1968). *Statistical theories of mental test scores*. Reading, MA: Addison-Wesley Publishing Company.
Meredith, W. (1993). Measurement invariance, factor analysis and factor invariance. *Psychometrika, 58*, 525–543.
Molenaar, P. C. M. (2004). A manifesto on psychology as idiographic science: Bringing the person back into scientific psychology—this time forever. *Measurement: Interdisciplinary Research and Perspectives, 2*(4), 210–218.
Molenaar, P. C. M., & Newell, K. M. (2003). Direct fit of a theoretical model of phase transition in oscillatory finger motions. *British Journal of Mathematical and Statistical Psychology, 56*, 199–214.
Nesselroade, J. R. (1991). Interindividual differences in intraindividual changes. In L. M. Collins & J. L. Horn (Eds.), *Best methods for the analysis of change: Recent advances,*

unanswered questions, future directions (pp. 92–105). Washington, D.C.: American Psychological Association.

Newtson, D. (1993). The dynamics of action and interaction. In L. B. Smith & E. Thelen (Eds.), *A dynamic systems approach to development: Applications* (pp. 241–264). Cambridge, MA: MIT Press.

Ong, A. D., Bergeman, C., & Bisconti, T. L. (2004). The role of daily positive emotions during conjugal bereavement. *Journal of Gerontology: Psychological Sciences, 59B*(4), 168–176.

Oud, J. H. L., & Jansen, R. A. R. G. (2000). Continuous time state space modeling of panel data by means of SEM. *Psychometrika, 65*(2), 199–215.

Singer, H. (1993). Continuous-time dynamical systems with sampled data, errors of measurement, and unobserved components. *Journal of Time Series Analysis, 14*, 527–545.

Stevens, S. S. (1946). On the theory of scales of measurement. *Science, 103*(2684), 677–680.

Tarvainen, M. P., Georgiadis, S. D., Ranta-aho, P. O., & Karjalainen, P. A. (2006). Time-varying analysis of heart rate variability signals with kalman smoother algorithm. *Physiological measurement, 27*(3), 225–239.

Weber, E. J. M., Molennar, P. C. M., & Van der Molen, M. W. (1992). A nonstationarity test for the spectral analysis of physiological time series with an application to respiratory sinus arrhythmia. *Psychophysiology, 29*(1), 55–65.

West, M., & Harrison, J. (1997). *Bayesian forecasting and dynamic models* (2nd ed.). New York: Springer.

Part I

Parametric and Exploratory Approaches for Extracting Within-Person Nonstationarities

2

Dynamic Modeling and Optimal Control of Intraindividual Variation: A Computational Paradigm for Nonergodic Psychological Processes

Peter C.M. Molenaar and Nilam Ram

2.1 INTRODUCTION

In psychology, data analysis proceeds according to a standard approach that is focussed on inferences about states of affairs obtained within a population of homogeneous human subjects. The information that is employed to infer about such states of affairs at the population level is of a particular type, namely interindividual variation (variation between subjects; individual differences). This approach underlies all standard statistical analysis techniques such as analysis of variance, regression analysis, path analysis, factor analysis, and multilevel and mixed modeling techniques. Whether the data are obtained in cross-sectional or longitudinal designs, the statistical analysis is always focussed on the structure of interindividual variation at the population level. Parameters and statistics of interest are estimated by pooling across subjects, which implies that these subjects are assumed to be homogeneous in all relevant respects. This is the hallmark of analysis of interindividual variation: the sums defining the estimators in statistical analysis are taken over different subjects randomly drawn from a population of presumably homogeneous subjects.

It would seem that inferences about states of affairs at the population level obtained by pooling across subjects constitute general findings that apply to each individual subject in the population. Yet, such applications to individual subjects involve a shift in level, namely from the level of interindividual variation in the population to the level of intraindividual variation characterizing the behavior of individual subjects. Is this shift between levels justified?

It has been shown that in general the answer is negative (Molenaar, 2004). Knowledge about the structure of interindividual variation in the population usually cannot be applied at the level of individual subjects making up this population, and vice versa. This is the direct consequence of abstract mathematical–statistical theorems—the so-called classical ergodic theorems. Only if a process is ergodic can one generalize results pertaining to the structure of interindividual variation at the population level to the level of intraindividual variation characterizing the behavior of individual subjects belonging to this population, and vice versa. If a process is nonergodic, then no *a priori* relationships exist between the structures of interindividual and intraindividual variation; hence one cannot generalize from the population level to the level of individual subjects and vice versa. So when is a process ergodic, and when is it nonergodic?

In what follows, we start with the specification of the important concept of ergodicity (Section 2.2). Section 2.3 presents a discussion of one of the two major causes of nonergodicity, namely heterogeneity of subjects. Section 2.4 focusses on the other major cause of nonergodicity, namely time variation of the statistical characteristics of a process (so-called nonstationarity). A new statistical technique (extended Kalman filtering with iteration and smoothing, EKFIS) is introduced to handle nonstationary time series. In Section 2.5, an illustrative application is given of the EKFIS; in Section 2.6, the results of a Monte Carlo study of the EKFIS are presented. Section 2.7 describes the possibility of applying optimal control once a valid process model has been obtained by means of, for example, the EKFIS.

2.2 ERGODICITY

To give a heuristic description of ergodicity, it is helpful to conceive of each human being as an integrated high-dimensional dynamic system, the behavior of which evolves in place and time. In psychology one usually does not consider place, leaving time as the dimension of main interest. The system includes important functional subsystems such as the perceptual, emotional, cognitive, and physiological systems, as well as their dynamic interrelationships. The complete set of measurable time-dependent variables characterizing the system's behavior can be represented as a high-dimensional space, which will be called the behavior space. According to de Groot (1954), the behavior space contains all the scientifically relevant information about a person. The realized values of all measurable variables for a particular individual at consecutive time points then constitute a trajectory (life history) in this behavior space. This trajectory in behavior space is our basic unit of analysis. Accordingly, the complete set of life histories of a population of human subjects can be represented as an ensemble of trajectories in the same behavior space.

We also need a definition of interindividual and intraindividual variation. A standard dictionary definition of variation is "The degree to which something differs, for example, from a former state or value, from others of the same type, or from a standard." The degree to which something differs implies a comparison, either between different replicates of the same type of entity (interindividual variation) or between temporal states of the same individual entity (intraindividual variation). With respect to an ensemble of trajectories in behavior space, interindividual variation is defined as follows: (i) select a fixed subset of variables; (ii) select one or more fixed time points as measurement occasions; and (iii) determine the variation of the scores on the selected variables at the selected time points by pooling across subjects. In contrast, intraindividual variation is defined as follows: (i) select a fixed subset of variables; (ii) select a fixed subject; and (iii) determine the variation of the scores of the single subject on the selected variables by pooling across time points.

We can now pose our main question in more precise terms. Given the same set of selected variables, under which conditions will an analysis of interindividual variation yield the same results as an analysis of intraindividual variation? The general answer to this question is provided by the classical ergodic theorems. The first ergodic theorem was proven by Birkhoff (1931) and can be summarized as follows.

Let (X, μ) be a probability space, where X is a sample space and μ a probability measure. A transformation $T: X \rightarrow X$ is measurable if $T^{-1}(E)$ is measurable for every measurable subset $E \subseteq X$. T is called measure preserving if $\mu(T^{-1}(E)) = \mu(E)$ for every measurable subset $E \subseteq X$. For $x \in X$, the sequence $x, T(x), TT(x) = T^2(x), T^3(x), \ldots,$ is called a trajectory. Birkhoff's ergodic theorem states that if a measure preserving transformation T is ergodic, then, for any integrable function f, the average of f along a trajectory of T is equal almost everywhere to the average of f over the sample space X (cf. Choe, 2005, p. 89; Losato & Mackey, 1994, p. 64). Hence a dynamic law (i.e., the transformation T) defines an ergodic process if it is measure-preserving and if averages taken along a single trajectory (time series analysis of intraindividual variation) equal averages over the sample space (analysis of interindividual variation by pooling across subjects).

More specifically, a Gaussian process is ergodic if it simultaneously obeys two criteria (cf. Hannan, 1970, p. 201). Firstly, it has to be stationary. That is, it has to have constant mean function and sequential covariance function that is invariant under time shifts. Secondly, the behavioral process of each subject in the population has to obey the same dynamic law. This criterion will be referred to as the homogeneity criterion.

In what follows, we will first consider some of the implications of the second homogeneity criterion. Then, in the remainder of this chapter, the focus is on the first stationarity criterion.

2.3 (LACK OF) HOMOGENEITY

The issue is whether populations really consist of members who are homogeneous in all relevant aspects. This issue does not exist in physics. For instance, each molecule in a homogeneous gas obeys the same dynamic laws. And in a finite mixture of ideal gases, each component again consists of identical elements obeying the same dynamic laws. But the issue definitely arises for populations of complex systems such as human beings.

One way in which the homogeneity issue has been addressed in the psychological literature is by scrutinizing the use of average learning curves. The nonequivalence of an individual's learning trend function and the corresponding average trend function pooled across subjects, for instance, is reviewed with several references to the older literature in Sidman (1960, pp. 52–54). From a more general point of view, the distorting effect of aggregation across individuals in linear regression modeling is thoroughly discussed in Hannan (1991). More recently, the topic of aggregation has become prominent in macro-economics (e.g., Aoki, 2002; Forni & Lippi, 1997). A general result of this line of research is that, given an ensemble of time series characterizing the behavior of heterogeneous economic agents, the ensemble average bears no relationship to the individual series making up the ensemble.

In this section, it will be conjectured that heterogeneity is a general characteristic of human populations. Our reasons for this expectation are theoretical, based on the way in which neural networks in human brains develop during embryogenesis and ontogenesis. But first, we concisely address a methodological issue, namely that standard techniques for the analysis of interindividual variation can be surprisingly insensitive to the presence of substantial heterogeneity. This insensitivity will be shown for the standard factor model. Hence, the upshot of this section is that while there are good theoretical reasons for there to be substantial heterogeneity present in human populations, this heterogeneity will remain invisible in standard analyses of interindividual variation. We will point out some serious implications of this state of affairs.

The equation for a standard, centered one-factor model is (henceforth vector-valued variables are denoted by boldface lowercase letters; matrices are denoted by boldface uppercase letters)

$$\mathbf{y}(i) = \mathbf{\Lambda}\eta(i) + \boldsymbol{\varepsilon}(i), \tag{2.1}$$

where $\eta(i) \sim \mathrm{N}(0, 1)$ and $\boldsymbol{\varepsilon}(i) \sim \mathrm{N}(0, \mathbf{\Sigma}_e)$. $x \sim \mathrm{N}(a, b)$ denotes that variable x has normal distribution with mean a and variance b. In this model, $\mathbf{y}(i)$ is the p-variate vector of observed scores for subject i. $\mathbf{\Lambda}$ is the fixed p-dimensional vector of fixed factor loadings. $\eta(i)$ is the factor score of subject i, and $\boldsymbol{\varepsilon}(i)$ is the p-variate vector of measurement errors for subject i. It is always assumed that Equation 2.1 is structurally identifiable by constraining $j - 1$ elements of the jth column of $\mathbf{\Lambda}, j = 2, \ldots, p$.

Notice that in the standard factor model, variables $\mathbf{y}(\mathrm{i})$, $\eta(i)$, and $\boldsymbol{\varepsilon}(i)$ are realizations of random variables having Gaussian distributions with parameters [means, (co-)variances] that are invariant across subjects. For instance, the measurement errors for each subject i are realizations of a p-variate Gaussian distribution with zero mean vector and diagonal covariance matrix $\mathbf{\Sigma}_e$, where both the mean vector and the covariance matrix are invariant across subjects in the population.

It is also assumed that the factor loadings in $\mathbf{\Lambda}$ are fixed; that is, they are invariant across all subjects. This assumption about the factor loadings being fixed is essential in the derivation of the maximum likelihood estimator for the model parameters. In contrast, the equation for a random factor model is shown here:

$$\mathbf{y}(i) = \mathbf{\Lambda}(i)\eta(i) + \boldsymbol{\varepsilon}(i), \tag{2.2}$$

where $\mathbf{\Lambda}(i) \sim \mathrm{N}(\mathbf{\Lambda}, \mathbf{\Sigma}_{\Lambda})$ and $\boldsymbol{\varepsilon}(i) \sim \mathrm{N}(0, \mathbf{\Sigma}_{\varepsilon(i)})$. The factor loadings in Equation 2.2 are no longer fixed, or invariant, across participants. Now $\mathbf{\Lambda}(i)$ has argument i, indicating that each subject has its own subject-specific values for the factor loadings. Instead of being fixed, as in the standard factor model, the factor loadings in the second model are assumed to have a p-variate Gaussian distribution across subjects with mean vector $\mathbf{\Lambda}$ and covariance matrix $\mathbf{\Sigma}_{\Lambda}$. Also, the measurement errors in Equation 2.2 have subject-specific p-variate Gaussian distributions with zero mean vector and diagonal covariance matrix $\mathbf{\Sigma}_{\varepsilon(i)}$.

Clearly, Equation 2.2 represents an extreme case of heterogeneity across subjects. According to Equation 2.2, each subject has an individual one-factor model with subject-specific factor loadings and subject-specific variances of the measurement errors. Yet it can be proven, using straightforward expansions of moments up to fourth order, that Equation 2.2 is indistinguishable from Equation 2.1 in analyses of interindividual variation (Kelderman & Molenaar, 2007). The proof easily generalizes to multi-factor models. Hence, standard factor analysis of intraindividual variation turns out to be insensitive to the presence of substantial degrees of heterogeneity in the population. This finding has been further confirmed in a series of simulation studies, employing longitudinal factor models (Molenaar, 1999) and genetic factor models (cf. Molenaar, 2008a).

To show that heterogeneity actually exists in real human populations, one needs to carry out replicated single-subject time series analysis of intraindividual variation. A principled exposition of the required methodology of replicated multivariate time series analysis is given in Hamaker, Dolan, and Molenaar (2005). Here, a more indirect, theoretical approach will be indicated, which implies that the presence of heterogeneity in psychologically relevant populations has high probability. The focus of this theoretical approach is on nonlinear epigenetic processes underlying the growth of neural networks. The mathematical–biological models explaining these epigenetic processes create endogenous variation that is due to neither genetic nor environmental influences, but is caused by the developmental process itself.

In mathematical biology, a class of successful models has been developed to explain self-organizing epigenetic processes: the class of nonlinear reaction–diffusion models of biological pattern formation. The first model of this kind was formulated by Turing (1952), followed by the classic paper of Gierer and Meinhardt (1972). Presently, the variety of applications of reaction–diffusion models is impressive; see Molenaar (2008a) for an overview. To give one example, Graham, Freeman, and Emlen (1993) present a reaction–diffusion model of developmental instability, which explains, among other things, the occurrence of differences between homologous structures on the left and right sides of bilaterally symmetric organisms. Edelman (1987) argues that left–right differences between homologous brain stem structures within an individual are of the same order of magnitude as analogous differences between subjects. Molenaar, Boomsma, and Dolan (1993) argued that the nonlinear epigenesis of neural growth based on reaction–diffusion models yields individual differences in cortical architecture that are not due to genetic or environmental influences, but are an inevitable outcome of the nonlinear self-organizing processes concerned. It was concluded from a review of inbreeding studies that a large part of what is commonly interpreted as the effect of nonshared environmental influences is in reality due to the effects of nonlinear epigenetics.

The evidence related to nonlinear epigenesis governed by self-organizing reaction–diffusion models suggests that at the microlevel, human brain architecture will be quite heterogeneous. Insofar as human behavior and information processing is dependent upon neural modules or networks, this heterogeneity can be expected to be reflected in psychological measurements. Stated more specifically, insofar as neural modules or networks underlie psychological faculties or factors, their heterogeneity emerging from nonlinear epigenetic processes will lead to factor models like Equation 2.2 with subject-specific factor loadings. Yet standard factor analysis based on models like Equation 2.1 will not detect the presence of such heterogeneity.

Standard factor analysis is often used in applied settings, such as constructing and validating psychological test inventories. The proven insensitivity to heterogeneity of this analysis has serious practical and ethical consequences. For instance, suppose that the items of a test inventory are shown to have high factor loadings in a standard factor analysis based on the first model equation. The test inventory is therefore considered to be reliable and is used in individual assessments. Decisions about individuals are based on the factor scores. Yet the actual factor loadings of individuals may obey the subject-specific factor model given by Equation 2.2, and may deviate substantially from the nominal factor scores obtained in the standard factor analysis. Evidently, this will yield individual assessments and decisions that are biased in arbitrary degrees (see Molenaar, 2008b, for further elaboration in the context of classical test theory).

2.4 NONSTATIONARITY

Having established the biological origins of heterogeneity, we now turn to the other criterion for nonergodicity: nonstationarity. We consider new developments in analyses of nonstationary time series, including some simple applications to simulated data. A general equation for a p-variate time series is as follows. Let $\mathbf{y}(t), t = 0, \pm 1, \pm 2, \ldots,$ denote a p-variate time series, defined as a p-variate random vector indexed by time t. The mean function of $\mathbf{y}(t)$ is in general a p-variate time-varying trend function: $E[\mathbf{y}(t)] = \mu(t)$. It is a function of time t. The sequential covariance function of $\mathbf{y}(t)$ is in general a $(p \times p)$ dimensional time-varying covariance matrix function: $\text{cov}[\mathbf{y}(t_1), \mathbf{y}(t_2)] = \mathbf{\Sigma}(t_1, t_2)$. It is a two-dimensional function of times t_1 and t_2.

In order to estimate the mean and covariance functions when only a single p-variate time series is available, the assumption of weak stationarity is introduced. The assumption of weak stationarity has the same conceptual status in analyses of intraindividual variation as the assumption of homogeneity in analyses of interindividual variation. Weak stationarity involves two assumptions. Firstly, it is assumed that the mean function is invariant in time. That is, $\mu(t) = \mu$. Secondly, it is assumed that the covariance function only depends on relative time differences, and hence reduces to a function of one-dimensional time. That is, $\mathbf{\Sigma}(t_1, t_2) = \mathbf{\Sigma}(t_2 - t_1)$, where the relative time difference $t_1 - t_2$ is called the "lag."

Most commercial software for time series analysis, and most textbooks on time series analysis, invoke the assumption of weak stationarity. In view of the criteria for nonergodicity, however, we need modeling techniques for nonstationary time series. Typical examples of nonstationary time series are repeated observations of learning processes, developmental processes, and transient brain responses. The EKFIS is a newly developed general technique for the statistical analysis of single-participant nonstationary time series (Molenaar, 2007). Although the EKFIS can handle arbitrary nonlinear state-space models with time-varying parameters, we will, for ease of presentation, confine our attention to linear state-space models with time-varying parameters.

Let $\mathbf{y}(t)$ denote a p-variate-observed time series. To ease the presentation, it will first be assumed that $\mathbf{y}(t)$ has zero mean function: $E[\mathbf{y}(t)] = 0$. Removing this assumption is straightforward, as will be indicated in what follows. The linear state-space model for $\mathbf{y}(t)$ can be shown in the following equations [diag-**A** denotes a square matrix **A** with zero off-diagonal elements; $\delta(u)$ is the Kronecker delta, which equals 1 if u is zero and equals zero if u is unequal zero]:

$$\mathbf{y}(t) = \mathbf{\Lambda}[\boldsymbol{\theta}(t)]\boldsymbol{\eta}(t) + \mathbf{v}(t), \tag{2.3a}$$

$$\text{cov}[\mathbf{v}(t), \mathbf{v}(t-u)] = \delta(u)\text{diag} - \mathbf{\Xi}, \tag{2.3b}$$

$$\boldsymbol{\eta}(t+1) = \mathrm{B}[\boldsymbol{\theta}(t)]\eta(t) + \boldsymbol{\zeta}(t+1), \tag{2.3c}$$

$$\text{cov}[\boldsymbol{\zeta}(t), \boldsymbol{\zeta}(t-u)] = \delta(u)\text{diag} - \mathbf{\Psi}, \tag{2.3d}$$

$$\boldsymbol{\theta}(t+1) = \boldsymbol{\theta}(t) + \boldsymbol{\xi}(t+1), \tag{2.3e}$$

$$\text{cov}[\boldsymbol{\xi}(t), \boldsymbol{\xi}(t-u)] = \delta(u)\text{diag} - \mathbf{\Phi}. \tag{2.3f}$$

The first pair of Equations 2.3a and 2.3b describes the way in which an observed p-variate time series $\mathbf{y}(t)$ is related to the latent r-variate state process $\boldsymbol{\eta}(t)$. The $(p \times r)$ dimensional matrix $\mathbf{\Lambda}[\boldsymbol{\theta}(t)]$ is akin to a matrix of factor loadings whose values may depend on a vector of time-varying parameters $\boldsymbol{\theta}(t)$. It describes the linear dependence of $\mathbf{y}(t)$ on $\boldsymbol{\eta}(t)$. The p-variate time series $\mathbf{v}(t)$ represents the measurement error process. Equation 2.3b specifies that the measurement error process consists of p component processes, which are mutually uncorrelated and lack any sequential dependency. We will refer to such a process as a white noise process [this denotation is standard in time series analysis and derives from the fact that the spectrum of $\mathbf{v}(t)$ is flat, like the spectrum of white light].

The second pair of Equations 2.3c and 2.3d describes the evolution of the state process $\boldsymbol{\eta}(t)$ in time. The $(r \times r)$ dimensional matrix $\mathbf{B}[\boldsymbol{\theta}(t)]$ is a matrix of regression coefficients whose values may depend on a vector of time-varying parameters $\boldsymbol{\theta}(t)$. The r-variate time series $\boldsymbol{\zeta}(t)$ represents process noise, which, according to Equation 2.3d, is a white noise process.

It is noted that all parameter matrices in this linear state-space model depend upon $\boldsymbol{\theta}(t)$, which is an s-variate time-varying vector of all unknown parameters. The third pair of Equations 2.3e and 2.3f describes the evolution in time of $\boldsymbol{\theta}(t)$ as a so-called first-order random walk. The s-variate time series $\boldsymbol{\xi}(t)$ represents the process noise in this random walk, which, according to Equation 2.3f, is a white noise process. It can be shown (cf. Young, 2000) that the random walk Equations 2.3e and 2.3f implies that $\boldsymbol{\theta}(t)$ depends only on the local data in the vicinity of t, thus guaranteeing its identifiability.

To fit a linear state-space model with time-varying parameters (Equation 3.3) to a single-subject observed time series $\mathbf{y}(t)$, we first define a new $(r + s)$-dimensional extended state process $\mathbf{x}(t)$ by adding the parameter process $\boldsymbol{\theta}(t)$ to the original state process $\boldsymbol{\eta}(t)$ ($\mathbf{a}'$ denotes the transpose of the column vector $\mathbf{a}$):

$$\mathbf{x}(t)' = [\boldsymbol{\eta}(t)', \boldsymbol{\theta}(t)'].$$

Next the original linear state-space model is rewritten as a nonlinear analog in order to accommodate the new extended state process $\mathbf{x}(t)$:

$$\mathbf{y}(t) = \mathbf{h}[\mathbf{x}(t), t] + \mathbf{v}(t),$$
$$\mathbf{x}(t + 1) = \mathbf{f}[\mathbf{x}(t), t] + \mathbf{w}(t + 1),$$

where $\mathbf{w}(t)' = [\boldsymbol{\zeta}(t)', \boldsymbol{\xi}(t)']$. Notice that $\mathbf{h}[\mathbf{x}(t), t]$ and $\mathbf{f}[\mathbf{x}(t), t]$ are vector-valued nonlinear functions of $\mathbf{x}(t)$. More specifically, each entry of $\mathbf{h}[\mathbf{x}(t), t]$ and $\mathbf{f}[\mathbf{x}(t), t]$ is a linear combination of constants, elements of $\mathbf{x}(t)$ and products of pairs of elements of $\mathbf{x}(t)$.

To fit the nonlinear state-space model with extended state process $\mathbf{x}(t)$ to the observed single-participant time series $\mathbf{y}(t)$, the EKFIS is used. The EKFIS is a recursive estimator in which the estimate of the state process at time $t + 1$, based on information up to and including time $t + 1$, is determined as a function of the estimated state process at the previous time t:

$$\mathbf{x}(t + 1 \mid t + 1) = \mathrm{EKF}[\mathbf{x}(t \mid t), \mathbf{y}(t + 1), \mathbf{P}(t \mid t), \mathbf{f}_x, \mathbf{F}_{xx}, \mathbf{h}_x, \mathbf{H}_{xx}].$$

Terms like $\mathbf{x}(a \mid b)$ denote the estimate of the state process at time a, based on information up to and including time b. $\mathbf{P}(t \mid t)$ is the covariance matrix of $\mathbf{x}(t \mid t)$. Additional terms are the Jacobian $\mathbf{h}_x$ of $\mathbf{h}[\mathbf{x}(t), t]$ [i.e., the matrix of first-order derivatives of $\mathbf{h}[\mathbf{x}(t), t]$ with respect to $\mathbf{x}(t + 1 \mid t)$]; the Jacobian $\mathbf{f}_x$ of $\mathbf{f}[\mathbf{x}(t), t]$ [i.e., the matrix of first-order derivatives of $\mathbf{f}[\mathbf{x}(t), t]$ with respect to $\mathbf{x}(t \mid t)$]; the Hessian $\mathbf{H}_{xx}$ of $\mathbf{h}[\mathbf{x}(t), t]$ [i.e., the tensor of second-order derivatives of $\mathbf{h}[\mathbf{x}(t), t]$ with respect to $\mathbf{x}(t + 1 \mid t)$]; and the Hessian $\mathbf{F}_{xx}$ of $\mathbf{f}[\mathbf{x}(t), t]$ [i.e., the tensor of second-order derivatives of $\mathbf{f}[\mathbf{x}(t), t]$ with respect to $\mathbf{x}(t \mid t)$].

There are several advantages of using EKFIS. First, EKFIS is exact for the linear state-space model with time-varying parameters because it keeps Taylor expansion terms up to second-order. Because the entries of $\mathbf{h}[\mathbf{x}(t), t]$ and $\mathbf{f}[\mathbf{x}(t), t]$ are at most products of pairs of elements of $\mathbf{x}(t)$, the second-order derivatives in $\mathbf{F}_{xx}$ and $\mathbf{H}_{xx}$ consist of constants. Derivatives of order higher than two are all zero. Also, EKFIS uses covariance resetting to make the recursive estimation more robust. Another advantage is that the EKFIS applies not only filtering or recursive estimation of the state process forward in time, but also smoothing or recursive filtering backwards in time. In this way, the information in the observed time series is used optimally. Additionally, EKFIS includes an iteration-within-recursion option, although we will not apply this option because in applications to the linear state-space model with time-varying parameters the second-order linearization of the EKFIS is exact.*

Notice that in Equation 2.3, the variances along the diagonal of $\boldsymbol{\Xi}$ in Equation 2.3b, the diagonal of $\boldsymbol{\Psi}$ in Equation 2.3d, and the diagonal of $\boldsymbol{\Phi}$ in Equation 2.3f do not belong to the parameter vector $\boldsymbol{\theta}(t)$. In principle, it is possible to estimate these variances by means of EKFIS (cf. Tucci, 2004, Chapter 4), but straightforward addition of these variances to $\boldsymbol{\theta}(t)$ is not advisable because then their estimates are not guaranteed to be nonnegative. Presently, we are elaborating an alternative recursive estimation technique for the variances in Equations 2.3b, 2.3d, and 2.3f, which guarantees their being nonnegative. But here we will treat these variances as hyperparameters and estimate them according to an algorithm similar to the one described in Shumway and Stoffer (2006, p. 340), although differing in computational detail. That is, for a given multivariate

* The nonlinear analog of Equation 2.3 only involves products of pairs of states, implying that the Hessian is constant.

time series $\mathbf{y}(t), t = 1, 2, \ldots, T$, starting with trial values for the variances, the following algorithm is carried out: (1) execute the EKFIS for $t = 1, 2, \ldots, T$, while keeping the variances in Equations 2.3b, 2.3d, and 2.3f fixed; (2) compute the Gaussian likelihood and carry out a few iterations to maximize this likelihood with respect to the variances; (3) go to (1) until there is no longer an improvement in the likelihood; (4) (optionally) execute the EKFIS in a final run using the fixed-interval smoothing option.

2.5 ILLUSTRATIVE EKFIS APPLICATION TO A NONSTATIONARY TIME SERIES

To illustrate the use of the EKFIS, we will describe in detail its application to a nonstationary time series that has been generated by the following specific instance of Equation 2.3. In Equation 2.3a, let $\mathbf{y}(t)' = [y_1(t), y_2(t)]$ be a bivariate nonstationary time series that is observed at $t = 1, 2, \ldots, 100$. Furthermore, let $\mathbf{\Lambda}[\boldsymbol{\theta}(t)] = \mathbf{I}_2$, the (2,2)-dimensional unit matrix; $\boldsymbol{\eta}(t)' = [\eta_1(t), \eta_2(t)]$, and $\mathbf{v}(t)' = [v_1(t), v_2(t)]$. This yields $\mathbf{y}(t) = \boldsymbol{\eta}(t) + \mathbf{v}(t), t = 1, 2, \ldots, 100$. In Equation 2.3b, let the diagonal elements of $\mathbf{\Xi}$ (the variances of the measurement errors) be diag-$\mathbf{\Xi} = [0.1, 0.1]$.

To model the evolution of the state process $\boldsymbol{\eta}(t)$, the influence of a univariate time-varying covariate process $u(t)$ is added to Equation 2.3c in the following way: $\boldsymbol{\eta}(t+1) = \mathbf{B}[\boldsymbol{\theta}(t)]\boldsymbol{\eta}(t) + \mathbf{\Gamma}[\boldsymbol{\theta}(t)]u(t) + \boldsymbol{\zeta}(t+1), t = 1, 2, \ldots, 100$. $\mathbf{\Gamma}[\boldsymbol{\theta}(t)]$ is a (2,1)-dimensional matrix (column vector) containing the regression coefficients of $\boldsymbol{\eta}(t+1)$ on $u(t)$. We will discuss this addition shortly. The entries of the (2,2)-dimensional matrix $\mathbf{B}[\boldsymbol{\theta}(t)]$ are chosen as follows: $\beta_{11}(t) = \theta_1(t) = 0.5$; $\beta_{12}(t) = \theta_2(t) = 0$; $\beta_{21}(t) = \theta_3(t) = 0.5$; and $\beta_{22}(t) = \theta_4(t) = 0.5$. Hence, all four parameters in $\mathbf{B}[\boldsymbol{\theta}(t)]$ are constant. The entries of the (2,1)-dimensional matrix $\mathbf{\Gamma}[\boldsymbol{\theta}(t)]$ are chosen as follows: $\gamma_{11}(t) = \theta_5(t) = -0.5$; $\gamma_{21}(t) = \theta_6(t) = 0.5 - 0.01t, t = 1, 2, \ldots, 100$. Hence $\gamma_{11}(t)$ is constant, but $\gamma_{21}(t)$ is time-varying according to a linear trend: $\gamma_{21}(0) = 0.5$ and $\gamma_{21}(100) = -0.5$. In Equation 2.3d, let the diagonal elements of $\mathbf{\Psi}$ (the variances of the state process noise) be diag-$\mathbf{\Psi} = [1.0, 1.0]$. The system of equations implied by the foregoing specifications is

$$
\begin{aligned}
y_1(t) &= \eta_1(t) + v_1(t),\\
y_2(t) &= \eta_2(t) + v_2(t),\\
\eta_1(t+1) &= 0.5\eta_1(t) - 0.5u(t) + \zeta_1(t+1),\\
\eta_2(t+1) &= 0.5\eta_1(t) + 0.5\eta_2(t) + 0.5u(t) + \zeta_2(t+1),\\
\theta_1(t+1) &= \theta_1(t) + \xi_1(t+1) \quad (\text{where } \theta_1(t) = \beta_{11}(t) = 0.5),\\
\theta_2(t+1) &= \theta_2(t) + \xi_2(t+1) \quad (\text{where } \theta_2(t) = \beta_{12}(t) = 0),\\
\theta_3(t+1) &= \theta_3(t) + \xi_3(t+1) \quad (\text{where } \theta_3(t) = \beta_{21}(t) = 0.5),\\
\theta_4(t+1) &= \theta_4(t) + \xi_4(t+1) \quad (\text{where } \theta_4(t) = \beta_{22}(t) = 0.5),\\
\theta_5(t+1) &= \theta_5(t) + \xi_5(t+1) \quad (\text{where } \theta_5(t) = \gamma_{11}(t) = -0.5),\\
\theta_6(t+1) &= \theta_6(t) + \xi_6(t+1) \quad (\text{where } \theta_6(t) = \gamma_{21}(t) = 0.5 - 0.01t),\\
t &= 1, 2, \ldots, 100.
\end{aligned}
$$

The time-varying covariate process $u(t)$ influences the state process. In this illustration $u(t)$ is univariate, but in general it can have arbitrary dimension. The dynamics of $u(t)$ itself are not modeled: $u(t)$ is taken to be given. In the next section, it will be explained how $u(t)$ can be chosen in such a way as to steer the state process $\boldsymbol{\eta}(t)$ in desired directions while optimizing a so-called cost function.

In the present illustration, the univariate covariate process $u(t)$ is generated according to the following model: $u(t+1) = 0.8u(t) + a(t+1)$, where $a(t)$ is Gaussian white noise with variance equal to 1.0. But $u(t)$ can be chosen arbitrarily. For instance, if $u(t) = 1.0$, and hence constant in time, the component $\boldsymbol{\Gamma}[\boldsymbol{\theta}(t)]u(t)$ would represent a possibly time-varying mean trend of the state process $\boldsymbol{\eta}(t)$. This is a standard way of handling arbitrary mean functions $E[\mathbf{y}(t)] = \boldsymbol{\mu}(t)$.

The bivariate observed time series $\mathbf{y}(t)$ is depicted in Figure 2.1. This "single-subject" time series, together with $u(t)$, constitutes the sole input to EKFIS. It is the task of EKFIS to determine which parameters are constant and which are time varying. And for those parameters that are time-varying, EKFIS has to estimate their time-dependent trajectories. In fact, EKFIS estimates time-dependent trajectories for each parameter according to the algorithm described at the end of Section 2.4.

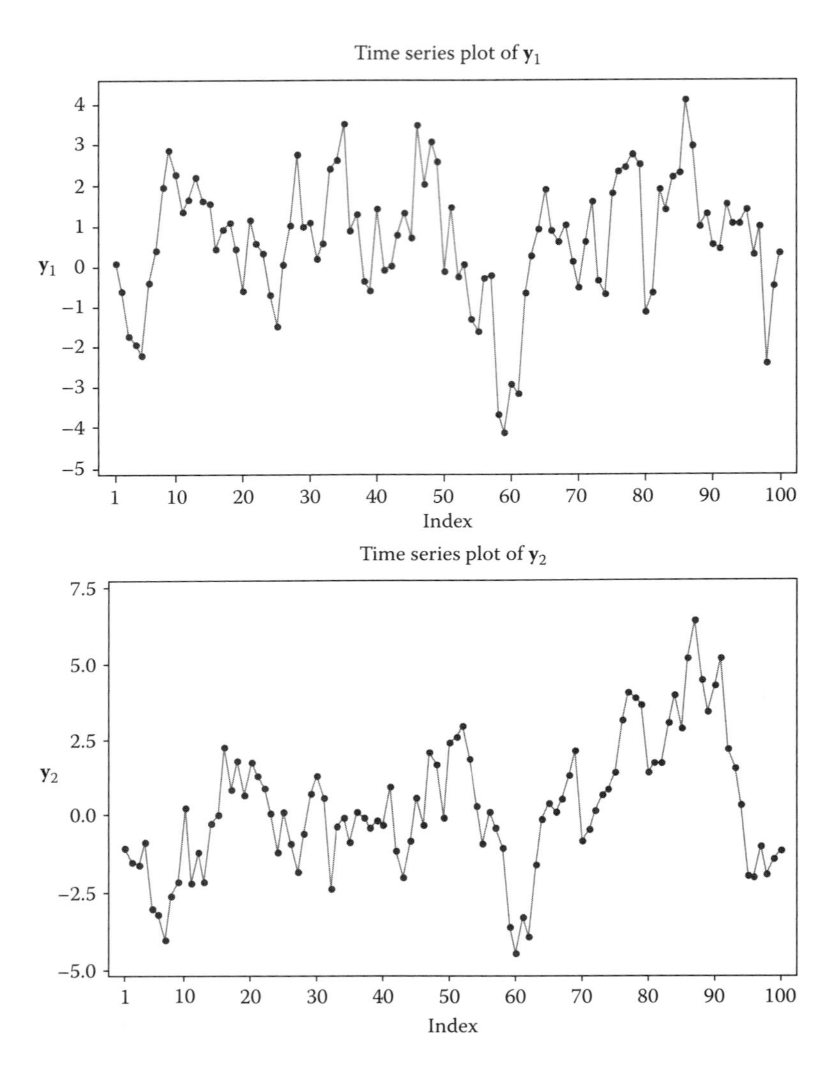

FIGURE 2.1 Single-subject bivariate nonstationary time series (simulated data).

The measurement error variances along the diagonal of $\boldsymbol{\Xi}$ in Equation 2.3b, the variances of the state process noise along the diagonal of $\boldsymbol{\Psi}$ in Equation 2.3d, and the variances of the process noise in the random walk models for the parameters along the diagonal of $\boldsymbol{\Phi}$ in Equation 2.3f are the hyperparameters that are estimated nonrecursively according to an algorithm similar to the one described in Shumway and Stoffer (2006, p. 340). Because the true parameters $\theta_i(t), i = 1, 2, \ldots, 5$, are constant, it is expected that the estimated variances of the process noise in their random walk models will be about zero. This is confirmed in the present application: the estimated variances of $\xi_i(t+1), i = 1, 2, \ldots, 5$, are all negligible. Only the estimated variance of the process noise in the random walk model for $\theta_6(t) = \gamma_{21}(t) = 0.5 - 0.01t, t = 1, 2, \ldots, 100$, is expected to be nonzero. Again, this is confirmed in the present application: the estimated variance of $\xi_6(t+1)$ is 0.006.

Figure 2.2 shows trajectories of two of the estimated parameters. Given the rather extreme shortness of the observed time series as well as the complexity of the fitted model, the estimates turn out to be surprisingly good. In particular, the true linearly time-varying trajectory of $\theta_6(t) = \gamma_{21}(t) = 0.5 - 0.01t$ is well recovered. Although the EKFIS also yields time-varying estimated standard errors for each of the parameter trajectories, we prefer not to present these because they appear to be biased upwards and perhaps have to be estimated by means of bootstrap techniques. This, as well as a host of other issues, will have to be addressed in a series of large scale Monte Carlo studies.

2.6 A MONTE CARLO STUDY

A first application of the EKFIS to empirical data [multivariate nonstationary time series of emotional reactions of (step-)sons to their (step-)fathers] is reported in Molenaar, Sinclair, Rovine, Ram, and Corneal (2009). In what follows, the results of a Monte Carlo study of the EKFIS will be reported in order to further chart the performance characteristics of this new technique.

We use the following simulation model. In Equation 2.3a, let: (1) $y(t)$ be a 5-variate nonstationary time series that is observed at $t = 1, 2, \ldots, 100$; (2) $\mathbf{\Lambda}[\boldsymbol{\theta}(t)]$ be the (5,2)-dimensional matrix of constant factor loadings, the first column of which is $[1.0, 0.8, 0.6, 0.0, 0.0]'$ and the second column of which is $[0.0, 0.0, 0.6, 0.8, 1.0]'$. In Equation 2.3b, let diag-$\mathbf{\Xi} = [0.5, 0.5, 0.5, 0.5, 0.5]$. In Equation 2.3c, let $\mathbf{B}[\boldsymbol{\theta}(t)]$ be the (2,2)-dimensional matrix, the first row of which is $[0.7, 0.0]$ and the second row of which is $[0.5 - 0.01t, 0.7]$. In Equation 2.3d let diag-$\mathbf{\Psi} = [1.0, 1.0]$.

Notice that the element $\beta_{21}(t)$ in $\mathbf{B}[\boldsymbol{\theta}(t)]$ is linearly decreasing between $\beta_{21}(0) = 0.5$ at $t = 0$ and $\beta_{21}(100) = -0.5$ at $t = 100$: $\beta_{21}(t) = 0.5 - 0.01t, t = 1, 2, \ldots, 100$. With this simulation model, 1000 replicates are

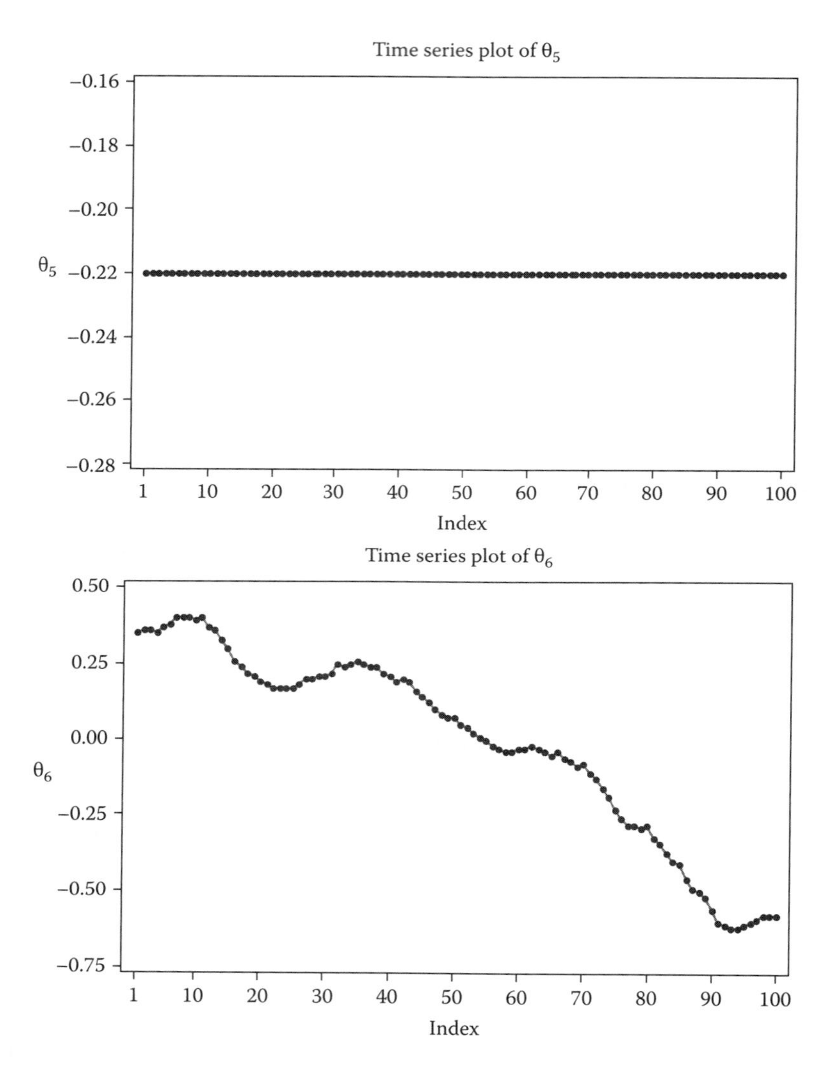

FIGURE 2.2 Estimated time-dependent trajectories of parameters $\theta_5(t)$ and $\theta_6(t)$ in the state-space model for the single-subject bivariate nonstationary time series.

generated. The true model structure is fitted to each replicate by means of the EKFIS, as described in Section 2.5.

The first panel in Figure 2.3 depicts the average of the estimated trajectory of $\beta_{21}(t)$ (solid line), surrounded by $\beta_{21}(t) \pm \sigma_{12}(t)$ (dotted lines), where $\sigma_{12}(t)$ is the standard deviation of estimated values of $\beta_{21}(t)$ at time t across the 1000 replicates. The average estimated trajectory of $\beta_{21}(t)$ appears to be

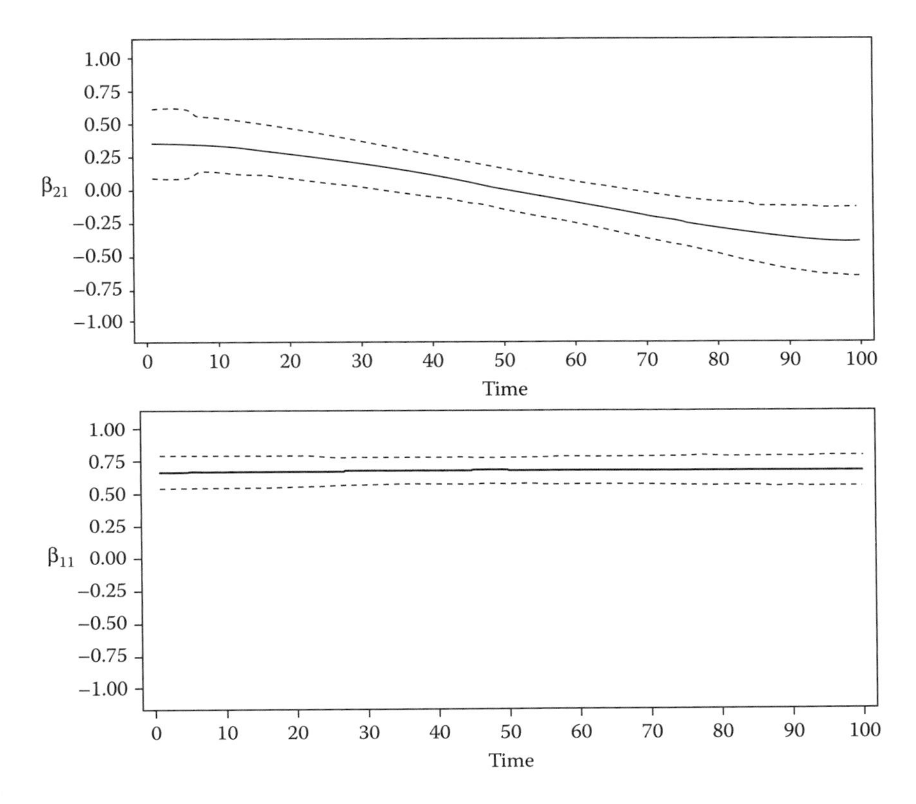

FIGURE 2.3 Averaged estimated trajectories of $\beta_{21}(t)$ and $\beta_{11}(t)$ across 1000 replications in Monte Carlo study of EKFIS.

linearly decreasing, but at a less steep rate than the true trajectory of $\beta_{21}(t)$. The average rate of linear decline of the estimated trajectories of $\beta_{21}(t)$ is -0.009 (standard deviation 0.004 across 1000 replications), whereas it is -0.01 for the true trajectory of $\beta_{21}(t)$.

The second panel in Figure 2.3 depicts the average estimated trajectory of $\beta_{11}(t)$ (same conventions as for the first panel). It appears to be constant in time and close to its true value of 0.7. The average estimated trajectories of the remaining free parameters in $\mathbf{\Lambda}[\boldsymbol{\theta}(t)]$ and $\mathbf{B}[\boldsymbol{\theta}(t)]$ (not shown here) also appear to be constant in time and close to their true values.

It was explained at the close of Section 2.4 that the variances along the diagonal of $\mathbf{\Xi}$ in Equation 2.3b, the diagonal of $\mathbf{\Psi}$ in Equation 2.3d, and the diagonal of $\mathbf{\Phi}$ in Equation 2.3f are treated as hyperparameters that are estimated off-line by means of an algorithm maximizing the likelihood, similar to the algorithm described in Shumway and Stoffer (2006, p. 340). The average estimates of the variances along the diagonal of Ξ in Equation 2.3b (standard deviations across 1000 replications within parentheses) are, respectively, 0.52 (0.16), 0.46 (0.13), 0.42 (0.13), 0.48 (0.12), and 0.49 (0.15). Their true values are 0.5. The average estimates of the variances along the diagonal of $\mathbf{\Psi}$ in Equation 2.3d are both 0.89 (0.23), which is somewhat smaller than their true values of 1.0.

Of special interest are the variances along the diagonal of $\mathbf{\Phi}$ in Equation 2.3f, associated with the random walk model for the time varying parameter vector $\boldsymbol{\theta}(t)$. If a variance along the diagonal of $\mathbf{\Phi}$ is (close to) zero, then this implies that the corresponding parameter is (about) constant in time. It is found that the average variance associated with the parameter $\beta_{21}(t)$ (i.e., the only parameter that is time varying in the true state-space model) is 0.0066. The next largest average variance is 0.0011 (six times smaller); it is associated with the parameter $\beta_{11}(t)$, the average estimated trajectory of which is depicted in the second panel of Figure 2.3 and appears to be constant in time.

The results obtained in this Monte Carlo study, which is part of an ongoing large-scale simulation study, are promising. The EKFIS has been applied to 5-variate manifest time series, corrupted by substantial measurement error and of limited length ($T = 100$), without any *a priori* information about which parameters are constant and which are time varying. Yet, the EKFIS detects which parameters are constant in time and which are time varying, yielding acceptable estimates of their trajectories even though a very preliminary implementation of the algorithm has been used. The implementation of the EKFIS used in this study (and made available to the readership of this book) is preliminary in several respects. For instance, it is computationally suboptimal, does not include robustness checks and options, still lacks the iteration option, and should be amended by adding an intelligent superstructure to further optimize parameter estimation and provide bootstrapped standard errors. Also, the ability to estimate time-varying measurement error variances and process noise variances has to be added. We expect that the development of the EKFIS program along these lines will further improve its fidelity. Last but not least, the present implementation of the EKFIS is not at all user-friendly, requiring writing and compiling separate Fortran subroutines implementing each particular variant of model Equations 2.3a and 2.3c.

2.7 OPTIMAL CONTROL

For quite a long time, there has been the continuing interest of theoretical psychologists in control theory, starting with Miller, Galanter, and Pribam (1960). More recent publications apply control theory for instance to depression (Hyland, 1987), self-regulation of behavior (Carver & Scheier, 1998), and cognition and behavior (Johnson, Chang, & Lord, 2006). As these applications demonstrate, control models have usually been considered in a theoretical context. To the best of our knowledge, control theory has never been used in psychology as a computational tool.

Computational control theory is a vast subject, ranging from simple proportional-integrative-derivative control to advanced techniques such as receding horizon control (Kwon & Han, 2005), neural network control of nonlinear systems (Sarangapani, 2006), or fuzzy control of chaotic systems (Li, 2006). Here, we only summarize the currently most often applied technique: linear–quadratic Gaussian (LQG) control.

Consider again the state-space model used in the illustration in the previous section: $\mathbf{y}(t) = \boldsymbol{\eta}(t) + \mathbf{v}(t), \boldsymbol{\eta}(t+1) = \mathbf{B}[\boldsymbol{\theta}(t)]\boldsymbol{\eta}(t) + \boldsymbol{\Gamma}[\boldsymbol{\theta}(t)]u(t) + \boldsymbol{\zeta}(t+1)$. To reiterate, $u(t)$ is a given (fixed) covariate process. In case it can be manipulated, one can manipulate $u(t)$ in such a way that $\boldsymbol{\eta}(t)$ stays as closely as possible to a desired level. Let $\boldsymbol{\eta}^*(t)$ denote the desired level of $\boldsymbol{\eta}(t)$ (recall that for ease of presentation it is assumed that $E[\mathbf{y}(t)] = E[\boldsymbol{\eta}(t)] = \mathbf{0}$). Because manipulations have their costs (e.g., medication), the desired level of $u(t)$, denoted by $u^*(t)$, is introduced. Based on these definitions, the linear–quadratic cost function $C(u, T)$ is defined (again, for ease of presentation we leave out the final boundary term) as follows:

$$C(u,T) = \sum_{t=1,T-1} \{[\boldsymbol{\eta}(t) - \boldsymbol{\eta}^*(t)]'\mathbf{R}_t[\boldsymbol{\eta}(t) - \boldsymbol{\eta}^*(t)] + [u(t) - u^*(t)]'Q_t[u(t) - u^*(t)]\},$$

where $\mathbf{R}_t$ and Q_t are (2,2)-dimensional and (1,1)-dimensional positive-definite weight matrices, respectively. T is the horizon of the control problem.

The controller chooses $\boldsymbol{\eta}^*(t), u^*(t), \mathbf{R}_t$, and Q_t. $\mathbf{R}_t$ and Q_t are called design parameters in the literature on control theory. These design parameters quantify the considered severity (cost) of deviations of $\boldsymbol{\eta}(t)$ and

$u(t)$ from $\boldsymbol{\eta}^*(t)$ and $u^*(t)$, respectively. Often, the design parameters are identity matrices of appropriate dimensions. The controller's main task is to determine $u(t)$ in such a way that $C(u, T)$ is minimized. For Gaussian $\mathbf{v}(t)$ and $\boldsymbol{\zeta}(t)$, the ensuing LQG control problem is solved (e.g., by means of dynamic programming; cf. Kwon & Han, 2005, Chapter 2) by the feedback relationship

$$u(t)_{\text{opt}} = F_t[\boldsymbol{\eta}(t) \mid \boldsymbol{\eta}^*(t), u^*(t), \mathbf{R}_t, Q_t, T].$$

It can be shown that this feedback law also applies if $\boldsymbol{\eta}(t \mid t)$, the Kalman filtered estimate of $\boldsymbol{\eta}(t)$, is substituted for $\boldsymbol{\eta}(t)$ in F_t. This is called the certainty equivalence principle (cf. Whittle, 1990, chapter 2). Sinclair and Molenaar (2007) present an application of optimal feedback control to an individual psychotherapeutic process.

Feedback–feedforward control: A further elaboration of LQG control is possible when the state process is subject to predictable perturbations. For instance, meals in diabetes patients constitute such predictable perturbations of the body glucose level. This opens up the possibility of applying feedback–feedforward control, where the feedforward part anticipates the predictable perturbations. To examine feedback–feedforward control, we use a simple, bivariate simulation model (cf. Sinclair & Molenaar, 2007, for a more elaborate presentation). Because we intend to apply feedback–feedforward control to optimize treatment of disease processes, such as diabetes type I and asthma, we call this the "patient model":

$$x_1(t+1) = 0.8x_1(t) - 0.3x_2(t) + 0.7u_1(t) + p_1(t),$$
$$x_2(t+1) = 0.5x_1(t) + 0.7x_2(t) + 0.4u_1(t) + p_2(t).$$

The simple illustrative model has constant coefficients and no process noise. The process variables describing the patient are a two-dimensional patient process, x_1 and x_2. For instance, x_1 is the body concentration of insulin and x_2 is the body concentration of glucose. The control variable, $u(t)$, is one-dimensional and could be, for example, the amount of insulin delivered by a pump. The events that can be anticipated are called "predictable perturbations" and are shown as two-dimensional, p_1 and p_2. This could be, for instance, the effects of taking the next meal on body insulin concentration and body glucose level. Again to ease the presentation, it is assumed that all process variables have been centered with respect to steady-state baselines. Hence, positive and negative deflections can be interpreted as fluctuations with respect to these baselines.

The aim of feedback–feedforward control is to minimize $C(u, T)$ defined in the previous section [substituting $\mathbf{x}(t)$ for $\boldsymbol{\eta}(t)$]. The process is started at the initial value of $x_1(0) = 5$ and $x_2(0)$ is 5. We use receding horizon control with a horizon of $T = 4$ time points. Receding horizon control is state of the art in modern control theory (cf. Kwon & Han, 2005). In the simulation, the desired levels of $x_1(t)$, $x_2(t)$, and $u(t)$ are chosen to be zero. $\mathbf{R}_t$ is chosen to be constant in time and diagonal: $\mathbf{R}_t = \mathbf{R} = \text{diag}[0.000001, 1.0]$. Also, Q_t is chosen to be constant in time: $Q_t = Q = 0.000001$. This implies that effectively only deviations of $x_2(t)$ from zero are penalized. That is, we penalize deviations of body glucose level from its baseline. We penalize neither deviations in body insulin nor external insulin delivery. We set predictable perturbations of x_1 to occur at times 3 and 6, denoted as $p_1(3) = 9$ and $p_1(6) = 9$. Predictable perturbations of x_2 occur at times 4, 6, and 8, denoted as $p_2(4) = 9, p_2(6) = 9$, and $p_2(8) = 9$. It is noted that all values used in this simulation model are entirely arbitrary. The only purpose of the simulation is to illustrate the effects of feedback and feedforward control.

Figure 2.4 shows the patient model under various conditions of control. The solid black line is x_1, or body insulin level, and the long dashed line is x_2, or body glucose level. The triangles and circles represent predictable perturbations of body insulin and body glucose, respectively. The short dashed line gives u_1, the optimal feedback control to counteract deviations of x_2 from zero. The top series in Figure 2.4 shows the patient model without exercising control [$u(t) = 0$ for all t]. Note that the short dashed line for the control variable, external insulin, remains at zero. The middle series shows the client process and the time course of optimal control using only feedback. Remember that only deviations of x_2, represented by the long dashed line, from zero are penalized. It is seen that x_2 starts at 5 at time 1. At the next time point, it is driven to zero and stays there until a perturbation occurs. When a predictable perturbation occurs, it momentarily deviates from zero, after which it is driven back again to zero by the feedback control. Meanwhile x_1, depicted by the solid line, and the control u, depicted by the short dashed line, show substantial deviations from zero. This is because these deviations are not penalized.

The bottom series in Figure 2.4 shows the effect of feedback–feedforward control of x_2, depicted by the long dashed line. It is driven to zero from its

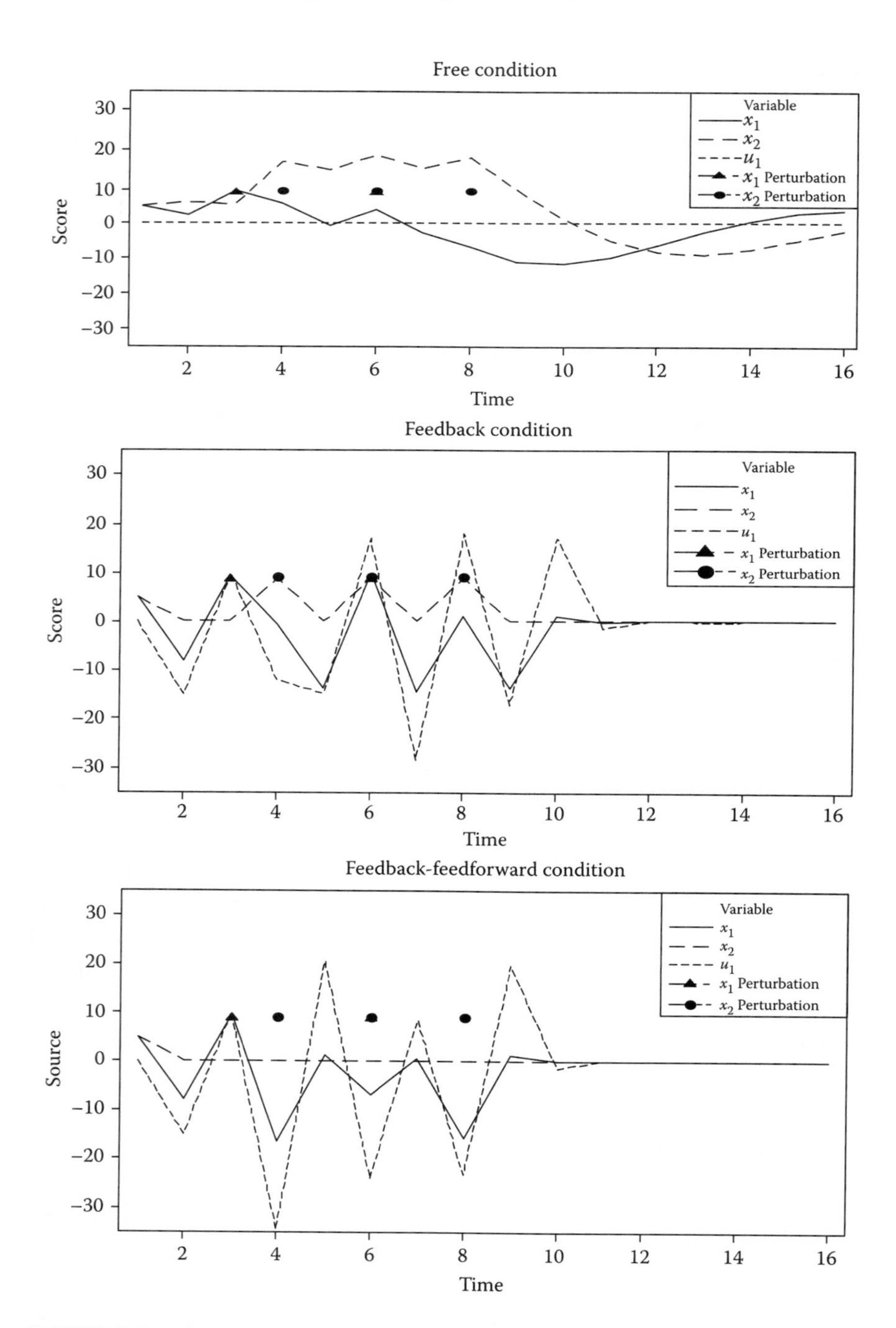

FIGURE 2.4 Behavior of patient model under different conditions of control: free condition (upper panel), feedback control (middle panel), and feedback–feedforward control (lower panel). See text for additional details.

starting value of 5 at time 1, and it stays at zero despite the occurrence of predictable perturbations. This is because the perturbations are anticipated by the model, and the values of x_1 and u adjust to compensate for them prior to their occurrence. Meanwhile x_1, depicted by the solid line, and the control u, depicted by the short dashed line, show substantial deviations from zero.

2.8 CONCLUSION

The classical ergodic theorems imply that single-subject time series analysis is necessary in order to obtain valid results for nonergodic psychological processes. One source of nonergodicity is subject-specificity of the dynamic laws characterizing a process. We have shown that standard factor analysis of interindividual variation is insensitive to the presence of wide-scale subject-specificity. Another source of nonergodicity is nonstationarity of a process. We have presented advanced computational techniques to model and control nonstationary processes.

REFERENCES

Aoki, M. (2002). *Modeling aggregate behavior and fluctuations in economics: Stochastic views of interacting agents*. Cambridge: Cambridge University Press.

Birkhoff, G. (1931). Proof of the ergodic theorem. *Proceedings of the National Academy of Sciences USA, 17*, 656–660.

Carver, C.S. & Scheier, M.F. (1998). *On the self-regulation of behavior*. New York: Cambridge University Press.

Choe, G.H. (2005). *Computational ergodic theory*. Berlin: Springer.

De Groot, A.D. (1954). Scientific personality diagnosis. *Acta Psychologica, 10*, 220–241.

Edelman, G.M. (1987). *Neural Darwinism: The theory of neuronal group selection*. New York: Basic Books.

Forni, M. & Lippi, M. (1997). *Aggregation and the microfoundations of dynamic macroeconomics*. Oxford: Clarendon Press.

Gierer, A. & Meinhardt, H. (1972). A theory of biological pattern formation. *Kybernetik, 12*, 30–39.

Graham, J.H., Freeman, D.C., & Emlen, J.M. (1993). Antisymmetry, directional asymmetry, and dynamic morphogenesis. *Genetica, 89*, 121–137.

Hamaker, E.L., Dolan, C.V., & Molenaar, P.C.M. (2005). Statistical modeling of the individual: Rationale and application of multivariate time series analysis. *Multivariate Behavioral Research, 40*, 207–233.

Hannan, E.J. (1970). *Multiple time series.* New York: Wiley.
Hannan, M.T. (1991). *Aggregation and disaggregation in the social sciences.* Lexington, MA.: Lexington Books.
Hyland, M.E. (1987). Control theory of psychological mechanisms of depression. *Psychological Bulletin, 102,* 109–121.
Johnson, R.E., Chang, C.H., & Lord, R.G. (2006). Moving from cognition to behavior: What the research says. *Psychological Bulletin, 132,* 381–415.
Kelderman, H., & Molenaar, P.C.M. (2007). The effect of individual differences in factor loadings on the standard factor model. *Multivariate Behavioral Research, 42,* 435–456.
Kwon, W.H. & Han, S. (2005). *Receding horizon control: Model predictive control for state models.* London: Springer.
Li, Z. (2006). Fuzzy chaotic systems: *Modeling, control and applications.* Berlin: Springer.
Losato, A., & Mackey, M.C. (1994). *Chaos, fractals, and noise: Stochastic aspects of dynamics.* Berlin: Springer.
Molenaar, P.C.M. (1999). Longitudinal analysis. In H.J. Ader & G.J. Mellenbergh (Eds.), *Research methodology in the social, behavioral and life sciences.* (pp. 143–167). London: Sage.
Molenaar, P.C.M. (2004). A manifesto on psychology as idiographic science: Bringing the person back into scientific psychology, this time forever. *Measurement, 2,* 201–218.
Molenaar, P.C.M. (2007). *EKFIS: Extended Kalman Filtering with Iteration and Smoothing* (computer program) (Technical Report). University Park: The Pennsylvania State University.
Molenaar, P.C.M. (2008a). On the implications of the classic ergodic theorems: Analysis of developmental processes has to focus on intraindividual variation. *Developmental Psychobiology, 50,* 60–69.
Molenaar, P.C.M. (2008b). Consequences of the ergodic theorems for classical test theory, factor analysis, and the analysis of developmental processes. In S.M. Hofer & D.F. Alwin (Eds.), *Handbook of cognitive aging* (pp. 90–104). Thousand Oaks, CA: Sage.
Molenaar, P.C.M., Boomsma, D.I., & Dolan, C.V. (1993). A third source of developmental differences. *Behavior Genetics, 23,* 519–524.
Molenaar, P.C.M., Sinclair, K.O., Rovine, M.J., Ram, N., & Corneal, S.E. (2009). Analyzing developmental processes on an individual level using nonstationary time series modeling. *Developmental Psychology, 45,* 260–271.
Miller, G.A., Galanter, E., & Pribam, K.H. (1960). *Plans and the structure of behavior.* New York: Holt.
Sarangapani, J. (2006). *Neural network control of nonlinear discrete-time systems.* Boca Raton, FL: CRC Press.
Shumway, R.S. & Stoffer, D.S. (2006). *Time series analysis and its applications. With R examples.* New York: Springer.
Sidman, M. (1960). *Tactics of scientific research: Evaluating experimental data in psychology.* New York: Basic Books.
Sinclair, K.O. & Molenaar, P.C.M. (2008). Optimal control of psychological processes: A new computational paradigm. *Bulletin de la Société des Sciences Médicales Luxembourg,* 13–33.
Tucci, M.P. (2004). *The rational expectation hypothesis, time-varying parameters and adaptive control: A promising combination?* Dordrecht: Springer.

Turing, A.M. (1952). The chemical basis of morphogenesis. *Philosophical Transactions of the Royal Society London, B237*, 37–72.

Whittle, P. (1990). *Risk-sensitive optimal control.* Chichester: Wiley.

Young, P. (2000). Stochastic, dynamic modeling and signal processing: Time variable and state dependent parameter estimation. In W.J. Fitzgerald, R.L. Smith, A.T. Walden, & P. Young (Eds.), *Nonlinear and nonstationary signal processing*. Cambridge: Cambridge University Press.

3

Dynamic Spectral Analysis of Biomedical Signals with Application to Electroencephalogram and Heart Rate Variability

Mika P. Tarvainen

3.1 INTRODUCTION

A biomedical signal or biosignal is any signal measurable from the human body. The measurable quantity can be electrical or, for example, changes in pressure or volume. The fundamental aim of biosignal analysis is to obtain information on the physiological or psychophysiological state of the subject or to improve the understanding of functioning and control mechanisms of the particular organ under investigation. Three different approaches to biosignal analysis can be distinguished: analysis of transient events related to some physical stimulus, analysis of spontaneous activity of the measured signal, and correlation analysis of two or more biosignals of different origin. The goal of event-related analysis is to analyze those parts of the signal that are related to some external stimulation. In the analysis of the spontaneous activity of the measured signal, on the other hand, the entire measurement sequence is analyzed. The characteristics of the signal are typically parametrized by calculating different statistics, and it is common to characterize the measurement in the frequency domain by calculating the spectrum of the signal. Finally, by means of correlation analysis it is possible to study the interdependencies between different physiological events.

An important issue in the analysis of biosignals is stationarity. A stationary signal is such that its statistical properties do not change over time. Stationarity is often a desired property since many of the analysis methods, especially the frequency-domain methods where the spectrum of the signal is calculated, require a stationary signal. Unfortunately, biosignals are rarely stationary in the long run. Sometimes the measured signal can, however, be assumed to be piecewise stationary. In such cases, the signal can be divided into stationary segments and each segment can be analyzed separately using traditional methods (Barlow, 1985). When the signal is notably nonstationary such a segmentation cannot be accomplished, and instead time-varying analysis methods are required.

The time-varying spectrum of the signal can be obtained, for example, with time–frequency representation (TFR) methods such as the traditional short-time Fourier transform (STFT) or the wavelet transform (WT), see for example, Akay (1998), Cohen (1989), and Hlawatsch and Boudreaux-Bartels (1992). An alternative approach for calculating TFR is to use time-varying parametric spectrum estimation methods (Haykin, 1991; Kitagawa & Gersch, 1996). A common approach for this method is to use an autoregressive (AR) or autoregressive moving average (ARMA) model with time-varying parameters for the signal. The most challenging task in parametric methods is the estimation of the time-varying model parameters. One solution for this is to use recursive algorithms such as Kalman filter or Kalman smoother (Kalman, 1960; Rauch, Tung, & Strieber, 1965). A detailed introduction to these algorithms can be found, for example, from Anderson and Moore (1979), Gelb (1974), Melsa and Cohn (1978), and Sorenson (1980).

The purpose of this chapter is to provide a brief introduction to dynamic spectral estimation methods and their application to biomedical signals. In this chapter, we will first introduce two different biomedical signals, that is, electroencephalogram (EEG) and heart rate variability (HRV), and provide a brief overview of them. Next, the two most commonly used TFRs, that is, STFT and WT, are described. Following this, the main focus of this chapter, parametric time-varying spectrum estimation methods, will be discussed. After this rather theoretical part, two illustrative case studies are presented. In the first case, the presented methodology is applied in the estimation of event-related sychronization dynamics of EEG. In the second, HRV dynamics during an orthostatic test are examined. Finally, conclusions about the presented dynamic spectrum estimation methods are drawn.

3.2 BIOMEDICAL SIGNALS

3.2.1 Electroencephalography

An EEG is a recording of the electrical activity of the brain. It has been found to be a useful tool for studying the functional state of the brain and for diagnosing certain neurophysiological disorders. In the following, a brief overview of EEG, its measurement and basic properties is given. A more extensive introduction to EEG can be found, for example, from Niedermeyer and Silva (1999).

EEG is usually recorded with Ag/AgCl electrodes. To reduce the contact impedance between the electrode–skin interface, the skin under the electrodes is abraded and a conducting electrode paste is used. The electrode placement should conform to the international 10–20 system (Klem et al., 1999) shown in Figure 3.1.

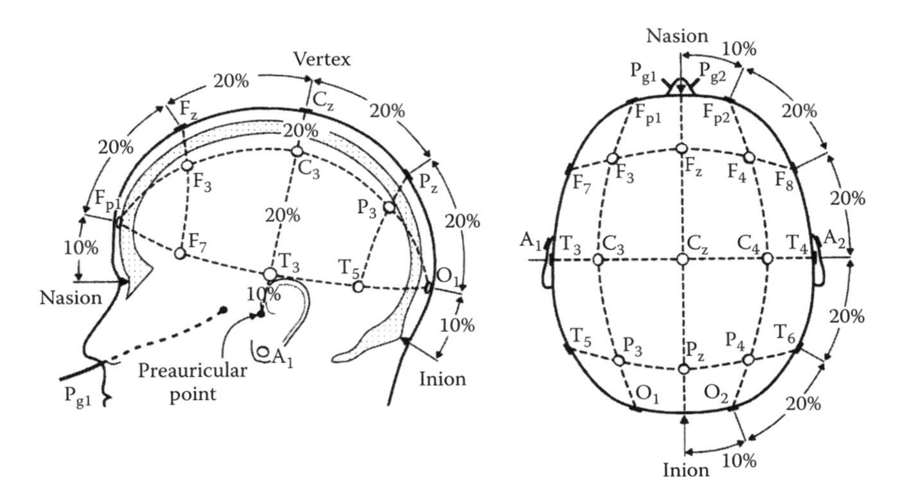

FIGURE 3.1 The international 10–20 electrode system. A = ear lobe, C = central, Pg = nasopharyngeal, P = parietal, F = frontal, Fp = frontal polar, and O = occipital. [Redrawn from Malmivuo, J., & Plonsey, R. (1995). *Bioelectromagnetism: Principles and applications of bioelectric and biomagnetic fields*. Oxford: Oxford University Press (Web Edition).]

One important issue in the recording is the selection of the reference electrode. In common reference recordings, the reference site should be as electrophysiologically inactive as possible. Another approach is to use bipolar recordings that allow EEG activity between two active sites to be recorded. From the EEG recording it is possible to distinguish δ, θ, α, and β waves (Figure 3.2). Both the frequency of the observed rhythm and the site of the synchronized region generating it determine the classification of the signal (Hari & Salmelin, 1997). The frequency content of EEG is confined below 70 Hz and, thus, the minimum sampling rate for acquisition is approximately 200 Hz.

The extent of different quantitative methods applied to EEG recordings is diverse (Jansen, 1991; Nuwer 1988a,b; Pivik et al., 1993). Usually,

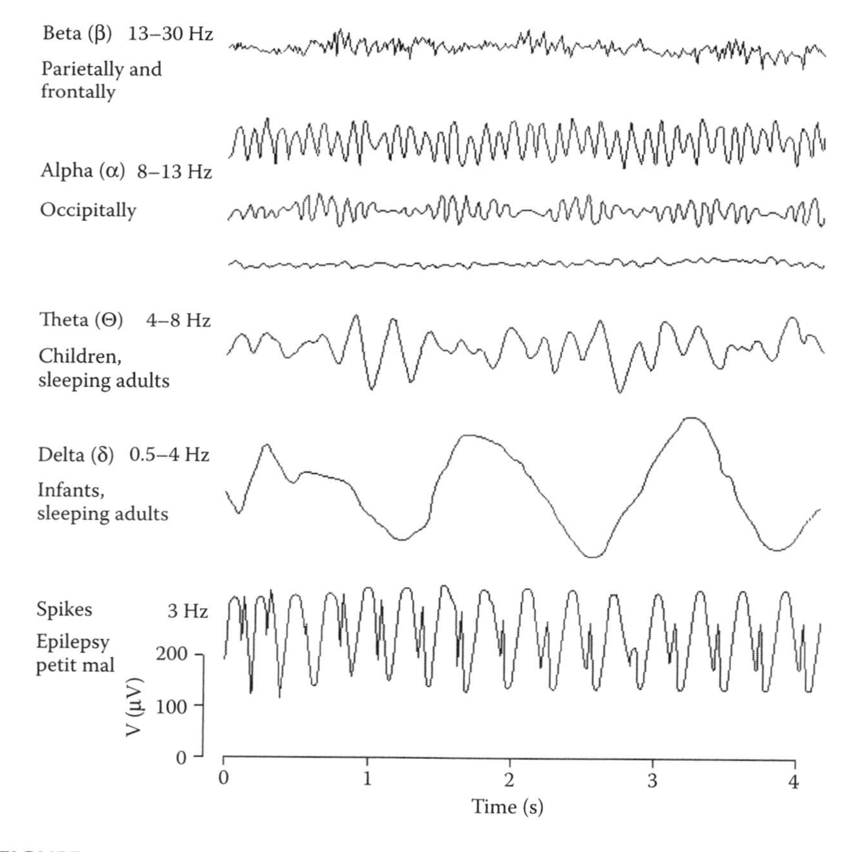

FIGURE 3.2 Some examples of EEG waves. [Redrawn from Malmivuo, J., & Plonsey, R. (1995). *Bioelectromagnetism: Principles and applications of bioelectric and biomagnetic fields.* Oxford: Oxford University Press (Web Edition).]

however, EEG activity is quantified in the frequency domain. Both power and amplitude spectrum representations have been used. The spectrum can be calculated using either nonparametric or parametric methods. In clinical evaluation of EEG, the spectrum is commonly calculated using the Fast Fourier transform (FFT). One important issue in the spectrum estimation is that of stationarity. Usually EEG can be considered to be stationary only within some short intervals. In the study by Cohen and Sances Jr (1977), it was suggested that EEG intervals shorter than 12 s may be considered stationary. In addition, EEG can exhibit several disruptive artifacts such as eye movement or eye blink artifacts. Therefore, the spectrum is usually obtained by averaging spectra computed from several short artifact-free stationary intervals that accurately describe the background activity. The variance of the resulting spectrum depends on the number of epochs.

In quantitative analysis, the EEG spectrum is divided into frequency bands. The classic frequency bands are 0–4 Hz (δ), 5–7 Hz (θ), 8–13 Hz (α), and 14–30 Hz (β) (Nuwer, 1988b). These divisions are not, however, always followed. It is also common to further divide some of the bands, for example, α band to α-I (8–10 Hz) and α-II (10–13 Hz) and β band to β-I (13–20 Hz) and β-II (20–30 Hz). For each band, measures such as absolute power and amplitude, relative power and amplitude, peak frequency, and mean frequency are extracted. In addition, power ratios between specific bands are often used.

The above-described quantitative analysis can be used to study the characteristics of the stationary background EEG activity. However, it is also known that EEG can exhibit considerable short-term nonstationarities, the analysis of which require time-varying spectrum estimation methods or TFRs. One such application is the estimation of event-related synchronization (ERS) and event-related desynchronization (ERD) dynamics of occipital α rhythm.

3.2.1.1 ERS/ERD

EEG activity at the 8–13-Hz frequency band is, in general, called α rhythm (Markand, 1990). To be precise, there are three physiologically distinct α rhythms, namely the classical posterior α occurring during relaxed wakefulness, the Rolandic or central μ rhythm reactive to motor actions, and the midtemporal third rhythm that might sometimes fall into the upper θ band (Niedermeyer, 1997). Here, only the classical posterior α rhythm will be considered.

The posterior α rhythm is best observed from parietal, posterior temporal, and occipital regions of the brain and is, thus, also referred to as occipital α rhythm. The occipital α rhythm is strongest with eyes closed during relaxed wakefulness. This rhythm is attenuated by attention and is usually completely blocked by visual stimulation (e.g., opening the eyes). Such a stimulus-induced attenuation or blocking is called ERD and the opposite phenomenon, ERS (Pfurtscheller & Lopes da Silva, 1999). The ERS/ERD has been differentiated to at least two α components with different spatial characteristics (Klimesch, 1999, Pfurtscheller, Neuper, & Mohl, 1994). In addition, the ERS after eye closure starts up at higher frequency and directly begins to shift to lower frequencies (Markand, 1990). This short-term phenomenon of occipital α rhythm has been called the "squeak" effect. It does not occur every time the eyes are closed, and even though it has not been reported to have any clinical significance (Westmoreland & Klass, 1990) it is a good test for resolution of the TFR analysis method (Tarvainen et al., 2004).

The changes in ERS/ERD are time but not phase-locked to the entailed stimulus, and cannot, therefore, be extracted by simple first-order methods such as averaging, but may be detected by frequency analysis (Pfurtscheller & Lopes da Silva, 1999). A traditional method, which has been used, for example, by Pfurtscheller (1992), Pfurtscheller et al. (1994), and Pfurtscheller and Lopes da Silva (1999), for quantifying ERD dynamics is as follows. First of all, the ERD trials for every stimulus are filtered with a bandpass filter centered at the desired frequency band. The filter outputs are then squared in order to obtain power values. The ERD time course is finally obtained by averaging the squared filter outputs over all trials. In addition, the obtained time courses can be smoothed by averaging over time samples. A drawback of this approach is the rather low-frequency (LF) resolution. Furthermore, the selection of the band limits can be problematic, even though the limits are nowadays usually adjusted individually based on some specific frequency. Another traditional ERD quantification method is the intertrial variance method proposed by Kalcher and Pfurtscheller (1995). In this method, each trial is bandpass filtered and the variance of the filtered trials is calculated for each time point.

An alternative approach is to use a high-resolution TFR method for representing the ERD in the time–frequency plane. This kind of a representation gives a comprehensive picture of the ERD dynamics and no prior frequency band selections are required. In addition, classical ERD parameters, such as power and mean or peak frequency within some specific frequency band, can be easily extracted from the TFR.

3.2.2 Heart Rate Variability

The main task of the heart and cardiovascular system is to provide a sufficient amount of blood delivering nutrients and oxygen to tissues and vital organs; it also participates in body temperature regulation. The work is mainly carried out by the left ventricle of the heart, which pumps blood through the aorta into greater circulation. In different conditions, sufficient blood flow is obtained due to elaborate interacting control systems. The rhythm of the heart is controlled by the sinoatrial (SA) node, which is modulated by both the sympathetic and parasympathetic branches of the autonomic nervous system (ANS). Sympathetic activity tends to increase heart rate (HR↑) and its response is slow (few seconds) (Berntson et al., 1997). Sympathetic innervation also covers the arterial walls and causes vasoconstriction, for example, in physical exertion the vessels of most internal organs contract. Parasympathetic activity, on the other hand, tends to decrease heart rate (HR↓) and mediates faster (0.2–0.6 s) (Berntson et al., 1997). In addition to central control, there are some feedback mechanisms that can provide quick reflexes. One such mechanism is the arterial baroreflex.

The continuous modulation of the sympathetic and parasympathetic innervations results in variation of HR. These variations are commonly analyzed by dividing them into three frequency bands: very low frequency (VLF, 0–0.04 Hz), LF (0.04–0.15 Hz), and high frequency (HF, 0.15–0.4 Hz). The HF band includes the most conspicuous periodic component of HRV, that is, the so-called respiratory sinus arrhythmia (RSA). In addition to the physiological influence of breathing on HRV, this HF component is generally believed to be of parasympathetic origin. Another widely studied component of HRV is the LF component, which includes the component referred to as the 10-s rhythm or the Mayer wave (Berntson et al., 1997). The rhythms within the LF band have been thought to be of both sympathetic and parasympathetic origin (Berntson et al., 1997). even though some researchers have suggested them to be mainly of sympathetic origin (Malliani et al., 1991). The fluctuations below 0.04 Hz, on the other hand, have not been studied as much as the higher frequencies. These frequencies are commonly divided into VLF (0.003–0.04 Hz) and ultra low frequency (ULF, 0–0.003 Hz) bands, but in case of short-term recordings the ULF band is generally omitted (Task Force of the European Society of Cardiology and the North American Society of Pacing and Electrophysiology, 1996). These lowest frequency rhythms are characteristic of HRV signals and have been related to, for example, humoral factors such as thermoregulatory processes and the renin–angiotensin system (Berntson et al., 1997).

Even though HRV has been studied extensively during the last decades, within which numerous research articles have been published, the practical use of HRV has reached some consensus in only two clinical applications (Task Force of the European Society of Cardiology and the North American Society of Pacing and Electrophysiology, 1996). That is, it can be used as a predictor of risk after myocardial infarction (Huikuri et al., 2003; Lombardi, Mäkikallio, Myerburg, & Huikuri, 2001) and as an early warning sign of diabetic neuropathy (Braune & Geisenörfer, 1995; Pagani, 2000). In addition, HRV has been found to correlate with, for example, age, mental and physical stress, and attention (Berntson et al., 1997; Pumprla et al., 2002).

3.2.2.1 Derivation of HRV Time Series

The aim in HRV analysis is to examine the sinus rhythm modulated by the ANS. Therefore, one should technically detect the occurrence times of the SA-node action potentials. This is, however, practically impossible, and thus the fiducial point for the heart beat is usually determined from the ECG recording. The nearest observable activity in the ECG compared to SA-node firing is the P-wave resulting from atrial depolarization (see Figure 3.3) and, thus, the heart beat period is generally defined as the time difference between two successive P-waves. The signal-to-noise ratio of the P-wave is, however, clearly lower than that of the strong QRS complex (a waveform consisting of Q, R, and S waves), which results primarily from ventricular depolarization. Therefore, the heart beat period is commonly evaluated as the time difference between the easily detectable QRS complexes.

Thus, the first step in HRV time series derivation is the detection of QRS complexes. Typically, a QRS detector consists of a preprocessing part followed by a decision-making part. Several different QRS detectors have been proposed within the last few decades (Friesen et al., 1990; Hamilton &

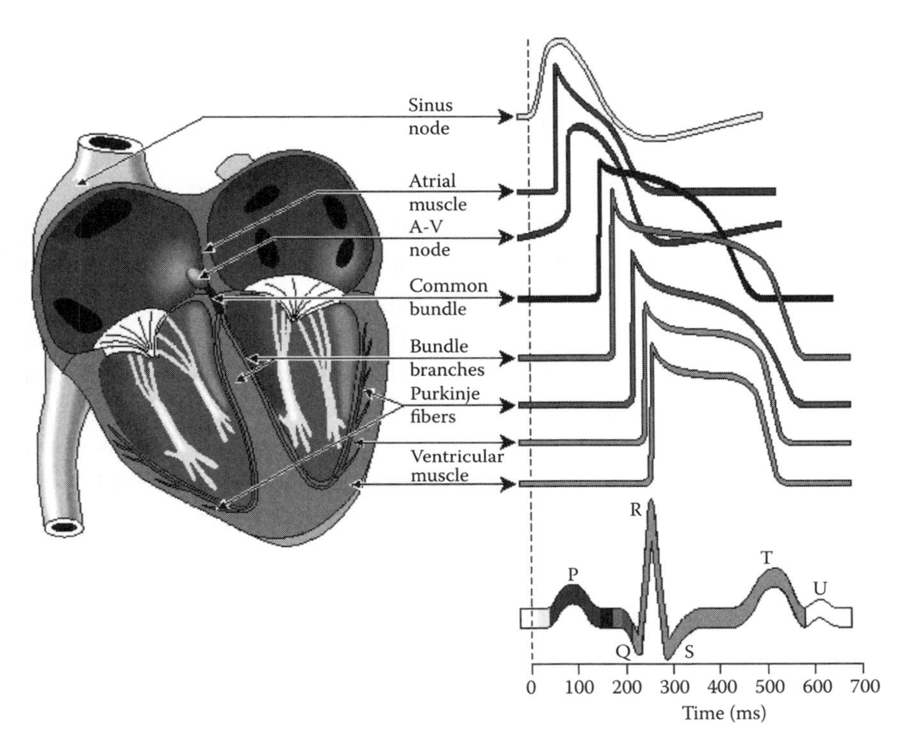

FIGURE 3.3 Electrophysiology of the heart. The different waveforms and their typical latency values for each of the specialized cells found in the heart are shown. [Redrawn from Malmivuo, J., & Plonsey, R. (1995). *Bioelectromagnetism: Principles and applications of bioelectric and biomagnetic fields.* Oxford: Oxford University Press (Web Edition).]

Tompkins, 1986; Pahlm & Sörnmo, 1984; Pan & Tompkins, 1985; Thakor, Webster, & Tompkins, 1983). For an easy-to-read review of these methods, see Afonso (1993). The preprocessing of the ECG usually includes at least bandpass filtering to reduce power line noise, baseline wander, muscle noise, and other interference components. The passband can be set to approximately 5–30 Hz, which covers most of the frequency content of the QRS complex (Pahlm & Sörnmo, 1984). In addition, preprocessing can include differentiation and/or squaring of the samples. After preprocessing, the decision rules are applied to determine whether or not a QRS complex has occurred. The decision rule usually includes an amplitude threshold, which is adjusted adaptively as detection progresses. In addition, the average heart beat period is often used in the decision-making. The fiducial point is generally selected to be the R-wave and the corresponding time instants are given as the output of the detector.

The accuracy of the R-wave occurrence time estimates is often required to be 1–2 ms, and thus the sampling frequency of the ECG should be at least 500–1000 Hz (Task Force of the European Society of Cardiology and the North American Society of Pacing and Electrophysiology, 1996). If the sampling frequency of the ECG is less than 500 Hz, the errors in R-wave occurrence times can cause critical distortion to HRV analysis results, especially to spectrum estimates (Merri et al., 1990). The distortion of the spectrum is even bigger if the overall variability in HR is small (Pinna, et al., 1994). The estimation accuracy can, however, be improved by using a model-based approach for QRS fiducial point correction (Bragge et al., 2005) or by interpolating the QRS complex, for example, by using a cubic spline interpolation (Daskalov & Christov, 1997). It should be, however, noted that when the SA-node impulses are of interest there is an unavoidable estimation error of approximately 3 ms due to fluctuations in the AV-nodal conduction time (Rompelman, 1993).

After the R-wave occurrence times have been estimated, interbeat intervals or RR intervals are obtained as differences between successive R-wave occurrence times, that is, $\mathrm{RR}_n = t_n - t_{n-1}$ (see Figure 3.4). The time series constructed from all available RR intervals is, clearly, not equidistantly sampled, but has to be presented as a function of time, that is as values (t_n, RR_n). This time series is often referred to as HRV time series, even though it contains RR interval values rather than HR values in beats/minute.

One characteristic property of the HRV time series that has to be considered prior to frequency-domain analysis is the fact that it is non-equidistantly sampled. In general, three different approaches have been used to get around this issue (Task Force of the European Society of Cardiology and the North American Society of Pacing and Electrophysiology, 1996). The simplest approach that has been adopted by, for example, Baselli et al. (1987) is to assume equidistant sampling and calculate the spectrum directly from the RR interval tachogram, that is, RR intervals as a function of beat number (see Figure 3.4). This assumption can, however, cause distortion in the spectrum (Mateo & Laguna, 2000). This distortion becomes substantial when the variability is large in comparison with the mean level. Furthermore, the spectrum cannot be considered to be a function of frequency but rather of cycles per beat (DeBoer, Karemaker, & Strackee, 1984). Another common approach adopted here is to use interpolation methods for converting the nonequidistantly sampled RR interval time series to the equidistantly sampled one (Task Force of the European Society of Cardiology and the North American Society of Pacing and Electrophysiology, 1996) (see Figure 3.4). One choice for the interpolation method is the cubic spline interpolation (Mateo & Laguna, 2000). After interpolation, regular spectrum estimation methods can be applied. The third general approach, called the spectrum of counts, considers a series of impulses (delta functions positioned at beat occurrence times) (DeBoer, Karemaker, & Strackee, 1985). This approach relies on the generally accepted integral pulse frequency modulator, which aims to model the neural modulation of the SA node (Rompelman, 1993). According to this model, the modulating signal is integrated until a reference level is achieved, after which an impulse is emitted and the integrator is set to zero. The spectrum of the

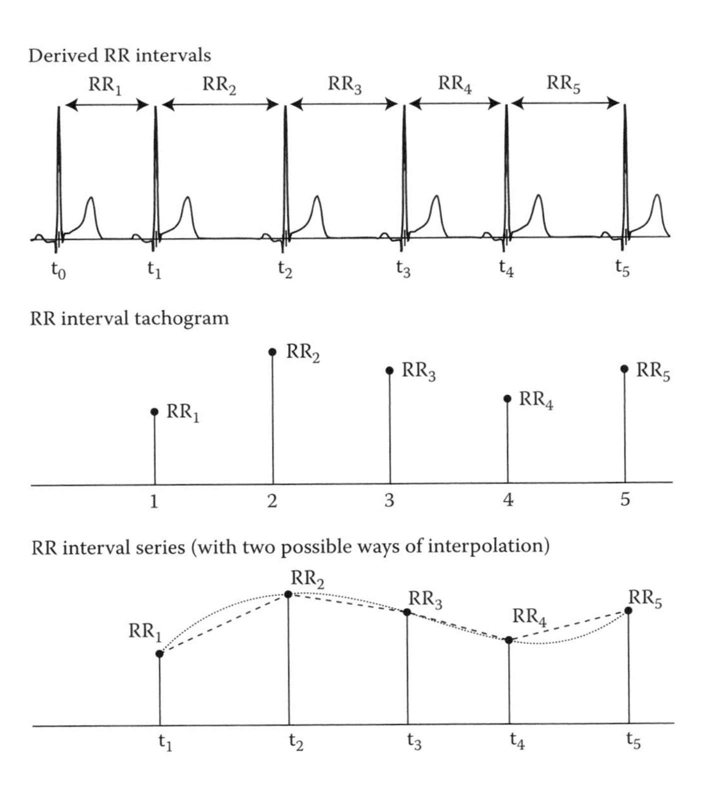

FIGURE 3.4 Derivation of RR interval time series: derivation of RR intervals from ECG (top panel), RR interval tachogram (middle panel), and interpolated RR interval series (bottom panel). In the bottom panel, the trajectories of two interpolation methods, namely cubic spline (dotted line) and linear interpolation (dash line), are illustrated.

series of events can be calculated, for example, by first lowpass filtering the event series and then calculating the spectrum of the resulting signal (DeBoer et al., 1984).

3.3 TIME–FREQUENCY REPRESENTATIONS

A TFR describes the energy density of the observed signal simultaneously in time and frequency. TFR methods can be divided into linear and quadratic methods based on how they depend on the observed signal (Hlawatsch & Boudreaux-Bartels, 1992). Here, two linear TFRs, namely the STFT and the WT, are considered briefly. In addition to these two linear TFRs, various quadratic TFRs such as the Wigner distribution and its numerous smoothed versions have been proposed. For good tutorials on TFR methods, see for example, Akay, (1998); Cohen (1989), and Hlawatsch and Boudreaux-Bartels (1992).

3.3.1 Short-Time Fourier Transform

The STFT consists simply of local spectra of the observation at different times. In the STFT the spectrum at time t is estimated by taking the Fourier transform of the observed signal x_t multiplied with an analysis window w_t centered at time t and the time variation is obtained by sliding the analysis window over the whole signal. In case of discrete time signals, the Fourier transform is computed as a discrete Fourier transform (DFT). The DFT of a signal x_t of N points at frequency f_k is defined as

$$X_{\mathrm{DFT}}(f_k) = \sum_{j=0}^{N-1} x_j \mathrm{e}^{-i2\pi jk/N}, \tag{3.1}$$

where $f_k = kf_s/N$, $k = 0, 1, \ldots, N-1$, and f_s is the sampling frequency. Accordingly, the STFT is obtained by multiplying the signal x_t with a sliding window as

$$X_{\mathrm{STFT}}(t, f_k) = \sum_{j=0}^{N-1} x_j w_{t-j} \mathrm{e}^{-i2\pi jk/N}, \quad f_k = kf_s/N, \tag{3.2}$$

where the analysis window is such that $w_{t-j} > 0$ for $|t-j| < D/2$ and $w_{t-j} = 0$ otherwise. The value $D \ll N$ is the effective length of the analysis window. The time-varying power spectrum estimate is then given as the squared magnitude of the STFT with proper power scaling, that is

$$P_{\mathrm{STFT}}(t, f_k) = \frac{1}{N f_s U} |X_{\mathrm{STFT}}(t, f_k)|^2, \tag{3.3}$$

where U is the energy of the analysis window given as $U = [1/(D+1)] \sum_{j=0}^{D} w_j^2$. The TFR given by the above equation is also commonly known as the spectrogram.

The time–frequency resolution of the spectrogram depends on length D of the analysis window. The frequency resolution is inversely proportional to the window length according to $\Delta f = f_s/D$, whereas the time resolution behaves vice versa. That is, an improvement in the time resolution is obtained by shortening the analysis window. This is demonstrated in Figures 3.5 and 3.6, where spectrograms with two different window lengths are presented for a simulated nonstationary signal. In addition to this trade-off between time and frequency resolutions, one should also notice that the accuracy of Fourier transform may suffer when estimating VLF values from a short sample. In order to get at least somewhat reliable power estimates for a frequency component, the component should have several full cycles within the analysis window.

The STFT given in Equation 3.2 has another useful interpretation as follows. Multiplying the STFT by $e^{i2\pi tk/N}$ on both sides yields

$$X_{\mathrm{STFT}}(t, f_k) = e^{-i2\pi tk/N} \sum_{j=0}^{N-1} x_j w_{t-j} e^{i2\pi(t-j)k/N} \tag{3.4}$$

$$= e^{-i2\pi tk/N} (x_t * w_t e^{i2\pi tk/N}), \tag{3.5}$$

where w_t is assumed to be symmetric. From the above presentation it is observed that STFT can also be interpreted as filtering the observation with a causal filter with impulse response

$$h_t = w_t e^{i2\pi tk/N} \tag{3.6}$$

and multiplying the filter output with phase shift factor $e^{-i2\pi tk/N}$. In frequency domain this filtering corresponds to windowing the

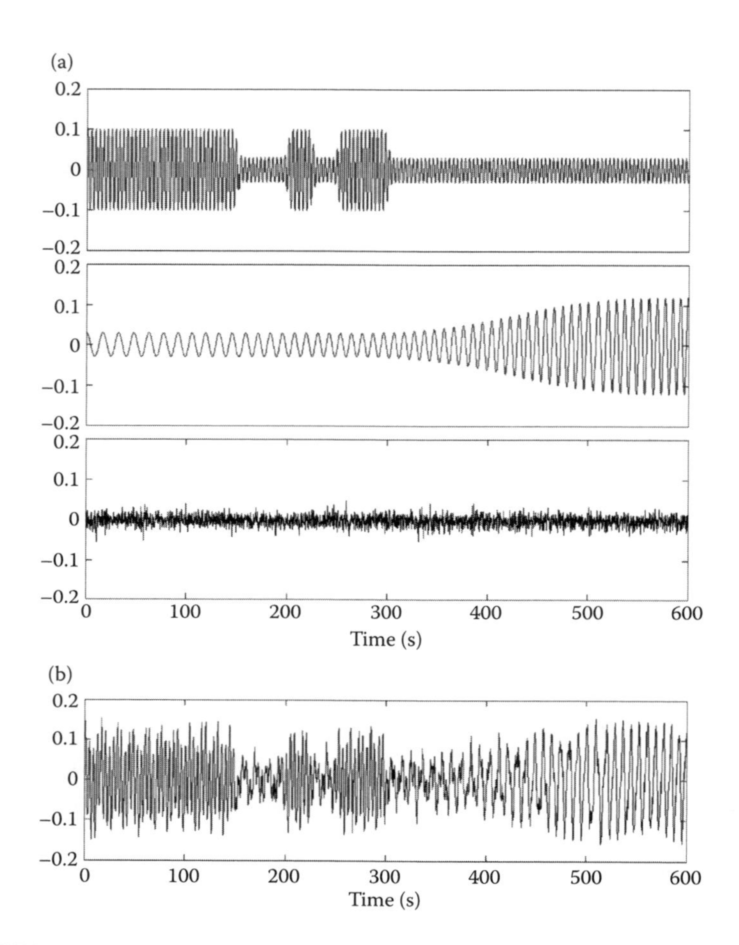

FIGURE 3.5 A simulated nonstationary signal. (a) The simulated signal contains 0.25-Hz sinusoid with varying amplitude (top), chirp signal (frequency shifting from 0.06 to 0.14 Hz) with an abrupt change in frequency (i.e., between 500 and 520 s the frequency is 0.1 Hz) and varying amplitude (middle), and random noise (bottom). (b) The simulated signal is obtained by summing the three signals.

observation spectrum with the window transform centered at frequency f_k. That is

$$x_t * w_t e^{i2\pi tk/N} \leftrightarrow X(f)W(f - f_k). \tag{3.7}$$

In other words, STFT can be interpreted as filtering the observation x_t with a bandpass filter having constant bandwidth for all frequencies f_k.

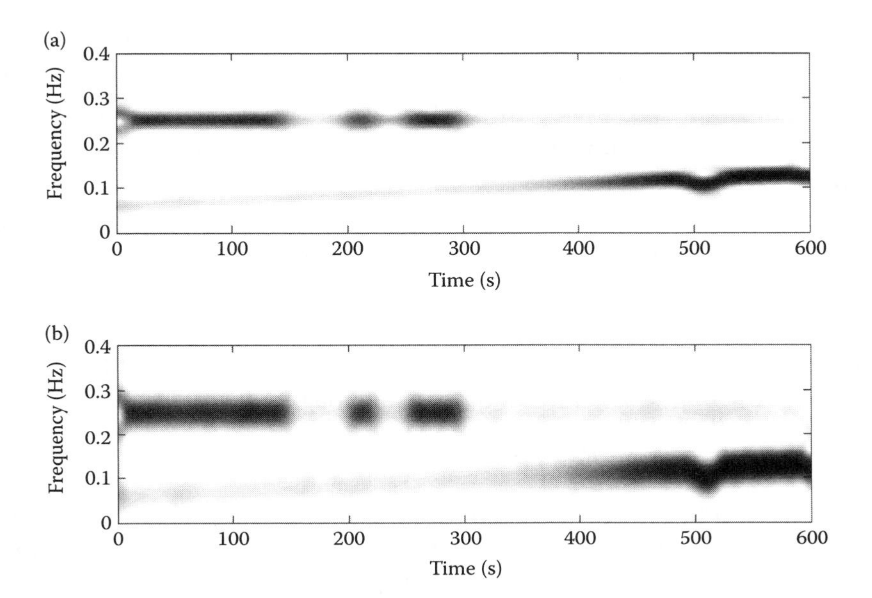

FIGURE 3.6 Spectrograms of the simulated signal shown in Figure 3.5 for (a) 60-s and (b) 30-s window lengths.

3.3.2 Wavelet Transform

The WT is a fairly new TFR method, originally introduced as a time-scale method (Rioul & Vetterli, 1991; Rioul & Flandrin, 1992; Vetterli & Herley, 1992). The WT has a clear interpretational connection to STFT. That is, the WT can also be interpreted as filtering the observed process with a bandpass filter centered at specific frequency. The fundamental difference to STFT is that in WT the bandwidth of the filter is proportional to frequency. The WT has also been termed as a constant-Q transform since the filter quality factor Q defined as the ratio of center frequency and bandwidth is constant (Rioul & Vetterli, 1991). Thus, the WT results in improved time resolution but decreased frequency resolution for higher frequencies and vice versa for lower frequencies.

The continuous wavelet transform (CWT) is defined as

$$X_{\mathrm{CWT}}(\tau, a) = \int x(t)h^*_{a,\tau}(t)\mathrm{d}t = \frac{1}{\sqrt{a}}\int x(t)h^*\left(\frac{t-\tau}{a}\right)\mathrm{d}t, \qquad (3.8)$$

where $h_{a,\tau}(t)$ is the wavelet prototype (of choice to the user) localized in time, a is a scale parameter, τ is a shifting factor, and * denotes complex conjugate. Thus, the wavelet basis is obtained by scaling and shifting in time the single wavelet prototype $h_{a,\tau}(t)$. For large values of a, the wavelet is a stretched LF version of the prototype and for small values of a, a contracted HF version is obtained. If compared to STFT given above, it is noted that in STFT the "analyzing wavelet" is a modulated version of the analysis window.

The CWT can also be seen as an orthonormal basis decomposition and, furthermore, it preserves energy (Rioul & Vetterli, 1991). Therefore, the CWT can be used to define a TFR. The frequency scale for the WT is obtained by substituting $a = f_0/f$, where f_0 is the center frequency of the wavelet (Rioul & Flandrin, 1992). The wavelet spectrum estimate, known as the scalogram, is obtained as the squared magnitude of the CWT

$$P_{\mathrm{CWT}}(\tau, f) = |X_{\mathrm{CWT}}(\tau, f)|^2. \tag{3.9}$$

In the discrete time case, the scale factor a and time shift τ are discretized. In the discretization corresponding to a dyadic time–frequency grid, this is done by setting $a = 2^m$ and $\tau = n2^m\Delta T$, where ΔT is the sampling interval of the discrete signal and m and n are integers (Vetterli & Herley, 1992). The discretized wavelet prototype can be written in the form

$$h_{m,n}(t) = 2^{-m/2}h(2^{-m}t - n\Delta T). \tag{3.10}$$

The fundamental decision in wavelet analysis is how to select the wavelet prototype. Numerous such prototypes have been proposed. One such prototype is the modulated Gaussian function known as Morlet wavelet, which is of the form

$$h(t) = \mathrm{e}^{-(1/2)t^2 + i\omega_0 t}, \tag{3.11}$$

where $\omega_0 = 5.33$. The scalogram of the simulated signal shown in Figure 3.5 obtained by using the Morlet wavelet is presented in Figure 3.7. This simulation shows clearly how the time–frequency resolution of the scalogram changes as a function of frequency.

3.4 PARAMETRIC TIME-VARYING SPECTRUM ESTIMATION

In parametric spectrum estimation, the observed signal is modeled with a parametric model of choice and the spectrum estimate is obtained from

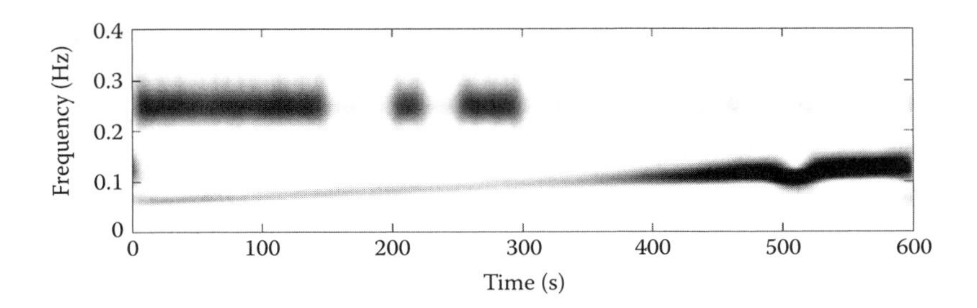

FIGURE 3.7 Scalogram of the simulated signal shown in Figure 3.5.

the estimated model parameters. In time-varying spectrum estimation, the model parameters are considered to be functions of time. The first steps in parametric spectrum estimation are to select the parameter model to be used and its order (i.e., number of parameters). After that, the time-varying parameters need to be estimated. This task can be accomplished by using recursive algorithms such as Kalman filter and Kalman smoother. The whole procedure for parametric time-varying spectrum estimation is presented in the following subsections.

3.4.1 Parametric Models

The most common parametric models used in biomedical signal analysis are the AR, moving average (MA), and mixed ARMA models. Let us start by defining these models for the stationary case.

First of all, the difference between a model and a process needs to be clarified. A signal x_t is said to be an AR process of order p, that is, an AR(p) process, if it satisfies the difference equation

$$x_t = -\sum_{j=1}^{p} a_j x_{t-j} + e_t, \tag{3.12}$$

where $a_1, a_2, \ldots, a_p$ are parameters of the AR model and e_t is a white noise process. A white noise process e_t is a random process with zero mean and its autocorrelation sequence $r_e(\tau) = \sigma_e^2$ when $\tau = 0$ and $r_e(\tau) = 0$ otherwise. In other words, the components of a white noise process are uncorrelated with variance σ_e^2. The correlation sequence can also be presented using the Dirac delta function as $r_e(\tau) = \sigma_e^2\delta(\tau)$. As the term "autoregressive" indicates, the present value of the process x_t is generated (regressed) on the

p previous values $x_{t-1}, \ldots, x_{t-p}$. In addition, randomness is introduced into the process by the noise term e_t.

In AR modeling, the observed signal x_t is technically assumed to be an AR process of some specific order p. Then, the model parameters a_j are estimated so that the prediction error or residual ϵ_t,

$$\epsilon_t = x_t + \sum_{j=1}^{p} a_j x_{t-j}, \tag{3.13}$$

is minimized in some sense. In the case of the AR model, the estimation of parameters is a linear problem. Two common approaches for estimating AR parameters are the Yule–Walker method. This method minimizes the residual variance and least squares methods, which minimize the residual norm (Marple, 1987). It should be noted that if the observed signal x_t is not an AR process, which is basically true for any real life biomedical signal, the residual ϵ_t is not a white noise process.

Another general class of time series models is the MA model. Time series x_t is called an MA process of order q, denoted by MA(q), if it satisfies

$$x_t = \sum_{k=0}^{q} b_k e_{t-k}, \tag{3.14}$$

where $b_0, b_1, \ldots, b_q$ are the MA parameters and e_t is a white noise process. By comparing the AR and MA models it is noted that the white noise process e_t is used in both models. The difference between the models is, however, that in the AR model the value of e_t influences the value x_t and, thereby, also all the future values $x_{t+1}, x_{t+2}, \ldots$. In the MA model, on the other hand, the value of e_t influences only a finite extent of future values of x_t, namely $x_{t+1}, \ldots, x_{t+q}$. This difference accounts for the fact that the autocorrelation function of an MA(q) process cuts off after lag q, whereas the autocorrelation function of an AR(p) process becomes extinct gradually (Priestley, 1981).

A natural generalization of AR and MA models is to combine them to yield a mixed ARMA model. The process x_t is called an ARMA(p, q) process if it satisfies the difference equation

$$x_t = -\sum_{j=1}^{p} a_j x_{t-j} + \sum_{k=0}^{q} b_k e_{t-k}, \tag{3.15}$$

where $a_1, a_2, \ldots, a_p$ and $b_0, b_1, \ldots, b_q$ are the AR and MA parameters, respectively. Clearly, AR and MA models are special cases of an ARMA model. The AR model is obtained by setting $q = 0$ and $b_0 = 1$ in the ARMA model and, correspondingly, the MA model by setting $p = 0$.

The above models were defined for the stationary case. All of these models can also be applied in the nonstationary case by allowing the model parameters to change in time. For example, the time-varying ARMA model is defined as

$$x_t = -\sum_{j=1}^{p} a_t^{(j)} x_{t-j} + \sum_{k=0}^{q} b_t^{(k)} e_{t-k}, \tag{3.16}$$

where $a_t^{(j)}$ is the value of the jth AR parameter at time t and $b_t^{(k)}$ the value of the kth MA parameter at time t. Usually it is assumed that $b_t^{(0)} = 1$.

3.4.2 Model Order Selection

The central problem in the model order determination is the tradeoff between the model fit (i.e., the residual variance) and the model complexity (i.e., the number of model parameters). Suppose that an AR model of order p is fitted into a realization of an AR process of finite order. If the order p is smaller than the true model order, the residual variance σ_ϵ^2 is expected to be larger than the true white noise variance σ_e^2. When p is increased over the true order, on the other hand, the residual variance is not expected to decrease significantly because a white noise process cannot be modeled. Thus, the optimal model order could be determined by plotting the residual variance σ_ϵ^2 as a function of the model order p and selecting the optimal order p from the point where the graph levels off. This method for AR model order determination was proposed by Whittle (1963) and is demonstrated in Figure 3.8.

Various refined versions of the above method have been proposed ever since, for example, the review by Gustafsson and Hjalmarsson (1995). Some of the well-known model order selection criteria are the two developed by Akaike. The first of these is the final prediction error (FPE) criterion, where the model order p is selected so that the term

$$\text{FPE}(p) = \sigma_\epsilon^2 \frac{N + (p+1)}{N - (p+1)}, \tag{3.17}$$

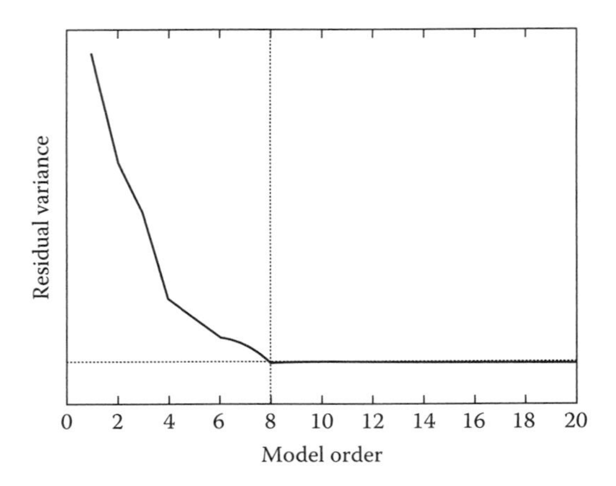

FIGURE 3.8 Residual variance as a function of model order for an AR(8) process. The vertical dotted line indicates the true model order and the horizontal dotted line indicates the variance of the true white noise process.

where N is the length of the signal, is minimized (Marple, 1987). The second criterion proposed by Akaike is Akaike's information criterion (AIC), which is of the form (Marple, 1987).

$$\mathrm{AIC}(p) = N \ln(\sigma_\epsilon^2) + 2p. \tag{3.18}$$

Again the optimal model order p is selected so that $\mathrm{AIC}(p)$ is minimized. AIC has also been used for estimating the AR and MA orders p and q of an ARMA model. This is done by simply replacing p with the sum $p + q$ and calculating $\mathrm{AIC}(p, q)$ for a finite combination of p and q values. Yet another criterion for model order selection is the so-called minimum description length (MDL) criterion, which is given by

$$\mathrm{MDL}(p) = N \ln(\sigma_\epsilon^2) + p \ln(N). \tag{3.19}$$

All the previous model order selection criteria are derived for true AR processes and are therefore known to work well for simulated AR processes. Actual measured biosignals are, however, hardly AR processes. In this case, the model bias increases the residual variance, and therefore affects the model order selection criteria. In other words, the suitability of the model order selection criteria depends on how well the signal is modeled by an AR process. Thus, the model order selection criteria can only be used as guidelines for the model order in real applications.

Basically, the above criteria are designed for the stationary case. The selection of the model order in the nonstationary case is not so straightforward. Some approaches for estimating the model order in the nonstationary case can be found, for example, in Goto, Nakamura, and Uosaki (1995) and Haseyama and Kitajima (2001). For example, in Goto et al. (1995), a modified AIC was used for estimating the order of the AR model along with the model parameters iteratively. In practice, however, the model order is usually fixed according to some prior knowledge or known guidelines. A fixed value for the model order can also be roughly estimated by using some of the criteria from the stationary case.

3.4.3 State-Space Formalism

Let x_t be an output of a time-varying ARMA(p,q) model given in Equation 3.16. The problem is then to estimate the $p + q$ unknown parameters $a_t^{(1)}, \ldots, a_t^{(p)}$ and $b_t^{(1)}, \ldots, b_t^{(q)}$ for each time instance t. This is clearly a highly undeterministic problem, but it can be solved recursively with Kalman filter and smoother algorithms. In the following, the solution of the time-varying parameters is presented only for the ARMA model. Time-varying AR or MA models are not considered separately because the revision of the results for these models is straightforward.

The formulation of Kalman filter and smoother equations is based on the state-space formalism, which is one of the fundamental models of systems theory. The general form of the state-space equations is as follows. Let x_t be the observed signal and θ_t a state vector including the parameters to be estimated. The evolution of the state θ_t is described with a linear equation

$$\theta_{t+1} = F_t\theta_t + G_t w_t, \tag{3.20}$$

where F_t and G_t are known matrices and w_t is a noise process. The observed signal x_t depends on the state θ_t according to the linear observation model

$$x_t = H_t\theta_t + e_t, \tag{3.21}$$

where H_t is a known observation matrix and e_t is a noise process. The observation and state noise processes e_t and w_t are assumed to be uncorrelated zero-mean white noise processes with covariances C_{e_t} and C_{w_t}.

Thus, in order to utilize Kalman filter or smoother algorithms, the time-varying ARMA(p,q) model given in Equation 3.16 needs to be written in the state-space form. This can be accomplished by denoting the AR and MA parameters at time t as

$$\theta_t = (-a_t^{(1)}, \ldots, -a_t^{(p)}, b_t^{(1)}, \ldots, b_t^{(q)})^{\mathrm{T}} \tag{3.22}$$

and the sequences of past observations and noise terms as

$$H_t = (x_{t-1}, \ldots, x_{t-p}, e_{t-1}, \ldots, e_{t-q}). \tag{3.23}$$

Using the above notations the time-varying ARMA(p,q) model can be written in the form

$$x_t = H_t\theta_t + e_t, \tag{3.24}$$

which is formally a linear observation model with H_t being the regression vector and e_t the observation error. Note that the sequence $e_{t-1}, \ldots, e_{t-q}$ in the regression vector is not measured unlike x_t, but it has to be estimated using the Kalman filter or other related smoother algorithms, to be described in the next section. The evolution of the state θ_t when no prior information is available is typically described with a random walk model (Haykin, 1991), yielding a state equation of the form

$$\theta_{t+1} = \theta_t + w_t. \tag{3.25}$$

Equations (3.24) and (3.25) form the state-space signal model for the time-varying ARMA process x_t.

3.4.4 Kalman Filter and Smoother Algorithms

Both Kalman filter and smoother algorithms are recursive algorithms that can be used to estimate the time-varying state vector (i.e., the time-varying ARMA model parameters). The Kalman filter is a real time processing algorithm in which the state estimate is updated immediately after a new observation is available. The Kalman smoother algorithm considered here consists of a Kalman filter algorithm and a fixed-interval smoother. Such a Kalman smoother algorithm estimates each state θ_t based on all the observations, and thus the estimates are expected to be more accurate than the filter estimates. Unlike the Kalman filter, the fixed-interval smoother cannot be used in applications where real time processing is required. In such applications, one might however want to use a different kind of smoother, such as the fixed-lag smoother, which is also suitable for real time processing by introducing only a pre-fixed time lag in the estimation. In addition to Kalman filter and smoother algorithms, there are also some other recursive algorithms that can be used in estimating time-varying parameters of an AR or ARMA model (Haykin, 1991). Two rather popular methods are recursive least squares (RLS) and least mean square (LMS). In fact, both RLS and LMS can be considered as specific versions of the Kalman filter algorithm because they can be derived from the Kalman filter with specific assumptions.

3.4.4.1 Kalman Filter Algorithm

The Kalman filtering problem is to find the linear mean square estimator $\hat{\theta}_t$ for state θ_t given the observations $x_1, x_2, \ldots, x_t$. It can be shown that such a mean square estimate is equal to the conditional mean

$$\hat{\theta}_t = E\{\theta_t | x_1, x_2, \ldots, x_t\}. \tag{3.26}$$

For the derivation of the Kalman filter equations see, for example, Melsa and Cohn (1978). For the state-space equations given in Equations 3.24 and 3.25 (corresponding to a time-varying ARMA model), Kalman filter equations can be written in the form

$$C_{\tilde{\theta}_{t|t-1}} = C_{\tilde{\theta}_{t-1}} + C_{w_{t-1}}, \tag{3.27}$$

$$K_t = C_{\tilde{\theta}_{t|t-1}} H_t^{\mathrm{T}} (H_t C_{\tilde{\theta}_{t|t-1}} H_t^{\mathrm{T}} + C_{e_t})^{-1}, \tag{3.28}$$

$$\epsilon_t = x_t - H_t \hat{\theta}_{t-1}, \tag{3.29}$$

$$\hat{\theta}_t = \hat{\theta}_{t-1} + K_t \epsilon_t, \tag{3.30}$$

$$C_{\tilde{\theta}_t} = (I - K_t H_t) C_{\tilde{\theta}_{t|t-1}}, \tag{3.31}$$

where $\tilde{\theta}_t = \theta_t - \hat{\theta}_t$ is the state estimation error, $\tilde{\theta}_{t|t-1} = \theta_t - \hat{\theta}_{t-1}$ is the state prediction error, and K_t is the Kalman gain vector. Note that the unknown observation noise term e_t is estimated as the one-step prediction error ϵ_t of the observation x_t in every step of the iteration.

3.4.4.2 Kalman Smoother Algorithm

The fixed-interval smoothing problem is to find estimates $\hat{\theta}_t^{\mathrm{S}}$ for each state θ_t given all the observations $x_1, x_2, \ldots, x_N$. The superscript S is used here to refer to smoothed estimates. The mean square estimate for this is equal to the conditional mean

$$\hat{\theta}_t^{\mathrm{S}} = E\{\theta_t | x_1, x_2, \ldots, x_N\}. \tag{3.32}$$

Different approaches for the derivation of the fixed-interval smoothing equations have been presented. Here, the so-called Rauch–Tung–Striebel form (Rauch et al., 1965) of the smoothing equations is adopted. In this approach, the Kalman filter estimates $\hat{\theta}_t$ are assumed to be already determined and the smoothed estimates are obtained by running the filtered estimates backwards in time by taking $t = N-1, N-2, \ldots, 1$. The smoothing recursions for the state estimate and error covariance are then given by

$$\hat{\theta}_t^{\mathrm{S}} = \hat{\theta}_t + A_t(\hat{\theta}_{t+1}^{\mathrm{S}} - \hat{\theta}_t), \tag{3.33}$$

$$C_{\tilde{\theta}_t^{\mathrm{S}}} = C_{\tilde{\theta}_t} + A_t(C_{\tilde{\theta}_{t+1}^{\mathrm{S}}} - C_{\tilde{\theta}_{t+1|t}})A_t^{\mathrm{T}}, \tag{3.34}$$

$$A_t = C_{\tilde{\theta}_t} C_{\tilde{\theta}_{t+1|t}}^{-1}, \tag{3.35}$$

where the filtered estimates are used for the initialization, that is, $\hat{\theta}_N^{\mathrm{S}} = \hat{\theta}_N$ and $C_{\tilde{\theta}_N^{\mathrm{S}}} = C_{\tilde{\theta}_N}$.

3.4.5 Initialization of the Algorithm

First of all, it should be noted that the smoother algorithm does not require any additional specifications, but the ones adopted for the filter algorithm act on the smoothed estimates as well. Thus, only the initialization and operation of the Kalman filter algorithm need to be considered.

To operate the Kalman filter algorithm, initial values for the state estimate $\hat{\theta}_t$ and its error covariance $C_{\tilde{\theta}_t}$ and for the noise covariances C_{w_t} and C_{e_t} need to be specified. In practice, the distribution of the initial state θ_0 is unknown and, therefore, the initial values $\hat{\theta}_0$ and $C_{\tilde{\theta}_0}$ are usually determined by some conventional means. A common approach for the initialization is to set the initial state estimate, for example, to $\hat{\theta}_0 = 0$ and its error covariance, for example, to $C_{\tilde{\theta}_0} = I$ and then to run a short segment from the beginning of data backwards in time. If the initial guess for the error covariance is far from the true one, the error covariance does not necessarily have enough time to converge on the true value. In this case, the backward run may be repeated until convergence is observed. The values obtained for the state estimate and error covariance in the backward run are then used as initial values in the actual forward run of the filter. This kind of initialization is not, however, needed if a sufficient amount of data before the time instant of interest is available.

The state noise covariance C_{w_t} and the observation noise covariance C_{e_t} are the terms that determine the adaptation of the Kalman filter (i.e., the speed of change of the state estimate) through the Kalman gain vector K_t. In the study by Isaksson and Wennberg (1976), $C_{w_t} = \sigma_w^2 I$ and $C_{e_t} = \sigma_e^2 = 1$, where σ_w^2 is the state noise covariance coefficient, I is an identity matrix, and σ_e^2 is the observation noise variance, were used. In this case, however, the observation noise variance has no relation to the true error variance, and thus the state estimates may become meaningless. Another option is to estimate the observation noise variance iteratively at every step of the Kalman filter equations (Tarvainen et al., 2006)

$$\hat{\sigma}_{e_t}^2 = \gamma\hat{\sigma}_{e_{t-1}}^2 + (1-\gamma)\epsilon_t^2, \tag{3.36}$$

where $\gamma < 1$ is an adaptation coefficient [in Tarvainen et al. (2006), $\gamma = 0.95$ was used] and ϵ_t is the one-step prediction error given by Equation 3.29. A similar approach for the observation error variance estimation was adopted at least by Schack et al. (1995).

The state noise covariance, on the other hand, is selected to be diagonal as in Isaksson and Wennberg (1976) and the covariance coefficient σ_w^2 can be adjusted at every step of the Kalman filter equations as

$$\hat{\sigma}_{w_t}^2 = \kappa\hat{\sigma}_{e_t}^2/\hat{\sigma}_{x_t}^2, \tag{3.37}$$

where $\hat{\sigma}_{x_t}^2$ is the estimated variance of the observed signal at time t and κ is an update coefficient through which the adaptation of the algorithm can be adjusted. The observation variance $\hat{\sigma}_{x_t}^2$ can be computed as the variance of n consecutive observations preceding the time instant t, that is the variance of $x_t, x_{t-1}, \ldots, x_{t-n+1}$. The observation variance is included in order to remove the influence of signal amplitude on the estimates (Bohlin, 1977). In this way, the update coefficient does not basically need to be selected separately for signals with different variance levels. The adaptation of the algorithm can be increased by increasing κ. The variance of the state estimates is, however, inversely proportional to the value of κ and, therefore, κ

should be specified in such a way that a desired balance between the filter adaptation and estimate variance is obtained.

3.4.6 Parametric Spectrum Estimates

Consider next that the observed signal x_t is a time-varying ARMA(p,q) process satisfying the difference equations given in Equation 3.16. That is, x_t is an output of a linear time-varying filter with white noise input. Then, the power spectrum of x_t at time t is given from the momentary system coefficients as

$$P_{\text{ARMA}}(t,f) = \sigma_{\text{e}}^2(t)/f_{\text{s}} \frac{|1 + \sum_{k=1}^{q} b_t^{(k)} \mathrm{e}^{-i2\pi kf/f_{\text{s}}}|^2}{|1 + \sum_{j=1}^{p} a_t^{(j)} \mathrm{e}^{-i2\pi jf/f_{\text{s}}}|^2}, \qquad (3.38)$$

where $a_t^{(j)}$ and $b_t^{(k)}$ are the time-varying AR and MA model coefficients and $\sigma_e^2(t)$ is the variance of the white noise process e_t at time t. By considering the form of (3.38), it is easily observed that the term $\sigma_e^2(t)/f_s$ corresponds to the power spectrum of the white noise process e_t and the rational function corresponds to the power spectrum of the linear filter.

An estimate of the time-varying ARMA spectrum is obtained by substituting the ARMA coefficient estimates $\hat{a}_t^{(j)}$ and $\hat{b}_t^{(k)}$ and the estimated white noise variance $\hat{\sigma}_e^2(t)$. The ARMA coefficient estimates are obtained from the state estimates $\hat{\theta}_t$ calculated with the Kalman filter of smoother algorithms. The variance of the unknown white noise process e_t, on the other hand, is approximated with the variance of the observation error term ϵ_t.

Note that Equation 3.38 is a continuous function of frequency and can, thus, be evaluated at any desired frequencies up to the Nyquist frequency $f_s/2$. However, the frequency resolution is naturally not infinite, but is determined by the underlying parametric model, that is, the model structure and model order. The characteristics of Kalman filter or smoother spectra depend strongly on the order of the parametric model. As a rule of thumb it can be said that a smaller model order results in a smoother spectrum and a too high model order can produce spurious peaks in the spectrum, but in any case the order of the AR part should be at least twice the number of expected peaks in the spectrum. When compared to classical FFT-based spectrum estimation methods, the resolution of parametric methods is in

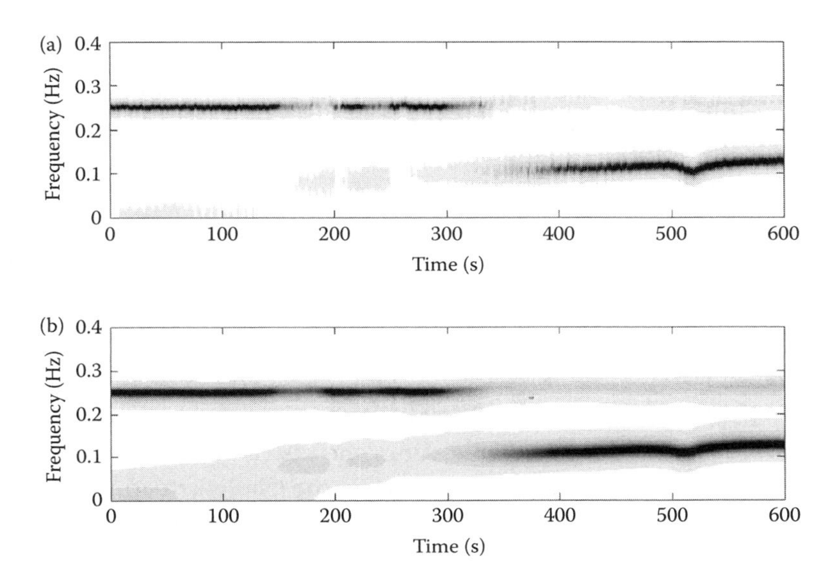

FIGURE 3.9 (a) Kalman filter and (b) Kalman smoother spectrum estimates for the simulated signal shown in Figure 3.5.

principle higher due to the implicit extrapolation of the observed signal (Marple, 1987).

Kalman filter and Kalman smoother spectrum estimates for the simulated signal shown in Figure 3.5 are presented in Figure 3.9. The initialization of the Kalman filter algorithm was made as described in the previous section. The observation and state noise covariance coefficients were computed as described in Equations 3.36 and 3.37, with observation noise adaptation coefficient $\gamma = 0.95$ and state noise update coefficient $\kappa = 5 \times 10^{-5}$. The essential difference between Kalman filter and smoother algorithms is easily observed from Figure 3.9. That is, the smoother algorithm eliminates the tracking lag present in the Kalman filter algorithm and gives overall an improved and smoother spectrum estimate. For a more detailed comparison of Kalman filter and smoother algorithms see, for example, Tarvainen et al. (2004).

3.4.7 Statistics of Parametric Spectrum Estimates

The statistics of parametric spectrum estimates can be rather easily evaluated because the covariance matrix of the state estimation error

$\tilde{\theta}_t$ (which provides a statistical measure of the uncertainty in $\hat{\theta}_t$) is calculated iteratively at every step of the Kalman filter or smoother algorithms. Basically there are at least two different approaches for evaluating the statistics of the spectrum estimates based on the estimated error covariances $C_{\tilde{\theta}_t}$.

One approach is to use a Monte Carlo type of method. In this approach, the parameter estimation errors at time t, denoted $\tilde{\theta}_t$, are assumed to be jointly Gaussian with mean zero and covariance $C_{\tilde{\theta}_t}$. Values from this distribution can be generated as follows. Let u be a Gaussian random variable with mean zero and variance 1, that is, $u \sim \mathcal{N}(0, 1)$, and assume that the covariance matrix $C_{\tilde{\theta}_t}$ can be written in the form $C_{\tilde{\theta}_t} = LL^{\mathrm{T}}$. Then according to probability theory, samples from the distribution of $\tilde{\theta}_t$ are given by Lu. The matrix L can be found by using the Cholesky decomposition. In this way, one can easily generate samples for the parameter estimation errors $\tilde{\theta}_t$, add these error values to the estimated parameter values, and calculate the corresponding spectrum estimates. By repeating this procedure many times, one can calculate statistical information, such as confidence intervals, for the spectrum estimates.

The second approach is to use an error propagation method. For the sake of simplicity, the derivation of this method is presented only for the AR model case. In this case, the state error covariance matrix $C_{\tilde{\theta}_t}$ includes variances and covariances of the AR parameter estimates at time t, and thus the variance of the spectrum estimate at time t can be evaluated by using the error propagation formula

$$\sigma^2_{P_{\mathrm{AR}}(t,f)} = \sum_{k=1}^{p} \left(\frac{\partial P_{\mathrm{AR}}(t,f)}{\partial \hat{a}_t^{(k)}} \right)^2 \sigma^2_{\hat{a}_t^{(k)}} + \sum_{k=1}^{p} \sum_{\substack{l=1 \\ l \neq k}}^{p} \frac{\partial P_{\mathrm{AR}}(t,f)}{\partial \hat{a}_t^{(k)}} \frac{\partial P_{\mathrm{AR}}(t,f)}{\partial \hat{a}_t^{(l)}} \sigma_{\hat{a}_t^{(k)} \hat{a}_t^{(l)}}, \tag{3.39}$$

where $\partial P_{\mathrm{AR}}(t,f)/\partial \hat{a}_t^{(k)}$ is the partial derivative of $P_{\mathrm{AR}}(t,f)$ with respect to $\hat{a}_t^{(k)}$, $\sigma^2_{\hat{a}_t^{(k)}}$ is the variance of the kth AR parameter estimate, and $\sigma_{\hat{a}_t^{(k)} \hat{a}_t^{(l)}}$ is the covariance of the kth and lth AR parameter estimates. In the case of the ARMA model, partial derivatives with respect to MA parameter estimates would be included in Equation 3.39. For the AR model case, the partial derivative of $P_{\mathrm{AR}}(t,f)$ with respect to $\hat{a}_t^{(k)}$ can be written in the form

$$\frac{\partial P_{\mathrm{AR}}(t,f)}{\partial \hat{a}_t^{(k)}} = \frac{-2\hat{\sigma}_e^2/f_s\left(\cos k\omega + \sum_{j=1}^{p} \hat{a}_t^{(j)} \cos(j-k)\omega\right)}{\left[\left(1+\sum_{j=1}^{p} \hat{a}_t^{(j)} \cos j\omega\right)^2 + \left(\sum_{j=1}^{p} \hat{a}_t^{(j)} \sin j\omega\right)^2\right]^2}, \tag{3.40}$$

where $\omega = 2\pi f/f_s$.

The further calculation of power and corresponding error variance for a specific band is straightforward. If the power spectrum is evaluated at discrete frequencies f_j, the power of band $f_1 < f < f_2$ at time t is obtained as

$$P_{[f_1,f_2]}(t) = \sum_{f_1<f_j<f_2} P_{\mathrm{AR}}(t,f_j)\Delta f, \tag{3.41}$$

where Δf is the frequency grid interval $\Delta f = f_j - f_{j-1}$. The partial derivative of the band power with respect to $P_{\mathrm{AR}}(t,f_j)$ is Δf and, thus the variance of the band power is obtained as

$$\sigma^2_{P_{[f_1,f_2]}(t)} = \sum_{f_1<f_j<f_2} \Delta f^2 \sigma^2_{P_{\mathrm{AR}}(t,f_j)}, \tag{3.42}$$

where the power values at different frequencies are treated as uncorrelated.

3.4.8 Spectral Decomposition of the AR Spectrum

One property of the AR spectrum estimation methods, which is sometimes advantageous in biomedical applications, is that the spectrum can be divided into separate components as follows. The AR spectrum estimate can also be written in the factored form

$$P_{\mathrm{AR}}(t,f) = \frac{\hat{\sigma}_e^2/f_s}{\prod_{j=1}^{p}(z-\alpha_t^{(j)})(1/z-\alpha_t^{(j)*})}, \tag{3.43}$$

where $z = e^{i2\pi f/f_s}$, $\alpha_t^{(j)}$ are the time-varying roots of the AR polynomial (also called poles), and * denotes the complex conjugate. Now, consider a pole $\alpha_t^{(j)}$ positioned at frequency f_j. The spectrum of this single component in the vicinity of f_j can be estimated as

$$P_{\text{AR}}^{(j)}(t,f) \approx \frac{c_t^{(j)}}{(z - \alpha_t^{(j)})(1/z - \alpha_t^{(j)*})}, \qquad z = e^{-i2\pi f/f_s}, \tag{3.44}$$

where the constant $c_t^{(j)}$ is given by

$$c_t^{(j)} \approx \frac{\hat{\sigma}_e^2/f_s}{\prod_{\substack{k=1\\k\neq j}}^{p} (z - \alpha_t^{(k)})(1/z - \alpha_t^{(k)*})}, \qquad z = e^{-i2\pi f_j/f_s}. \tag{3.45}$$

That is, the part $c_t^{(j)}$ of the AR spectrum estimate is assumed to be constant when $f \approx f_j$. The sum of the component spectra is approximately equal to the AR spectrum estimate, that is, $P_{\text{AR}}(t,f) \approx \sum_{j=1}^{p} P_{\text{AR}}^{(j)}(t,f)$.

The powers of the components can be estimated, for example, by using the method proposed by Johnsen and Andersen (1978). This method for component power estimation works for well-separated poles, but for poles close to each other power estimates can yield even negative values. A more robust way of estimating the powers is to simply calculate the areas of the spectral components.

3.5 CASE STUDY I: ESTIMATION OF ERS OF EEG

In this section, the Kalman smoother spectrum estimation method is applied for the evaluation of ERS and ERD dynamics.

The ERS/ERD of the occipital α rhythm was studied with an eyes open/closed procedure. In the test procedure, subjects closed and opened the eyes in accordance with auditory stimuli (beeps) at 15-s intervals. While in the eyes open state, the subject was instructed to focus the eyes to a fixed point. During the test procedure a total of 19 ERS/ERD samples were obtained for each subject. As a recording device a Braintronics CNV/ISO-1032 amplifier (sampling frequency 256 Hz and bandpass 0.3–70 Hz) with international 10–20 electrode coupling with the right mastoid as common reference was used. The ERS/ERD for visual stimulation is best seen in the posterior and occipital regions of the brain. Therefore, the occipital O2 channel was selected for the analysis. The sampling frequency of the selected

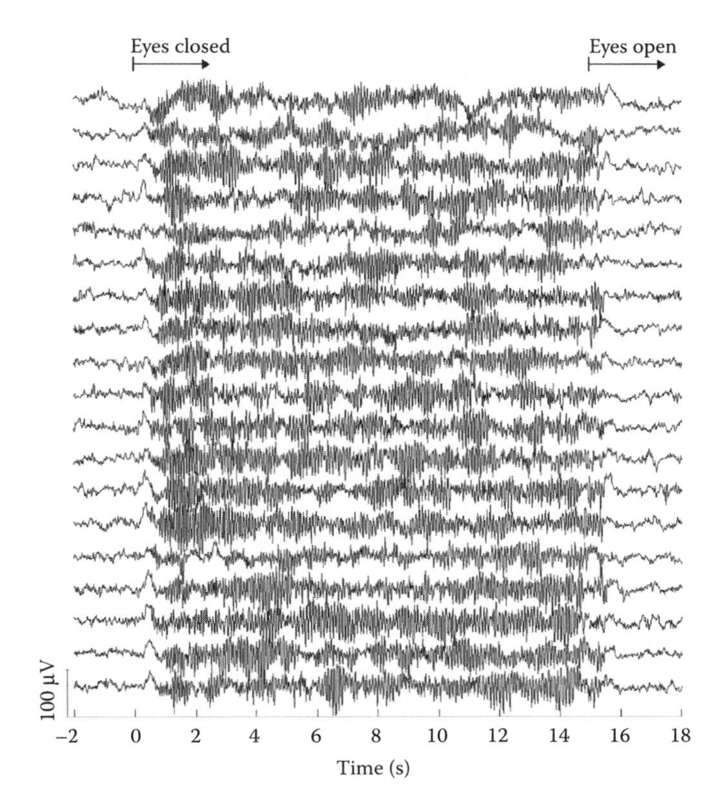

FIGURE 3.10 Measured ERS/ERD samples from O2 channel for one subject. A total of 19 samples were measured, the first one presented at the bottom. Auditory stimuli instructing the subject to close or open the eyes are presented at time instants 0 and 15 s.

channel was reduced after low-pass filtering to 64 Hz. The measured ERS/ERD trials for one of the subjects are presented in Figure 3.10.

In order to illustrate the performance of the Kalman smoother spectrum estimate on real EEG data it was compared with some commonly used spectrum estimation methods. The analyzed ERS/ERD sample and different dynamic spectrum estimates are shown in Figure 3.11. In addition to the Kalman smoother method, two rather popular parametric methods, namely RLS and LMS were considered. In all three parametric methods, an ARMA(6,2) model was used and the adaptation coefficients in each algorithm were selected based on subjective evaluation. In addition to parametric methods, commonly used spectrogram and scalogram TFRs were also computed. In the spectrogram a 1-s time-window was used and the scalogram was computed using the Morlet wavelet as described by Muthuswamy and Thakor (1998).

Time instance 0 in Figure 3.11 corresponds to the stimulus occurrence instructing the subject to close the eyes. Shortly after the eyes are closed, a substantial increase in α band power is observed in all spectra. The resolution of the spectrogram seems to be lower when compared to the three

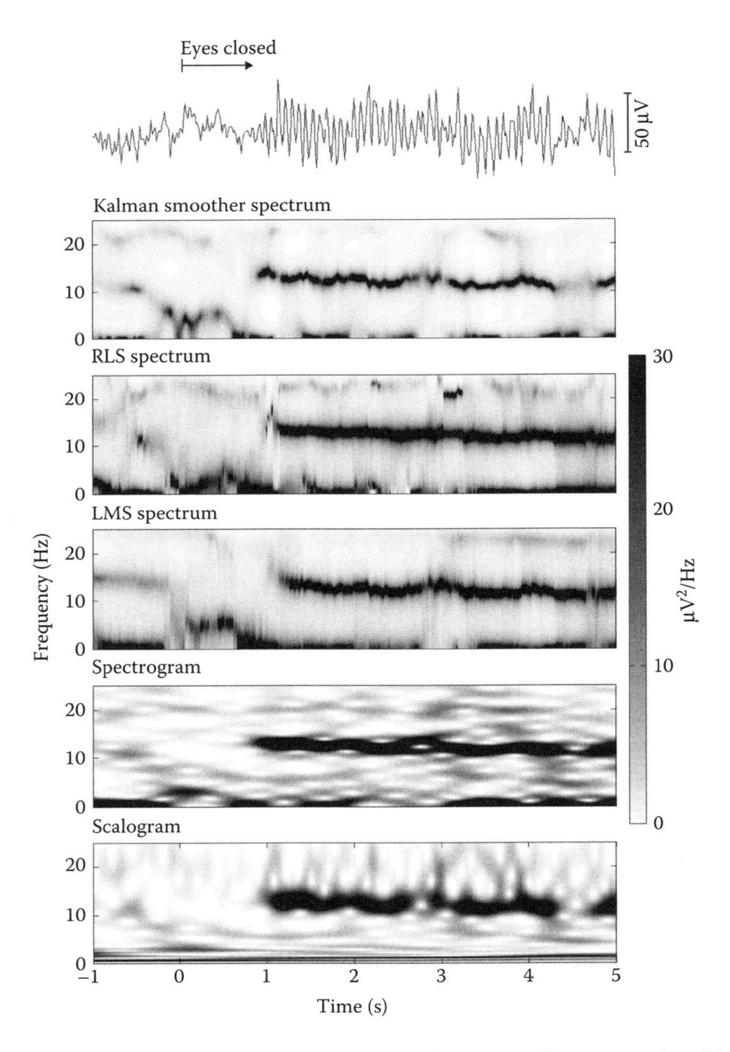

FIGURE 3.11 Estimation of time-varying PSD for a typical ERS sample with different methods. The measured ERS sample is presented on top and the different spectrum estimates underneath it.

parametric methods and the WT does not produce remarkable improvement. The main drawback of RLS and LMS is the unavoidable tracking lag clearly seen in both spectra. The observed time–frequency resolution of the Kalman smoother is, on the other hand, extremely high. Even the short-term changes in α rhythm, for example, the interval approximately from 4.3 to 4.7 s with decreased power in the α frequency band, are detected reliably.

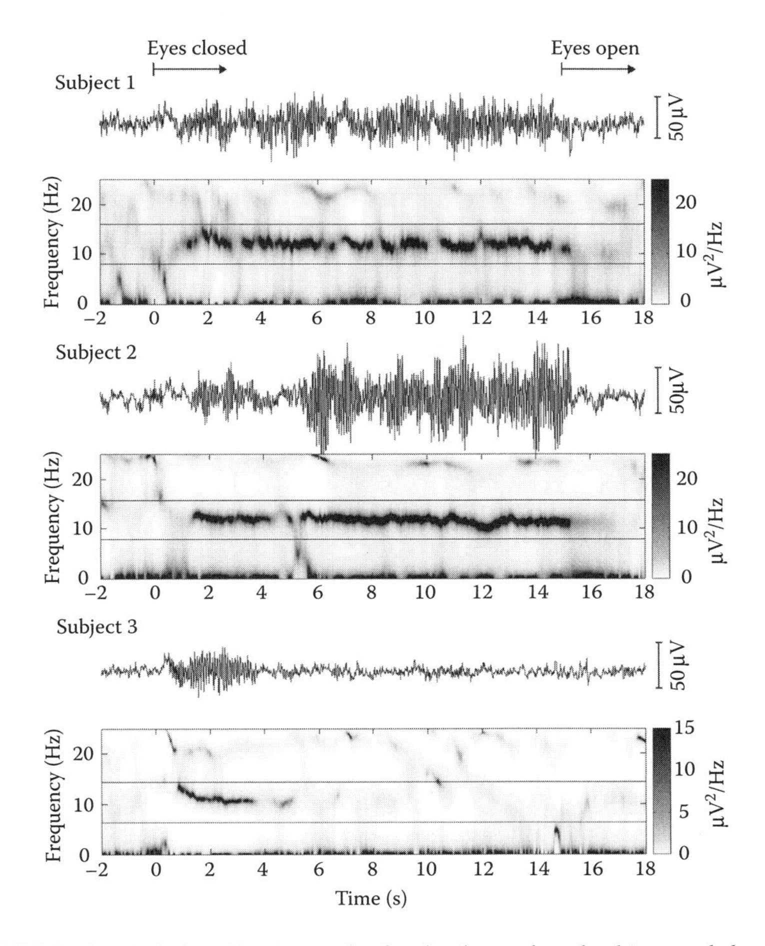

FIGURE 3.12 Typical ERS/ERD samples for the three selected subjects and the corresponding time-varying Kalman smoother spectra. Stimulus occurrence times (0 and 15 s) instructing subjects to close and open their eyes are marked on the top. Individually adjusted α frequency bands are marked with horizontal lines on top of each spectrum. The bandwidth is set to 8 Hz.

The ERS/ERD dynamics of occipital α rhythm can have different characteristics between individuals. Figure 3.12 shows typical ERS/ERD samples and the corresponding Kalman smoother spectra for three different subjects, which all had different characteristic patterns of α rhythms. For subject 1 the power of the α rhythm is quite invariant during the whole eyes closed period while for subject 3 the α power attenuates within a few seconds after eye closure. For subject 2, on the other hand, a slow increase of α power after eye closure seems to be characteristic. The center frequency of the α rhythm was also different between subjects (center frequencies were 12.06, 11.69, and 10.69 Hz for subjects 1, 2, and 3, respectively). In all spectra shown in Figure 3.12, the α rhythm seems to start at higher frequencies and shifts to lower frequencies within a few seconds. This is the well-known "squeak" phenomenon of occipital α rhythm (Westmoreland & Klass, 1990).

3.6 CASE STUDY II: ESTIMATION OF HRV DYNAMICS DURING AN ORTHOSTATIC TEST

In this section, the Kalman smoother spectrum estimation method is applied for estimating time-varying characteristics of HRV during an orthostatic test. The original study related to this topic was published by Tarvainen et al. (2006).

As an experimental protocol, an orthostatic test including a 30-s breath hold at the end was performed. In the experiment, the subject first lay supine for over 5 min and then stood up. After standing for about 5 min the subject held his breath for 30 s. The ECG signal was measured using a Neuroscan system (Compumedics Limited). ECG electrodes were placed according to the conventional 12-lead system with the Mason–Likar modification. For analysis, lead II was chosen. The sampling rate of the ECG signal was 1000 Hz. The QRS fiducial points were then extracted from the ECG signal by using an adaptive QRS detection algorithm and the RR interval series was formed. The RR interval series was further transformed to evenly sampled time series by using a 4-Hz cubic spline interpolation.

Altogether five healthy young male subjects were measured, but here only one of the subjects is analyzed as an illustrative example. The obtained RR

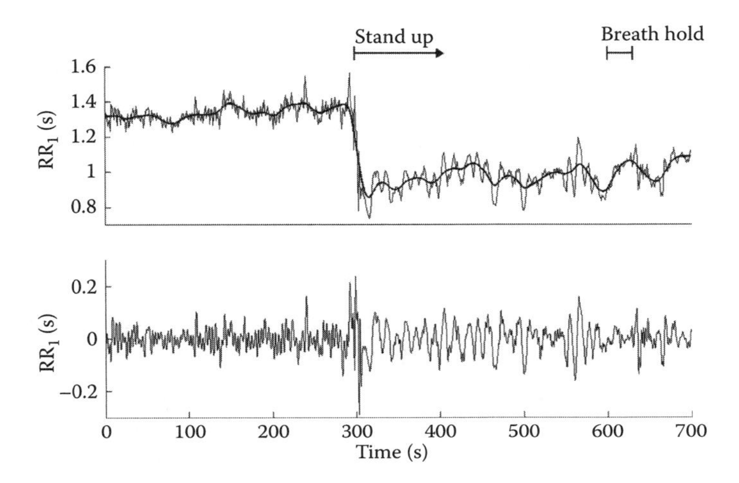

FIGURE 3.13 An orthostatic test recording with a 30-s breath hold at the end: RR interval series with the estimated trend (top) and detrended RR interval series (bottom).

interval series for the subject is presented on top of Figure 3.13. The time instance of standing up and the breath holding period are indicated on top. The LF trend components of HRV can distort parametric spectrum estimates as was shown by Tarvainen, Ranta-aho, and Karjalainen (2002). Thus, the trend was removed by using a smoothness priors-based method described by Tarvainen, Ranta-aho, and Karjalainen (2002). The estimated trend is presented with a bold line on top and the detrended RR interval series on the bottom of Figure 3.13. The changes between the HF and LF variability due to the posture change at about 300 s are evident. In addition, a decrease in HR is observed for the breath holding.

The first decision in the use of the Kalman smoother spectrum estimation method is the selection of the model type and order. Here an AR model was selected and the model order was estimated based on three different model order selection criteria: that is, FPE, AIC, and MDL. All of these criteria are functions of model order and the corresponding prediction error variance. It should be noted that all these criteria apply only for estimating the model order of a time-invariant AR model. Thus, the model order selection here is based on a time-invariant model. For the estimation of the prediction error variance of the time-invariant AR model, a forward–backward least-squares method, also known as the modified covariance method (Marple, 1987), was applied. Each model order selection criterion was evaluated separately for supine and standing periods. The FPE, AIC, and MDL criteria as functions of model order p for supine and standing periods are presented in Figure 3.14a. As a good compromise a model order $p = 16$ indicated with vertical lines in Figure 3.14a was selected for analysis. The stationary AR spectrum estimates (with the selected model order) for supine and standing periods are presented on top of Figure 3.14b. For comparison the spectrum estimates were also calculated with the Welch's periodogram method (Marple, 1987), shown on the bottom of Figure 3.14b. By comparing the two spectrum estimates, the model order $p = 16$ seems reasonable.

The Kalman smoother spectrum estimate was then calculated by using the time-varying AR(16) model for the RR interval series. The detrended RR interval series and the corresponding Kalman smoother spectrum are presented in Figure 3.15. The Kalman smoother algorithm was initialized according to Equations 3.36 and 3.37, with $\gamma = 0.95$ and $\kappa = 1 \times 10^{-5}$. The decision of update coefficient κ was made as a compromise between the adaptation speed of the algorithm and the statistics of the resulting spectrum estimate.

The LF and HF band powers and the LF/HF ratio as functions of time were then calculated. The band limits were set to 0.04–0.15 Hz (LF) and 0.15–0.4 Hz (HF) according to the recommendations given in Task Force of the European Society of Cardiology and the North American Society of Pacing and Electrophysiology (1996). The band powers are simply obtained by integrating the spectrum over the specific frequency band according to Equation 3.41. The variance of the Kalman smoother spectrum estimate was evaluated according to Equations 3.39 and 3.40 and the variance of the band powers according to Equation 3.42. The variance of the LF/HF ratio was evaluated correspondingly by using the error propagation formula. The obtained band powers and LF/HF ratio with ±2SD intervals are presented in Figure 3.16.

One advantage of parametric spectrum estimation methods is that the spectrum estimates can be divided into separate spectral components as described earlier in this chapter. Here the spectral decomposition is adopted to divide the Kalman smoother spectrum into separate LF and HF components. The spectral components are extracted by using Equations 3.44 and 3.45. The obtained LF and HF components are presented in Figure 3.17. The decomposition of the spectra at $t = 200$ and 400 s is illustrated on top of the figure. The powers of the LF and HF components can be evaluated simply by calculating the areas of the spectral components or by using

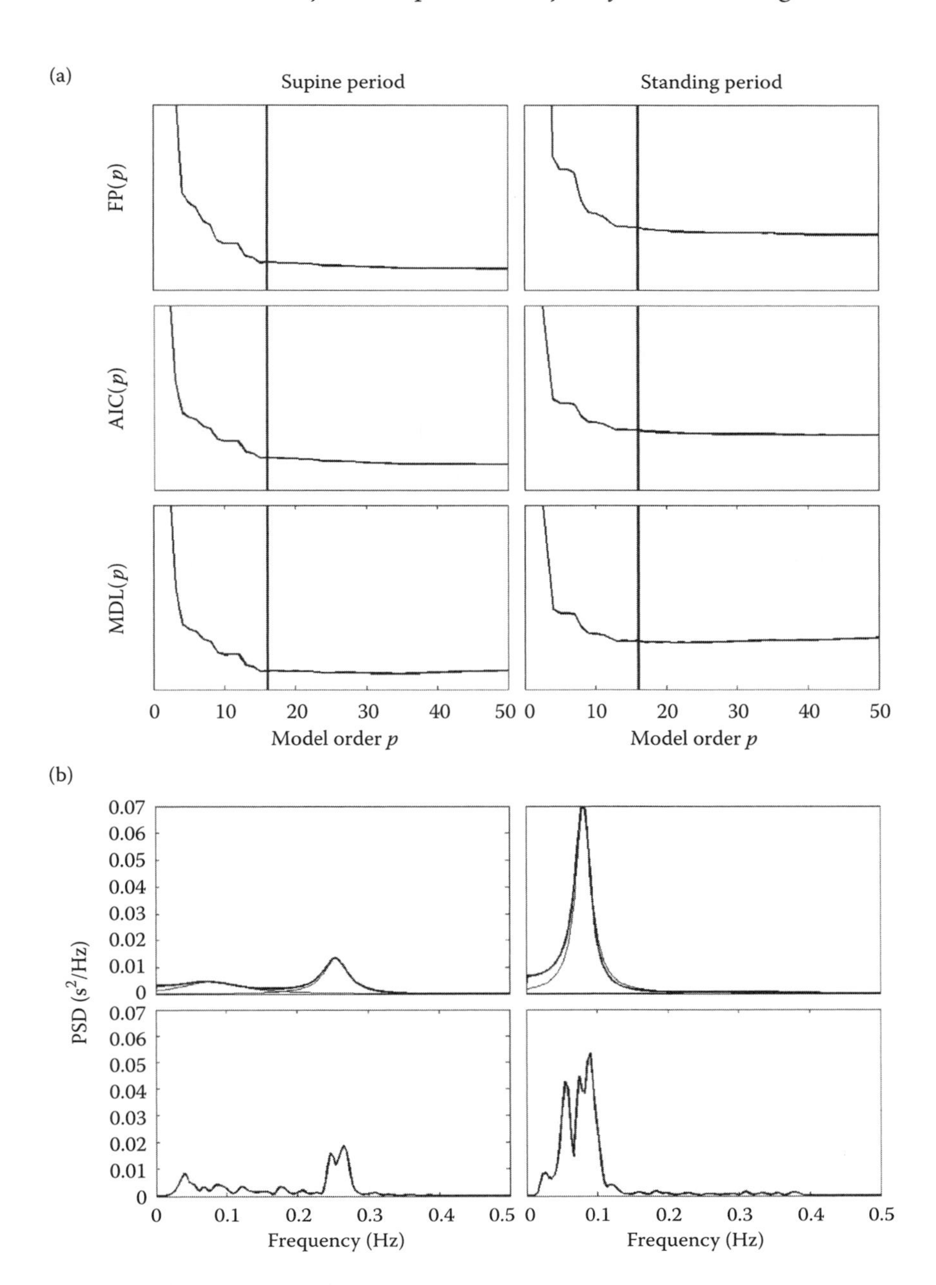

FIGURE 3.14 Selection of the AR model order. (a) FPE, AIC, and MDL criteria as functions of model order p for supine (left) and standing (right) periods. The selected model order $p = 16$ is indicated with vertical lines. (b) The AR spectrum for the selected order $p = 16$ (top) compared to Welch's periodogram (bottom) for supine (left) and standing (right) periods.

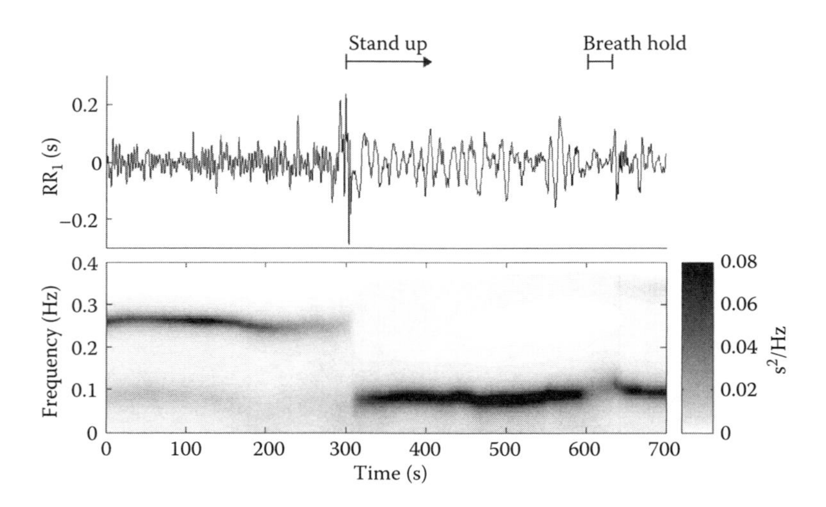

FIGURE 3.15 Time-varying spectrum estimation of HRV. The detrended RR interval series (top) and the corresponding Kalman smoother spectrum estimate (bottom).

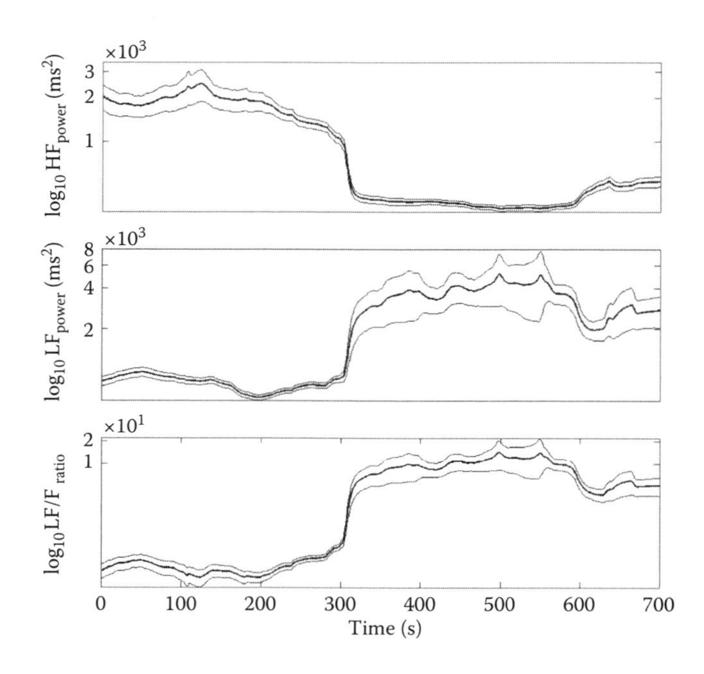

FIGURE 3.16 Estimated dynamics of LF and HF band powers and LF/HF ratio (bold line) with ±2SD intervals (thin line).

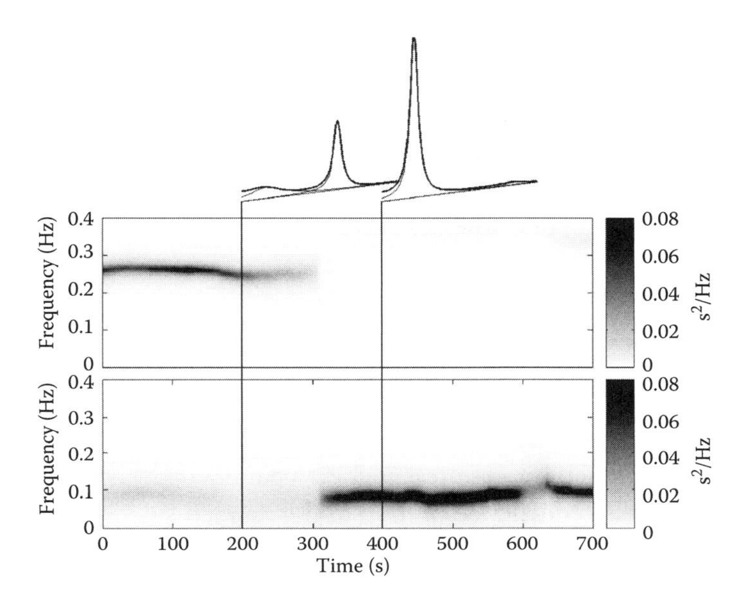

FIGURE 3.17 Decomposition of the Kalman smoother spectrum into LF (bottom) and HF (top) spectral components.

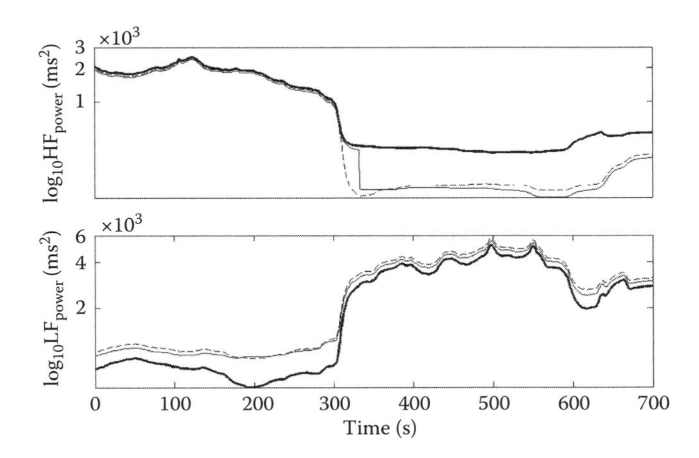

FIGURE 3.18 LF and HF component powers as band powers from nondecomposed spectrum (bold line), areas of corresponding decomposed spectral components (thin line), and by using the residue method (dashed line).

a residue-based method proposed by Johnsen and Andersen (1978). The component power estimates with the two different methods are presented in Figure 3.18 with comparison to the corresponding band powers already presented in Figure 3.16. The two component power estimates give quite similar results. However, the important observation is that the HF band power is much higher than component powers for the standing period when the HF power is much lower than the LF power. The reason for this is that the strong LF component overlaps with the HF band. For the supine period, the LF band power is lower than the two component powers. The reason for this is that the rather low and wide LF component overlaps with the VLF and HF bands.

3.7 DISCUSSION

In this chapter, a Kalman smoother algorithm-based time-varying spectrum estimation method was presented. As a parametric spectrum estimation method, the frequency resolution of the Kalman smoother spectrum estimates is in principle better than that of FFT-based spectrum estimates due to implicit extrapolation of the observed signal. In addition, Kalman smoother as a recursive algorithm is statistically recommendable because it is theoretically an optimal linear mean square estimator and it can be derived from the Bayes theorem (Anderson & Moore, 1979; Melsa & Cohn, 1978). Overall, the time–frequency resolution of the Kalman smoother spectrum is highly competent. The main advantage of the Kalman smoother approach when compared to other recursive algorithms such as RLS, LMS, or Kalman filter is that the lag error can be avoided (Tarvainen et al., 2004).

The adaptation of the Kalman smoother spectrum estimation method can in practice be adjusted with a single parameter. The adaptation of the algorithm is basically controlled by the ratio of the state noise and observation noise covariance coefficients, that is, σ_w^2/σ_e^2, which can be seen more easily from an alternative Kalman filter formulation used, for example, in Young, Pedregal, and Tych (1999). Thus, one easy way to operate the algorithm is to keep the observation noise covariance as constant and adjust only the state noise covariance. A more realistic approach is to estimate the observation noise covariance iteratively and update state noise covariance accordingly as in Equations 3.36 and 3.37. The latter approach may yield quicker convergence and more meaningful parameter estimates. The selection of the adaptation coefficient should be done by compromising between the adaptation speed of the algorithm and the variance of the parameter estimates. One advantage of the Kalman smoother-based spectrum estimation method is that the covariance of the parameter estimation errors is evaluated iteratively at every step of the algorithm. Thus, the uncertainty of the estimated parameters and also of the spectrum estimate computed from these parameters can be evaluated as described in this chapter.

Another advantage of the Kalman smoother spectrum estimation method is that the spectrum can be divided into separate frequency components. This is especially advantageous in some biomedical signal analysis applications where specific frequency components are analyzed. For example, in HRV analysis, LF and HF components can be extracted from the spectrum. The powers of the extracted components can be estimated by directly evaluating the area of the spectral components or by using the residue-based method proposed by Johnsen and Andersen (1978). When the component powers were compared to the corresponding band powers in Figure 3.18, it was observed that the two component power estimates gave quite similar results, but the band power values were quite different. The main reason for the difference in band power and component powers was that the LF component seemed to overlap with the VLF and HF bands. When computing band powers, this overlap tends to decrease LF band power and increase VLF and HF band powers. The level of this overlap naturally depends on the central frequency of the LF component. The central frequencies of both the LF and HF components are highly individual and may also vary according to the physical circumstances. Thus, it is reasonable to argue that in some cases the LF and HF powers can be evaluated more accurately from the decomposed spectrum. The component-wise power estimation may, however, yield highly distorted results when the decomposition of the LF and HF components is not clear and, thus, this kind of power estimation should be used with care.

One important practical issue of parametric time-varying spectrum estimation methods is the goodness-of-fit of the model and potential unrealistic inferences related to this. In the case of the time-varying AR/ARMA model, the goodness-of-fit depends on two things. Firstly, the order of the AR/ARMA model should be selected large enough to model the correlations within the data, but small enough to avoid overfitting. If too big a model order is selected, the resulting spectrum may include spurious peaks and lead to unrealistic inferences. In the selection of the model order, one may utilize the selection criteria given in Equations 3.17 through 3.19 or, alternatively, one may attempt to estimate the "optimal" model order dynamically as in Goto et al. (1995) and Haseyama and Kitajima (2001). Secondly, the adaptation coefficient controlling the convergence of the Kalman smoother influences the goodness-of-fit. The adaptation of the algorithm should be adjusted large enough to follow the dynamics of the data, but small enough to maintain eligible confidence limits for the estimated parameters. By adjusting the adaptation large enough, even highly "irregular" dynamics can be tracked, but at the same time the uncertainty of the estimates is increased and in the worst case the algorithm may become "unstable." Thus, the adaptation of the algorithm must be selected by compromising between the tracking capability and the accuracy of the estimates.

In conclusion, Kalman filter and smoother algorithms enable high-quality dynamic spectral analysis of biosignals. These algorithms are theoretically sound and their adaptation can be adjusted with a single parameter. In general, these algorithms can be used in any dynamical estimation problem (linear or nonlinear), which can be presented in the state-space formalism. In this chapter, only the linear case was considered. In the non-linear case, one can apply the well-known extended Kalman filter or the more recently proposed unscented Kalman filter (Julier & Uhlmann, 2004).

ACKNOWLEDGMENTS

This work was performed at the Biosignal Analysis and Medical Imaging Group (http://bsamig.uku.fi), Department of Physics, University of Kuopio, Finland and was supported by the Academy of Finland (projects 123579 and 126873). Portions of this chapter are based on the work of Tarvainen et al. (2004, 2006) and the author wants to acknowledge the contribution of his co-authors in these references. In addition, the author wants to thank Stefanos Georgiadis, PhD, and Professor Pasi Karjalainen, PhD, for all the helpful suggestions and discussions related to the topic of this chapter.

REFERENCES

Afonso, V. (1993). ECG QRS detection. In W. Tompkins (Ed.), *Biomedical digital signal processing* (pp. 237–264). Englewood Cliffs, NJ: Prentice-Hall.

Akay, M. (Ed.). (1998). *Time frequency and wavelets in biomedical signal processing*. New York: IEEE Press.

Anderson, B., & Moore, J. (1979). *Optimal filtering*. Englewood Cliffs, NJ: Prentice-Hall.

Barlow, J. (1985). Methods of analysis of nonstationary EEGs, with emphasis on segmentation techniques: A comparative review. *Electroencephalography Clinical Neurophysiology, 2*(3), 267–304.

Baselli, G., Cerutti, S., Civardi, S., Lombardi, F., Malliani, A., Merri, M., et al. (1987). Heart rate variability signal processing: A quantitative approach as an aid to diagnosis in cardiovascular pathologies. *International Journal of Bio-Medical Computing, 20*, 51–70.

Berntson, G., Jr., J. B., Eckberg, D., Grossman, P., Kaufmann, P., Malik, M., et al. (1997). Heart rate variability: Origins, methods, and interpretive caveats. *Psychophysiology, 34*, 623–648.

Bohlin, T. (1977). Analysis of EEG signals with changing spectra using a short-word Kalman estimator. *Mathematical Biosciences, 35*, 221–259.

Bragge, T., Tarvainen, M., Ranta-aho, P., & Karjalainen, P. (2005). High-resolution QRS fiducial point corrections in sparsely sampled ECG recordings. *Physiological Measurement, 26*(5), 743–751.

Braune, H.-J., & Geisenörfer, U. (1995). Measurement of heart rate variations: Influencing factors, normal values and diagnostic impact on diabetic autonomic neuropathy. *Diabetes Research and Clinical Practice, 29*, 179–187.

Cohen, B. C., & Sances Jr, A. (1977). Stationarity of the human electroencephalogram. *Medical Biological Engineering Computing, 15*, 513–518.

Cohen, L. (1989). Time-frequency distributions—A review. *Proceedings of the IEEE, 77*(7), 941–981.

Daskalov, I., & Christov, I. (1997). Improvement of resolution in measurement of electrocardiogram RR intervals by interpolation. *Medical Engineering Physics, 19*(4), 375–379.

DeBoer, R., Karemaker, J., & Strackee, J. (1984). Comparing spectra of a series of point events particularly for heart rate variability data. *IEEE Transactions on Biomedical Engineering, 31*(4), 384–387.

DeBoer, R., Karemaker, J., & Strackee, J. (1985). Spectrum of a series of point events, generated by the integral pulse frequency modulation model. *Medical Biological Engineering Computing, 23*, 138–142.

Friesen, G., Jannett, T., Jadallah, M., Yates, S., Quint, S., & Nagle, H. (1990). A comparison of the noise sensitivity of nine QRS detection algorithms. *IEEE Transactions on Biomedical Engineering, 37*(1), 85–98.

Gelb, A. (1974). *Applied optimal estimation*. Cambridge/London: The MIT Press.

Goto, S., Nakamura, M., & Uosaki, K. (1995, June). On-line spectral estimation of nonstationary time series based on AR model parameter estimation and order selection with a forgetting factor. *IEEE Transactions on Signal Processing, 43*(6), 1519–1522.

Gustafsson, F., & Hjalmarsson, H. (1995). Twenty-one ML estimators for model selection. *Automatica, 31*, 1377–1392.

Hamilton, P., & Tompkins, W. (1986, December). Quantitative investigation of QRS detection rules using the MIT/BIH arrhythmia database. *IEEE Transactions on Biomedical Engineering, 33*(12), 1157–1165.

Hari, R., & Salmelin, R. (1997). Human cortical oscillations: A neuromagnetic view through the skull. *Trends in Neuroscience, 20*(1), 44–49.

Haseyama, M., & Kitajima, H. (2001). An ARMA order selection method with fuzzy reasoning. *Signal Processing, 81*, 1331–1335.

Haykin, S. (1991). *Adaptive filter theory* (2nd ed.). Englewood Cliffs, NJ: Prentice-Hall.

Hlawatsch, F., & Boudreaux-Bartels, G. (1992). Linear and quadratic time-frequency signal representations. *IEEE Signal Processing Magazine*, 21–67.

Huikuri, H., Mäkikallio, T., Raatikainen, P., Perkiömäki, J., Castellanos, A., & Myerburg, R. (2003). Prediction of sudden cardiac death: Appraisal of the studies and methods assessing the risk of sudden arrhythmic death. *Circulation*, *108*(1), 110–115.

Isaksson, A., & Wennberg, A. (1976). Spectral properties of nonstationary EEG signals, evaluated by means of Kalman filtering: Application examples from a vigilance test. In P. Kellaway & I. Petersen (Eds.), *Quantitative analytic studies in epilepsy* (pp. 389–402). New York: Raven Press.

Jansen, B. (1991). Quantitative analysis of electroencephalograms: Is there chaos in the future? *International Journal of Bio-Medical Computing*, *27*, 95–123.

Johnsen, S., & Andersen, N. (1978, June). On power estimation in maximum entropy spectral analysis. *Geophysics*, *43*, 681–690.

Julier, S., & Uhlmann, J. (2004). Unscented filtering and nonlinear estimation. *Proceedings of the IEEE*, *92*(3), 401–422.

Kalcher, J., & Pfurtscheller, G. (1995). Discrimination between phase-locked and non-phase-locked event-related EEG activity. *Electroencephalography and Clinical Neurophysiology*, *94*, 381–384.

Kalman, R. (1960). A new approach to linear filtering and prediction problems. *Transactions of the ASME Journal Basic Engineering*, *82*, 35–45.

Kitagawa, G., & Gersch, W. (1996). *Smoothness priors analysis of time series*. Springer-Verlag.

Klem, G., Lüders, H., Jasper, H., & Elger, C. (1999). The ten-twenty electrode system of the international federation. In G. Deuschl & A. Eisen (Eds.), *Recommendations for the practice of clinical neurophysiology: Guidelines of the international federation of clinical neurophysiology* (pp. 3–6). Amsterdam: Elsevier.

Klimesch, W. (1999). EEG α and theta oscillations reflect cognitive and memory performance: A review and analysis. *Brain Research Reviews*, *29*, 169–195.

Lombardi, F., Mäkikallio, T., Myerburg, R., & Huikuri, H. (2001). Sudden cardiac death: Role of heart rate variability to identify patients at risk. *Cardiovascular Research*, *50*, 210–217.

Malliani, A., Pagani, M., Lombardi, F., & Cerutti, S. (1991). Cardiovascular neural regulation explored in the frequency domain. *Circulation*, *84*(2), 482–492.

Malmivuo, J., & Plonsey, R. (1995). *Bioelectromagnetism: Principles and applications of bioelectric and biomagnetic fields*. New York/Oxford: Oxford University Press (Web Edition).

Markand, O. (1990). α rhythms. *Journal of Clinical Neurophysiology*, *7*, 163–189.

Marple, S. (1987). *Digital spectral analysis*. Englewood Cliffs, NJ: Prentice-Hall International.

Mateo, J., & Laguna, P. (2000). Improved heart rate variability signal analysis from the beat occurrence times according to the IPFM model. *IEEE Transactions of Biomedical Engineering*, *47*(8), 985–996.

Melsa, J., & Cohn, D. (1978). *Decision and estimation theory*. Tokyo: McGraw-Hill.

Merri, M., Farden, D., Mottley, J., & Titlebaum, E. (1990). Sampling frequency of the electrocardiogram for spectral analysis of the heart rate variability. *IEEE Transactions in Biomedical Engineering*, *37*(1), 99–106.

Muthuswamy, J., & Thakor, N. (1998). Spectral analysis methods for neurological signals. *Journal of Neuroscience Methods*, *83*, 1–14.

Niedermeyer, E. (1997). α rhythms as physiological and abnormal phenomena. *International Journal of Psychophysiology, 26*, 31–49.
Niedermeyer, E., & Silva, F. da (Eds.). (1999). *Electroencephalography: Basic principles, clinical applications, and related fields* (4th Ed.). Baltimore: Williams & Wilkins.
Nuwer, M. (1988a). Quantitative EEG: II. Frequency analysis and topographic mapping in clinical settings. *Journal of Clinical Neurophysiology, 5*(1), 45–85.
Nuwer, M. (1988b). Quantitative EEG: I. Techniques and problems of frequency analysis and topographic mapping. *Journal of Clinical Neurophysiology, 5*(1), 1–43.
Pagani, M. (2000). Heart rate variability and autonomic diabetic neuropathy. *Diabetes Nutrition & Metabolism, 13*(6), 341–346.
Pahlm, O., & Sörnmo, L. (1984). Software QRS detection in ambulatory monitoring—A review. *Medical Biological Engineerings Computing, 22*, 289–297.
Pan, J., & Tompkins, W. (1985). A real-time QRS detection algorithm. *IEEE Transactions on Biomedical Engineering, 32*(3), 230–236.
Pfurtscheller, G., (1992). Event–related synchronization (ERS): An electrophysiological correlate of cortical areas at rest. *Electroencephalography and Clinical Neurophysiology, 83*, 62–69.
Pfurtscheller, G., & Lopes da Silva, F. (1999). Event-related EEG/MEG synchronization and desynchronization: Basic principles. *Clinical Neurophysiology, 110*, 1842–1857.
Pfurtscheller, G., Neuper, C., & Mohl, W. (1994). Event-related desynchronization (ERD) during visual processing. *International Journal of Psychophysiology, 16*, 147–153.
Pinna, G., Maestri, R., Cesare, A. D., Colombo, R., & Minuco, G. (1994). The accuracy of power-spectrum analysis of heart-rate variability from annotated RR lists generated by Holter systems. *Physiological Measurement, 15*, 163–179.
Pivik, R., Broughton, R., Coppola, R., Davidson, R., Fox, N., & Nuwer, M. (1993). Guidelines for the recording and quantitative analysis of electroencephalographic activity in research contexts. *Psychophysiology, 30*, 547–558.
Priestley, M. (1981). *Spectral analysis and time series*. London: Academic Press.
Pumprla, J., Howorka, K., Groves, D., Chester, M., & Nolan, J. (2002). Functional assessment of heart arte variability: Physiological basis and practical applications. *International Journal of Cardiology, 84*, 1–14.
Rauch, H., Tung, F., & Striebel, C. (1965). Maximum likelihood estimates of linear dynamic systems. *AIAA Journal, 3*, 1445–1450.
Rioul, O., & Flandrin, P. (1992). Time-scale energy distributions: A general class extending wavelet transforms. *IEEE Transactions on Signal Processing, 40*(7), 1746–1757.
Rioul, O., & Vetterli, M. (1991). Wavelets and signal processing. *IEEE Signal Processing Magazine*, 14–38.
Rompelman, O. (1993). Rhythms and analysis techniques. In J. Strackee & N. Westerhof (Eds.), *The physics of heart and circulation* (pp. 101–120). Bristol: Institute of Physics Publishing.
Schack, B., Bareshova, E., Grieszbach, G., & Witte, H. (1995). Methods of dynamic spectral analysis by self-exciting autoregressive moving average models and their application to analysing biosignals. *Medical Biological Engineering Computing, 33*, 492–498.
Sorenson, H. (1980). *Parameter estimation: Principles and problems*. Marcel Dekker.
Tarvainen, M., Georgiadis, S., Ranta-aho, P., & Karjalainen, P. (2006). Time-varying analysis of heart rate variability signals with Kalman smoother algorithm. *Physiological Measurement, 27*(3), 225–239.

Tarvainen, M., Hiltunen, J., Ranta-aho, P., & Karjalainen, P. (2004). Estimation of non-stationary EEG with Kalman smoother approach: An application to event-related synchronization (ERS). *IEEE Transactions on Biomedical Engineering, 51*(3), 516–524.

Tarvainen, M., Ranta-aho, P., & Karjalainen, P. (2002). An advanced detrending method with application to HRV analysis. *IEEE Transactions on Biomedical Engineering, 49*(2), 172–175.

Task Force of the European Society of Cardiology and the North American Society of Pacing and Electrophysiology (1996). Heart rate variability—standards of measurement, physiological interpretation, and clinical use. *Circulation, 93*(5), 1043–1065.

Thakor, N., Webster, J., & Tompkins, W. (1983). Optimal QRS detector. *Medical Biological Engineering Computing, 21*, 343–350.

Vetterli, M., & Herley, C. (1992). Wavelets and filter banks: Theory and design. *IEEE Transactions on Signal Processing, 40*(9), 2207–2232.

Westmoreland, B., & Klass, D. (1990). Unusual EEG patterns. *Journal of Clinical Neurophysiology, 7*(2), 209–228.

Whittle, P. (1963). *Prediction and regulation by linear least squares methods*. Princeton.

Young, P., Pedregal, D., & Tych, W. (1999). Dynamic harmonic regression. *Journal of Forecasting, 18*(6), 369–394.

4

Cluster Analysis for Nonstationary Time Series

Bing Gao, Hernando Ombao, and Moon-ho Ringo Ho

4.1 INTRODUCTION

The general goal of clustering is to identify structure in an unlabeled data set by organizing the data into homogeneous groups with maximum similarity within a group and the largest dissimilarity between groups. There has been growing interest in using time series clustering as a data mining tool in natural, life, and social sciences. In this chapter, we present a methodology that can choose a set of relevant spectral (spectrum-related) features for clustering segments of time series with similar characteristics in an automatic manner and determine the optimal number of clusters at the same time. In our application, we use electroencephalogram (EEG) signals collected from a patient with epilepsy. Our method is able to distinguish the epileptic seizure EEG signals from the normal state EEG signals.

4.1.1 Overview of Cluster Analysis

The general objective of cluster analysis is to group "objects," which are usually people but can also be channels, voxels or even brain states in neuroimaging applications, into clusters such that the objects within the same cluster are more similar to each other than to those in other clusters. The three major approaches to cluster analysis are hierarchical, partition, and model-based clustering. For the former two approaches, proximity measures such as the Euclidean distance (L_2 norm), the Manhattan distance (L_1 norm), the maximum distance (L_∞ norm), or user-defined distance are first computed among all pairs of objects. For hierarchical clustering, initially each cluster only contains a single object. Progressively, at each stage, the two "nearest" clusters determined from the proximity measures are combined to form one bigger cluster until a single cluster is formed at the end. The result is the construction of a hierarchy, or a tree-like structure called the dendrogram that depicts the information on clusters.

In partitional (or nonhierarchical) clustering, the objects are partitioned into a prespecified number of groups. The most common partitional method is k-means clustering (McQueen, 1967), which aims to find a partition that minimizes the within group's sum of squares. The procedure starts with a preliminary random partition of the objects into J groups (specified by the users), and the mean for each group is calculated. Then the object is reassigned to the group with the closest mean, and the group mean is recalculated, followed by reassigning the objects. These steps are repeated until no more new reassignments can be made. Interested readers may refer to Arabie, Hubert, and De Soete (1996), which contains excellent reviews on these two types of clustering methods and related topics. The two clustering methods above are popular in practice. They are heuristic, easily implemented, and available in most of the statistical packages. However, they do not include a formal statistical procedure for determining the number of clusters within the data, and do not provide a measure of the uncertainty associated with the cluster membership. In the model-based clustering approach (Fraley & Raftery, 2002; Raftery & Dean, 2006), the data are assumed to arise from a mixture of different distributions, each distribution representing a cluster. The maximum likelihood criterion is used to estimate the parameters of the distributions via the expectation-maximization (EM) algorithm (Dempster, Laird, & Rubin, 1977). Once the parameters have been estimated, each observation is placed in the cluster with the largest conditional probability. The Bayesian Information Criterion (BIC) is used to determine the optimal number of clusters for the data.

It is often the case that not all features (or variables) are useful for uncovering the true structure of the data. In fact, the irrelevant variables often hinder the clustering performance. Therefore, identifying the most effective variables for clustering, referred to as the variable or feature selection process, is necessary. One common approach for variable selection is to fit univariate models to each variable and select a small subset that passes some prespecified thresholds (McLachlan, Bean, & Peel, 2002; Meyer, 2003). Another approach is to simultaneously consider the problem of variable selection and optimal clustering. Fowlkes, Gnanadesikan, and Kettenring (1988) used a forward selection approach in the context of complete linkage hierarchical clustering. Variables are selected depending on the information on the between-cluster and total sum-of-squares, and their significance is judged based on graphical information. Friedman and Meulman (2004) proposed a procedure that assigns the different variables with different weights instead of selecting variables explicitly, such that different clusters can be separated by different subsets of variables. Raftery and Dean (2006) recast the problem as a model comparison by comparing two nested subsets of variables. They developed a stepwise algorithm to select variables that can best improve the BIC for clustering purposes. Tadesse, Sha, and Vannucci (2005) proposed a Bayesian clustering approach in which they search through all possible 2^p feature subsets through the introduction of a latent p-vector with binary entries, and used a stochastic search method to explore the space of possible values for this latent vector.

4.1.2 Clustering Methods for Time Series

For clustering time series data, Kakizawa, Shumway, and Taniguchi (1998) developed a method for multivariate stationary time series using the Kullback–Leibler (KL) divergence information and the Chernoff information as measures of disparity between spectra. A formal definition of stationarity requires that all parameters of the time series (such as the mean, the variance, the lagged autocorrelations, etc.) be constant over time. Denote the value of the time series at some time point t as x_t. A *strictly stationary* time series is one for which the probabilistic behavior of $x_{t_1}, x_{t_2}, \ldots, x_{t_k}$ is identical to that of the shifted set $x_{t_1+h}, x_{t_2+h}, \ldots, x_{t_k+h}$ for any collection of time points $t_1, t_2, \ldots, t_k$, for any number $k = 1, 2, \ldots,$ and for any shift $h = 0, \pm 1, \pm 2, \ldots$. In other words, the joint distribution of any subset of variables is the same as their counterparts in the shifted set. This version of stationarity is too strong for most applications. Instead, we shall consider a milder version, which imposes conditions only on the first two moments of a time series. A *weakly stationary* time series satisfies: (i) the expectation of x_t is constant over time [i.e., $E(x_t) = \mu$]; and (ii) the auto-covariance between x_t and x_{t+h}, $\gamma(t+h, t)$, depends only on their lag difference h, that is, $\gamma(t+h, t) = E[(x_{t+h} - \mu)(x_t - \mu)]$ for all time t and is often abbreviated as $\gamma(h)$. Note that (ii) implies that the variance of a weakly stationary process (obtained by setting $h = 0$) does not change with time. For a Gaussian process, weakly stationarity implies strong stationarity although this is not true for all purposes in general.

For a zero mean weakly stationary process (in practice, time series can be detrended such that its mean is equal to zero) with autocovariance sequence satisfying the summability condition: $\sum_{h=-\infty}^{\infty} |\gamma(h)| < \infty$, one can then define the spectrum $f(\omega) = (1/2\pi) \sum_{h=-\infty}^{\infty} \gamma(h) \exp(-i\omega h)$, $-\pi < \omega < \pi$, where $\exp(i\omega h) = \cos(\omega h) + i \sin(\omega h)$ and $i = \sqrt{-1}$. When the spectrum is known, its autocovariance is completely determined: $\gamma(h) = \int_{-\pi}^{\pi} f(\omega) \exp(i\omega h)\, d\omega$. Interested readers may refer to Brockwell and Davis (2002) or Shumway and Stoffer (2000) for more details. By setting $h = 0$, one obtains the variance $\gamma(0) = \int_{-\pi}^{\pi} f(\omega)\, d\omega$. Thus, the spectrum can be viewed as a decomposition of variance into frequency bands. The spectrum characterizes a time series in a unique manner and hence can be used as a "signature" of the given time series. Our method attempts to extract this signature from the time series data and utilize this to cluster time series accordingly.

The assumption of stationarity may not be satisfied in practice. That is, the spectrum (variance decomposition across frequency) may change over time. Using the Dahlhaus (1997) model for nonstationary time series, Shumway (2003) developed a novel methodology for time series clustering using the symmetrized KL divergence between clusters' time-varying spectra generated through the sliding window method. Our proposed methodology is similar to the Shumway (2003) method in a sense that it takes into account the time-varying spectral features of the time series. However, it differs from the Shumway (2003) method because it incorporates the selection of both time-varying spectral features and the number of groups in the clustering algorithm. In this chapter, the spectral features are extracted, not via the local Fourier transform as in Shumway (2003), but through the wavelet packet (WP) transform. Before we discuss the WP transform, we will first review the spectral analysis for stationary signals by Fourier transform in the next section.

4.2 FOURIER ANALYSIS

The primary goal of spectral analysis is to determine the frequency content in a time series. Spectral analysis is now widely used in cognitive neuroscience to gain a deeper understanding of the human brain function. Individual neurons and neural networks exhibit oscillatory activity over a wide range of frequencies: from delta-band activity (0–4 Hz) to at least gamma-band activity (~30–50 Hz), with recent evidence of activity well above 100 Hz. Oscillatory activity observed in EEG/magnetoencephalography (MEG) recordings often reflects synchronized neural activity that occurs over relatively short time periods (milliseconds). Oscillatory activity within specific frequency bands is one of the most promising candidate mechanisms associated with information processing (see Basar et al., 2001; Klimesch et al., 2005). For example, whereas cortical oscillations in the 30–50 Hz gamma-band [generated by specific neural subtypes (Gray & McCormick, 1996) and networks of interconnected inhibitory interneurons (Whittington et al., 1995)] are thought to reflect early states of sensory perception [e.g., see Pantev et al. (1991)], later 14–30 Hz beta-band activity is thought to be associated with encoding the sensory percept (Kopell et al., 2000; Traub et al., 1999). Thus, a starting point for understanding brain implementations of cognitive phenomena is to examine the frequency components of brain processes across time, obtained through the spectral analysis of brain signals. Fourier analysis is the classic approach for investigating the spectral properties of stationary time series signals. In a typical Fourier analysis, two steps are involved. The first step involves expressing a given time series in terms of the weighted sum of sinusoidal basis functions (known as Fourier waveforms), and determining these random weights, known as Fourier coefficients, through the Fourier transform. In the second step, these coefficients are used to compute the periodogram—the sample estimator for the spectrum of the time series. As demonstrated in Equation 4.2 below, periodogram analysis of time series can be viewed as the decomposition of variance of the dependent variable (time series) according to the variance explained by the "predictors" (the sinusoidal waveforms).

Consider a time series sequence $\mathbf{Y} = [Y_1, \ldots, Y_T]'$ with zero mean. (If a trend is present in the time series, one should remove the trend, prior to performing spectral analysis, by filtering the time series or by fitting some parametric or nonparametric model.) A real-valued time series sequence can be regarded as an element in the T-dimensional Euclidean space, denoted as $\mathcal{R}^T$. One can construct a basis for $\mathcal{R}^T$—a basis consists of linearly independent vectors that spans $\mathcal{R}^T$ (so that every vector in the space can be written as a linear combination of the elements of the basis). One basis for the Euclidean space $\mathcal{R}^T$ is the trigonometric or sinusoidal waveforms so that any time series Y_t can be represented as

$$Y_t = \sum_{k=-[(T-1)/2]}^{[T/2]} c_k \exp(i\omega_k t), \tag{4.1}$$

where $\omega_k = 2\pi k/T$ are called the Fourier or fundamental frequencies, $\exp(i\omega_k t) = \cos\omega_k t + i\sin\omega_k t$ and the notation $[x]$ is the greatest integer less than or equal to x. Equation 4.1 gives the Fourier representation of time series Y. Denote $\mathbf{e_k} = [\exp(i\omega_k), \exp(2i\omega_k), \ldots, \exp(Ti\omega_k)]'$, and $\{\mathbf{e_k}, k = -[(T-1)/2], \ldots, [T/2]\}$ forms the Fourier basis. The c_k's are called Fourier coefficients. The equation above is, in fact, a linear regression model with random coefficients and the columns of the design matrix are composed of the Fourier waveforms, $\{\mathbf{e_k}\}$. The Fourier coefficients are obtained via the Fourier transform

$$c_k = \frac{1}{T}\sum_{t=1}^{T} Y_t \exp(-i\omega_k t).$$

The sample variance of the time series can be expressed in terms of the Fourier coefficients as:

$$\frac{1}{T}\sum_{t=1}^{T} Y_t^2 = \sum_{k=-[(T-1)/2]}^{[T/2]} |c_k|^2. \tag{4.2}$$

A major goal in Fourier analysis is to identify those Fourier waveforms (or frequencies) that are major contributors to the total variance of the time series. This is synonymous to identifying the frequencies corresponding to coefficients with the largest magnitudes (or equivalently, $|c_k|^2$). Interested readers may refer to Bloomfield (2000), Brockwell and Davis (1991), Brillinger (1981), and Shumway and Stoffer (2000) for more details on Fourier analysis.

Fourier transform is typically applied to the *entire* time series and thus gives a decomposition of variance that is global in time. In some applications such as those in cognitive neuroscience, scientists are interested in how brain processes evolve over time. When the statistical properties of the time series change over time (e.g., variance changes with time), the Fourier system is no longer suitable. To illustrate this idea, two nonstationary signals were simulated (see Figure 4.1, left panel). Whereas both signals contained high- and low-frequency activities, the two signals differ in the timing of these activities. The time series in the top left panel shows slower oscillations followed by faster oscillations. The time series in the bottom left panel shows the reverse—faster oscillations followed by slower oscillations. Using the Fourier transform, the spectra of these two nonstationary time series are identical (see the right panel) and cannot be distinguished! An accurate representation for the spectra of these two time series should reflect changes in the distribution of variance across frequencies and time (see the right panel in Figure 4.2). Thus, in many instances, standard Fourier analysis techniques are not adequate for estimating the

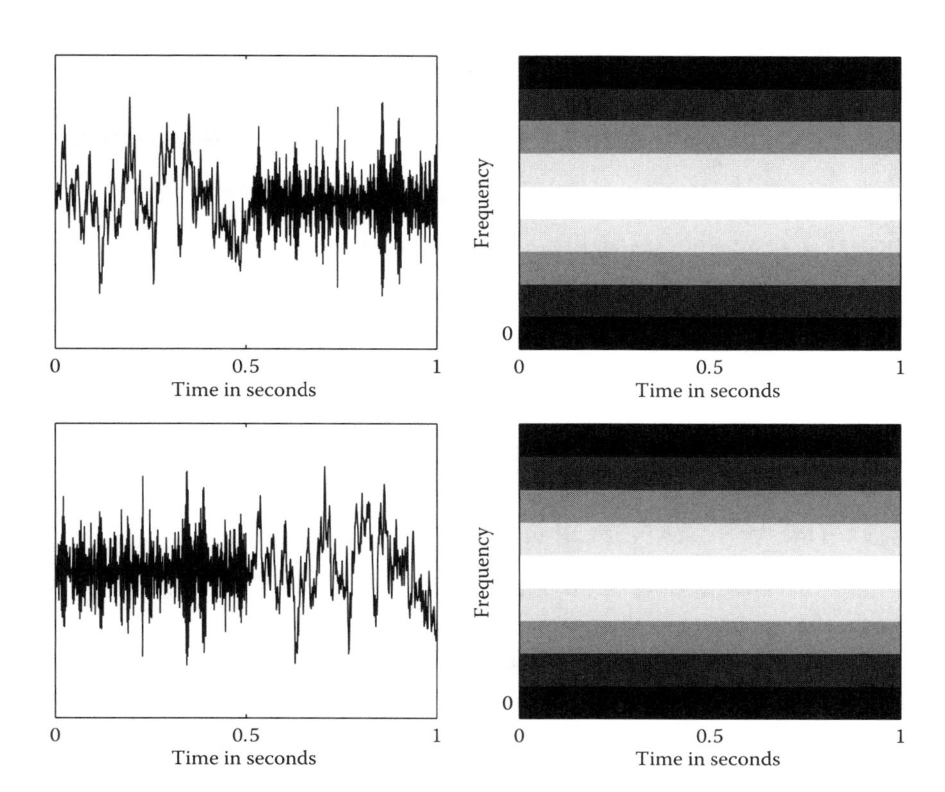

FIGURE 4.1 Left: Two nonstationary signals. Right: The spectra of the two signals derived from the classical Fourier analysis. Darker shades represent higher power.

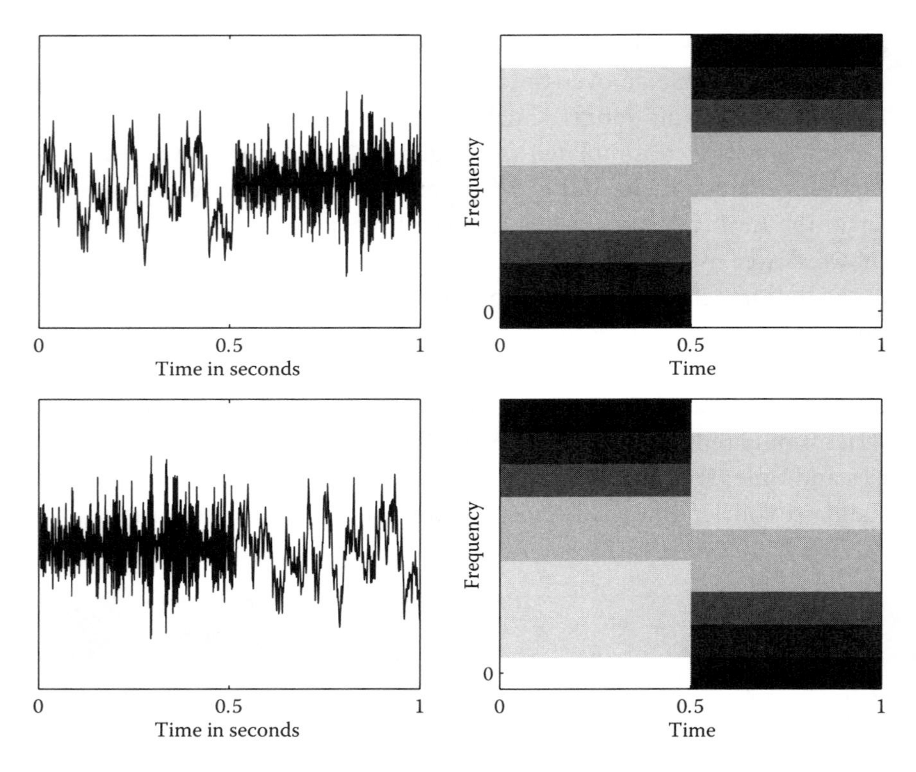

FIGURE 4.2 Left: Two nonstationary signals. Right: The true time-varying spectrum. Darker shades represent higher power.

spectra of nonstationary time series signals. The WP transform can be used to overcome this limitation, which will be discussed in the next section.

4.3 THE WP TRANSFORM

Under the assumption of stationarity, the auto-covariance and, equivalently, the spectrum of the time series does not change with time. However, the assumption of stationarity may not be satisfied in practice. For example, the difference in EEG signals before and during the epileptic seizure in Figure 4.3 suggests a time-varying spectrum. To analyze nonstationary time series, it is more appropriate to use time-localized transforms such as WP. These localized transforms give time-dependent decomposition of variance of a nonstationary time series. A brief introduction on WP will

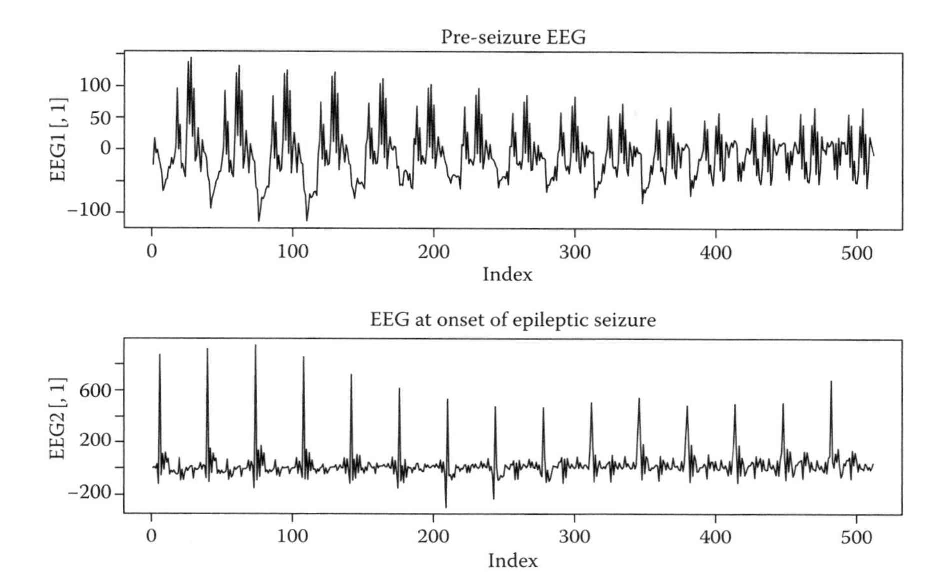

FIGURE 4.3 EEGs. Top: EEG signal recorded prior to an epileptic seizure. Bottom: EEG signal recorded during seizure onset.

be presented next. Interested readers may refer to Bruce and Gao (1996) and Vidakovic (1999) for an excellent treatment of wavelet theory and its applications to statistical problems.

WP analysis is a generalization of wavelet analysis (Wickerhauser, 1994). It is useful for analyzing nonstationary time series because it can provide decomposition of the variance (spectra) of a signal varying over time. Such a decomposition is achieved through the use of the WP basis function. In general, a basis function system is a set of known functions $\phi_k(t)$ that are mathematically independent of each other and that have the property that we can approximate arbitrarily well for any function by taking a weighted sum or linear combination of a sufficiently large number of these functions: $y(t) = \sum_{k=1}^{K} c_k \phi_k(t)$. Fourier basis functions discussed in the previous section and cubic splines are examples of basis function systems. Here, we focus on the WP basis system for representing nonstationary time series signals.

Each WP basis function consists of a set of orthonormal WP waveforms, $\psi_{j,b,k}(t)$, which are indexed by the triplet (j, b, k), where level j $(j = 0, 1, \ldots, J)$ indicates the resolution level in frequency (the larger the value of j, the finer the frequency resolution); b $(b = 0, 1, \ldots, 2^j - 1)$

indicates the rapidness of the oscillation of the WP (larger value of b corresponding to higher frequency and more oscillations) and k ($k = 0, \ldots, T/2^j - 1$) indicates the time shift or location. Each $\psi_{j,b,k}(t)$ associates with a (dyadic) frequency interval $[b/2^{j+1}, (b+1)/2^{j+1})$ and time interval $[k \times 2^j, (k+1) \times 2^j)$ at a specific resolution level j. Figure 4.4 (top panel) shows two examples of WP waveform at the same resolution level but oscillating at different frequencies. Using the WP basis function system, a given signal Y_t can be represented as a series sum of orthogonal WP waveforms, $\psi_{j,b,k}(t)$, at different oscillations, resolution scales, and time locations:

$$Y_t \approx \sum_j \sum_b \sum_k d_{j,b,k} \cdot \psi_{j,b,k}(t).$$

Analogous to the computation of the Fourier coefficient, the WP coefficient ($d_{j,b,k}$) corresponding to the WP waveform $\psi_{j,b,k}(t)$ is equal to the inner product between $\mathbf{Y} = [Y_1, \ldots, Y_T]'$ and $\psi_{j,b,k}$, that is, $d_{j,b,k} = \sum_{t=1}^{T} Y_t \psi_{j,b,k}(t)$. This is known as the *wavelet packet transform*. The WP coefficients can then be used to compute the signal's time-varying spectrum. Squaring the modulus of the WP coefficients gives the WP periodogram, the sample counterpart of the spectrum: $I_{j,b,k} = |d_{j,b,k}|^2$, which computes the amount of sample variance in the time series localized at the frequency band $[b/2^{j+1}, (b+1)/2^{j+1})$ during time interval $[k \cdot 2^j, (k+1) \cdot 2^j)$ at the resolution level j. The bottom panel in Figure 4.4 shows the WP periodograms corresponding to the two WP functions in the top panel.

By changing the resolution level j, scaling the oscillation b, and shifting the time location t, we can obtain a rich family of WP waveforms. Depending on the nature of the nonstationarity of a given signal (see Figure 4.2 again), we can select a set of suitable WP waveforms and hence the WP spectra to represent the time-varying properties of the signal. The WP coefficients associated with the corresponding WP waveforms are usually collectively indexed in a tabular form, known as the *WP table*. For a given signal $\mathbf{Y}$ of length T, where T is a multiple of 2^J, and J is the maximum resolution level, the corresponding WP table has $J + 1$ resolution levels. At each resolution j, there are T WP coefficients (and waveforms), divided into 2^j coefficient blocks. Stacking these coefficients from each resolution level on top of one another, we obtain the $(J+1) \times T$ table of WP coefficients. We illustrate this idea in Table 4.1, where the maximal resolution level is set to 2 (i.e., $J = 2$). At level $j = 0$, there is only one block with T WP coefficients.

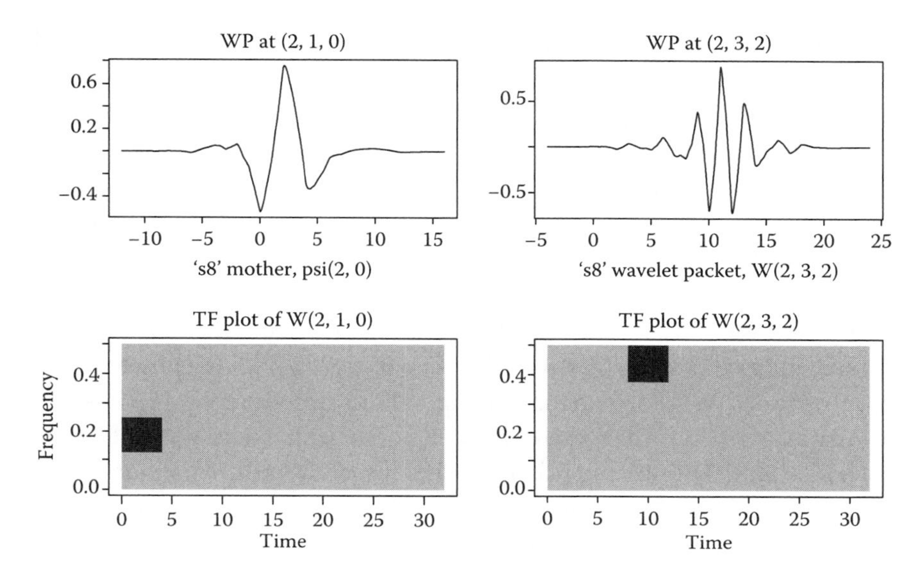

FIGURE 4.4 WP functions and their time–frequency representations. Left: WP function indexed by $(2, 1, 0)$ is oscillating at resolution level $j = 2$, has frequency concentrated at around $(1/8, 1/4]$, and has time shift index $k = 0$. Right: WP function indexed by $(2, 3, 2)$ is oscillating at resolution level $j = 2$, has frequency concentrated at $(3/8, 1/2]$, and has time shift index $k = 2$.

At level $j = 1$, there are $2^1 = 2$ blocks and each block contains $T/2$ WP coefficients. At level $j = 2$, there are $2^2 = 4$ blocks and each block contains $T/2^2 = T/4$ WP coefficients. Each of these coefficients is associated with one WP function ($\psi_{j,b,k}$). Each WP coefficient block [denoted as $B(j, b)$] covers a specific frequency band. The coefficient block at level 0, denoted as the block $B(0, 0)$, covers the frequency band $(0, \frac{1}{2})$ (where $\frac{1}{2}$ corresponds to Nyquist frequency). The magnitude of the T WP coefficients reflects how

TABLE 4.1

Wavelet Packet Library with $J = 2$

$B(0,0)$			
$B(1,0)$		$B(1,1)$	
$B(2,0)$	$B(2,1)$	$B(2,2)$	$B(2,3)$

Note: At level $j, j = 0, 1, 2$, there are 2^j blocks. Each block has $T/2^j$ WP coefficients. The coefficients in block $B(j, b)$ correspond to the wavelet packets with frequency concentrated on the interval $(b/2^{j+1}, b + 1/2^{j+1}]$. Moreover, these coefficients are indexed by time shifts $k = 0, \ldots, T/2^j$.

the spectra vary over this frequency band over time. The aforementioned frequency band is halved at the resolution $j = 1$. There are altogether two coefficient blocks, namely, $B(1, 0)$ and $B(1, 1)$. The block $B(1, 0)$ covers the frequency band $(0, \frac{1}{4}]$ and there are a total of $T/2$ WP coefficients within this block. The block $B(1, 1)$ covers the frequency band $(\frac{1}{4}, \frac{2}{4}]$ and there are also a total of $T/2$ WP coefficients within this block. At level 2, there are $2^2 = 4$ blocks of WP coefficients, $B(2, 0), B(2, 1), B(2, 2)$, and $B(2, 3)$, covering the frequency bands $(0, \frac{1}{8}]$, $(\frac{1}{8}, \frac{2}{8}]$, $(\frac{2}{8}, \frac{3}{8}]$, and $(\frac{3}{8}, \frac{4}{8}]$, respectively. Within each block, there are $T/2^j$ WP coefficients and each coefficient corresponds to time interval $[k \times 2^j, (k + 1) \times 2^j), k = 0, \ldots, T/2^j - 1$. Thus, at $j = 0$, each of the T WP coefficients corresponds to time interval $[k, (k + 1))$. Similarly, at $j = 1$ and 2, each of the T coefficients corresponds to time intervals $[2k, 2(k + 1))$ and $[4k, 4(k + 1))$, respectively. It is obvious that as j increases, the time resolution decreases (the width of the time interval to each of the WP coefficients correspondingly increases) but the frequency resolution increases (the frequency ranges become narrower to each WP coefficient block correspondingly).

The WP table provides a highly redundant representation of a signal of length T with $(J + 1) \times T$ WP coefficients (and waveforms). Depending on the nature of nonstationarity of a given signal (see, e.g., Figure 4.1, left panel), we can choose a total of T coefficients from the WP table to best represent the signal. These coefficients can be taken from different resolution levels (different values of j) and thus allow a *multiresolution* representation of the signal. For the sake of computational efficiency, coefficients are chosen in blockwise fashion as defined in the WP table rather than in an individual manner. Two rules are followed to pick the coefficient blocks in the WP table. First, every column in the WP table is covered by one block. This ensures that the WP transform can be converted to reconstruct the signal. Second, no column in the WP table has more than one block. This ensures that the transform is orthogonal. Following these rules, there are five possible ways to pick the coefficient blocks in a WP table with $J = 2$ (see Table 4.1), namely, (1) $B(0, 0)$ (no segmentation in the frequency axis, no change in the contribution of this frequency band in accounting for the variance of the given signals over time); (2) $B(1, 0)$ and $B(1, 1)$ (change in the contribution of the frequency range $(0, \frac{1}{4}]$ and $(\frac{1}{4}, \frac{1}{2}]$ over time); (3) $B(2, 0)$, $B(2, 1)$, $B(2, 2)$, and $B(2, 3)$ (change in the contribution of the frequency range $(0, \frac{1}{8}]$, $(\frac{1}{8}, \frac{2}{8}]$, $(\frac{2}{8}, \frac{3}{8}]$, and $(\frac{3}{8}, \frac{4}{8}]$ over time); (4) $B(1, 0)$, $B(2, 2)$, and $B(2, 3)$ (change in the contribution of the frequency range $(0, \frac{1}{4}]$, $(\frac{1}{4}, \frac{3}{8}]$, and $(\frac{3}{8}, \frac{1}{2}]$ over time); or (5) $B(2, 0)$, $B(2, 1)$, and $B(1, 1)$ (change in the contribution of the frequency range $(0, \frac{1}{8}]$, $(\frac{1}{8}, \frac{1}{4}]$, and $(\frac{1}{4}, \frac{1}{2}]$ over time).

Each one of the collection of WP coefficients above is referred to as a *basis* of a given time series signal Y. The question remains how to choose the "best" basis (denoted as $\mathcal{B}$) out of these five bases. As our goal in this paper is to group a set of time series into homogeneous subsets, the "best" basis is chosen that gives the best clustering power. The details will be presented in the next section. The WP coefficients $(d_{j,b,k})$ in the best basis can be used to compute the WP periodograms, the sample counterparts of the spectra, as $I_{j,b,k} = |d_{j,b,k}|^2$. By Parseval's theorem, $\sum_t Y_t^2 = \sum_{(j,b,k)\in\mathcal{B}} I_{j,b,k}$. Thus, for any time series Y_t with mean zero, its sample variance can be decomposed in terms of a set of WP periodograms: $\frac{1}{T}\sum_{(j,b,k)\in\mathcal{B}} I_{j,b,k} = \frac{1}{T}\sum_{(j,b,k)\in\mathcal{B}} |d_{j,b,k}|^2$ (analogous to Equation 4.2 in Fourier analysis). The bottom panel in Figure 4.4 shows the WP periodograms corresponding to the two WP functions in the top panel.

Percival (1995) and Percival and Walden (2000, pp. 306–313) showed that the WP coefficient is distributed asymptotically normal and the WP periodogram follows a chi-squared distribution, $I_{j,b,k} \sim f_{j,b,k} \cdot \chi_1^2$, where $f_{j,b,k}$ is the expected value of the WP coefficient, $d_{j,b,k}$, and it can be viewed as the approximate variance contribution of the time series at frequency band $((b-1)/2^{j+1}, b/2^{j+1}]$ and time support around $[k \cdot 2^j, (k+1) \cdot 2^j)$. Analogous to Fourier periodograms, WP periodograms are noisy since $\mathbb{V}\text{ar}(I_{j,b,k}) = 2f_{j,b,k}^2$. Thus, one may smooth the WP periodograms across a time window to obtain an averaged WP periodogram: $\alpha(j, b, k) = \sum_{|k'|\leq m_T/2} W(k') \cdot I_{j,b,k+k'}$, where m_T is the size of the smoothing window which depends on the length of time series T and $W(k')$ is the weight function which satisfies $\sum_{|k'|\leq m_T/2} W(k') = 1$. For data analysis in this chapter, we use the averaged WP periodogram $\alpha(j, b, k) = (1/m_T)\sum_{|k'|\leq m_T/2} I_{j,b,k+k'}$, which can be shown to be asymptotically distributed as $\alpha(j, b, k) \sim f_{j,b,k} \cdot \chi_\nu^2/\nu$ with effective degrees of freedom $\nu = m_T$. In the above formulation, for simplicity, it is assumed that the WP periodograms are independent. To the best of our knowledge, there are no known results on the asymptotic joint distribution of the WP periodograms, which might be quite difficult to derive. The only existing work that sets a rigorous framework for setting asymptotic decorrelation of between-scale wavelet coefficients is given in Craigmile and Percival (2005).

In summary, the WP periodograms give a time-varying decomposition of variance of the time series. They can be viewed as signatures or features of time series upon which we can perform clustering. As shown in Figures 4.3 and 4.11, the spectral features of epileptic seizure EEG signals are quite different from those of the normal state EEG. For normal EEG, only low frequencies contribute to the variance. On the other hand, for epileptic EEG, both low, middle, and high frequencies are present and contribute to the variance.

4.4 CLUSTERING NONSTATIONARY TIME SERIES

As discussed in the previous section, depending on the spectral trend of the nonstationary signal under consideration, one can choose the "most suitable" WP basis vector known as the *best basis vector* from the WP table to capture time-varying spectral features of the signals. In this chapter, a criterion for selecting the WP basis vector from the WP table that "best" distinguishes (clusters) between groups is provided.

Consider a data set consisting of information: $\{(Y_i, g_i), i = 1, \ldots, n\}$ where for the ith object, Y_i is the nonstationary signal with length T; g_i is the group index where $g_i \in \{2, \ldots, G\}$, and G is the total number of groups. In most of the clustering applications, the group index g_i is unobserved and the total number of groups G may be unknown. In this chapter, we present an automatic statistical procedure for clustering the signals into homogeneous groups and estimating the number of clusters simultaneously based upon the WP periodograms which define the "signature" of the time series. Our method consists of three major steps. The first step selects the best basis for clustering from the WP table. Out of the T WP coefficients in the best basis, not all of them are equally important or useful and may be removed without affect the clustering results. This is the major purpose of step 2, which selects the most useful features (WP coefficients) from the best basis. In cluster analysis, the number of groups is usually unknown; we will present a scheme to choose the optimal number of clusters through iterating step 1 and step 2. When the number of clusters is determined, the time series are classified into one of these groups in the last step. The details of each step are presented next.

4.4.1 Step 1: Select the Best Clustering Basis

We will assume that the true number of groups G is known for now. When it is not known, we can use BIC to find the optimal G. The details are given in Section 4.4.3. The first step in our proposed method is to choose a basis from the WP table that can best separate clusters in the data set. To select the best basis, we perform the following steps:

1. Compute the smoothed WP periodograms $\{\alpha_i(j, b, k)\}$ for all subjects and across all resolution levels and time blocks, $i = 1, \ldots, n$; $j = 0, \ldots, J$; $b = 0, \ldots, 2^j - 1$; $k = 0, \ldots, T/2^j - 1$.*
2. For each feature $\alpha(j, b, k)$, fit a finite mixture model and estimate the posterior probability of group membership for each object, denoted as $p_{ig}(j, b, k)$. The computational details for estimating the posterior probability are outlined in Appendix 4.1.
3. Compute the clustering power at each resolution level j, frequency index b and time location k:

$$\mathcal{D}(j, b, k) = \sum_{i=1}^{n} \sum_{g=1}^{G-1} \sum_{g'=g+1}^{G} p_{ig}(j, b, k) \log \frac{p_{ig}(j, b, k)}{p_{ig'}(j, b, k)} + p_{ig'}(j, b, k) \log \frac{p_{ig'}(j, b, k)}{p_{ig}(j, b, k)}. \tag{4.3}$$

4. Compute the total clustering power at each block $B(j, b)$: $\mathcal{D}(j, b) = \sum_k \mathcal{D}(j, b, k)$.
5. Choose the best basis based on the total clustering power by the best basis algorithm (BBA) of Coifman and Wickerhauser (1992), which is given in Appendix 4.2.

Intuitively, a best basis for clustering is the one which gives features that provide the "most definitive" clustering, that is, the one that gives values of the conditional probability p_{ig} in Equation 4.3 that are close to either 1 or 0. This point of view is slightly different from the traditional approach of computing some "disparity" measure between cluster centroids. Meyer (2003), for example, used the weighted average as the cluster centroid and

* For a time series signal of length T, the smallest blocks in the WP table have length $T/2^J$. Smaller blocks can give better frequency resolution for representing the local spectra. However, one should be careful about making the blocks too small. Blocks have to be large enough to give reliable estimates for the local spectra.

the Mahalonobis distance between centroids as the measure of disparity. Huang, Ombao and Stoffer (2004), under the context of supervised learning, uses the KL divergence. To motivate our clustering criterion in Equation 4.3, consider the case where there are only $G = 2$ groups. For a fixed object i and feature $\alpha(j, b, k)$, the clustering power criterion attains its minimum value of 0 when $p_{i1}(j, b, k) = p_{i2}(j, b, k) = 0.5$. In this situation, the feature $\alpha(j, b, k)$ is unable to make a definitive classification for object i. This can happen when the two groups have identical spectra at feature $\alpha(j, b, k)$, that is, $f_1(j, b, k) = f_2(j, b, k)$. Consequently, feature $\alpha(j, b, k)$ is unable to separate the two groups. In this situation, we expect the clustering power criterion to be close to 0 because the posterior probability that each object i belongs to either group is close to 0.5.

The proposed procedure above selects the best clustering basis (blocks of features with large clustering power values) from the WP table and eliminates those blocks that do not give definitive clustering. For the sake of computational efficiency, features are chosen in a *blockwise* manner in this step. Once the best clustering basis is chosen, individual features within this basis will be selected in step 2 next.

4.4.2 Step 2: Model-Based Selection of Features for Clustering

In the previous section, a data-adaptive procedure that gives us the best clustering basis $\mathcal{B}$ is developed. However, it may be the case that only a subset of features in $\mathcal{B}$ is relevant for clustering. We adapt the model-based variable selection scheme proposed by Raftery and Dean (2006) for extracting a subset of features in $\mathcal{B}$ that are critical for clustering.

Consider $X = \{\alpha_i(j, b, k) | i = 1, \ldots, n \text{ and } (j, b, k) \in \mathcal{B}\}$, which collects all the "features" in the chosen best basis. At any stage in our variable selection algorithm, Y is partitioned into three sets of variables, $X^{(1)}, X^{(2)}$, and $X^{(3)}$, namely,

- $X^{(1)}$: The set of already selected clustering variables
- $X^{(2)}$: The variable being considered for inclusion into or exclusion from the set of clustering variables
- $X^{(3)}$: The remaining variables.

The decision to include or exclude $X^{(2)}$ from the set of clustering variables is taken by comparing two models M_1 and M_2 where model M_1 specifies that given $X^{(1)}, X^{(2)}$ gives no additional information about the clustering. On the other hand, model M_2 implies that $X^{(2)}$ gives information about clustering membership, in addition to the clustering information provided by $X^{(1)}$. For instance, when $X^{(2)}$ consists of only one variable, the likelihood for the two models is given by

$$\begin{aligned} M_1 : p_{M_1}(X|g) &= p(X^{(3)}|X^{(2)}, X^{(1)})p(X^{(2)}|X^{(1)})p(X^{(1)}|g) \\ &= p(Y^{(3)})p(Y^{(2)})p(Y^{(1)}|g), \\ M_2 : p_{M_2}(X|g) &= p(X^{(3)}|X^{(2)}, X^{(1)})p(X^{(2)}, X^{(1)}|g) \\ &= p(Y^{(3)})p(Y^{(2)}|g)p(Y^{(1)}|g), \end{aligned}$$

where g is the unobserved set of cluster memberships. Models M_1 and M_2 are compared using the Bayes factor, which is difficult to evaluate analytically but can be approximated by BIC (Fraley & Raftery, 2002). Hence, we compare the BICs of the two models instead. In other words, the feature selection problem is recast into the model comparison framework.

4.4.2.1 *Summary of the Algorithm for Feature Selection*

Here we only summarize the major steps for selecting the critical features from the best clustering basis. The details can be found in Appendix 4.3.

1: Select the feature in $\mathcal{B}$ that shows the best evidence of clustering according to the BIC in Equation 4.19 (see Appendix 4.3). Denote this feature to be $\alpha^*(j_1, b_1, k_1)$.
2: Select feature $\alpha^*(j_2, b_2, k_2)$ to be the one so that the pair of features $\{\alpha^*(j_1, b_1, k_1), \alpha^*(j_2, b_2, k_2)\}$ shows most evidence of bivariate clustering, again according to BIC.
3: Select the next feature from the best clustering basis but excluding $\alpha^*(j_1, b_1, k_1)$ and $\alpha^*(j_2, b_2, k_2)$, denoted as $\mathcal{B} \setminus \{\alpha^*(j_1, b_1, k_1), \alpha^*(j_2, b_2, k_2)\}$ that shows most evidence of multivariate clustering including the previous variables selected. Accept the feature $\alpha^*(j_3, b_3, k_3) \in \mathcal{B} \setminus \{\alpha^*(j_1, b_1, k_1), \alpha^*(j_2, b_2, k_2)\}$ as a clustering variable if the evidence of clustering is stronger than of not clustering; in other words, the BIC of including the feature $\alpha^*(j_3, b_3, k_3)$ is larger than that of not including it.

4: Consider removal of a feature from $\{\alpha^*(j_1, b_1, k_1), \alpha^*(j_2, b_2, k_2), \alpha^*(j_3, b_3, k_3)\}$ to be the one that shows least evidence of multivariate clustering. Remove this feature from the set of clustering features if the evidence of clustering is weaker than of not clustering; that is, the BIC of including this feature is smaller than that of not including it.
5: Iterate steps 3 and 4 above until no more new features can be added in step 3 and also no feature can be dropped in step 4.

The procedure above is analogous to variable selection by a stepwise method in multiple regression analysis.

4.4.3 Criterion for Selecting the Optimal Number of Clusters

When the number of clusters G is unknown, it can be estimated by iterating the two steps in Sections 4.1 and 4.2. For each candidate, the number of clusters $g \in \{2, \ldots, G_{\max}\}$: (i) first, select the best basis; (ii) second, select the best subset of features, denoted as $\mathcal{F}_g$; (iii) compute $\mathrm{BIC}_g(\mathcal{F}_g)$ and choose G^* that satisfies

$$G^* = \arg\max_{g \in \{2,\ldots,G_{\max}\}} \mathrm{BIC}_g(\mathcal{F}_g). \tag{4.4}$$

For different numbers of groups g, the model-based feature selection method may select a different number of features. Let $\mathcal{F}_{G_1}$ be the subset selected when the number of clusters is G_1, and $\mathcal{F}_{G_2}$ be the subset of features selected when the number of clusters is G_2. To make the BICs comparable, we define

$$\mathrm{BIC}_{G_1} = \mathrm{BIC}_{\mathrm{c}}(\mathcal{F}_{G_1}) + \mathrm{BIC}_{\mathrm{nc}}(\mathcal{F}_{G_2} \setminus \mathcal{F}_{G_1}),$$
$$\mathrm{BIC}_{G_2} = \mathrm{BIC}_{\mathrm{c}}(\mathcal{F}_{G_2}) + \mathrm{BIC}_{\mathrm{nc}}(\mathcal{F}_{G_1} \setminus \mathcal{F}_{G_2}),$$

where

$$\mathrm{BIC}_{\mathrm{c}}(\mathcal{F}) = \sum_{(j,b,k)\in\mathcal{F}} \mathrm{BIC}_{\mathrm{c}}[(j,b,k)], \tag{4.5}$$

$$\mathrm{BIC}_{\mathrm{nc}}(\mathcal{F}) = \sum_{(j,b,k)\in\mathcal{F}} \mathrm{BIC}_{\mathrm{nc}}[(j,b,k)], \tag{4.6}$$

where $\mathrm{BIC}_{\mathrm{c}}[(j,b,k)]$ and $\mathrm{BIC}_{\mathrm{nc}}[(j,b,k)]$ are defined in Equations 4.19 and 4.20, respectively, in Appendix 4.3, and $\mathbf{F}_2 \setminus \mathbf{F}_1$ means the variables in $\mathbf{F}_2$ but not in $\mathbf{F}_1$.

If $\text{BIC}_{G_1} > \text{BIC}_{G_2}$, then the model with G_1 groups is superior to the model with G_2 groups. Otherwise the model with G_2 groups is better. We start the cluster number selection process by comparing the model with one cluster versus two clusters; then we use the model with bigger BIC to compare to the model with three clusters and so on until comparison to the model with $G_{\max}$ groups. The model returned at the end is the best model, which tells us what the most critical frequency features localized at a specific time interval that best distinguish the groups are.

4.4.4 Step 3: Clustering Based on the Selected Features

The proposed methodology selects the optimal number of clusters (if it is not known *a priori*) and the best subset of features $\mathcal{F}$ (selected from the best clustering WP basis). The last step is to assign each object to a cluster. The assignment or clustering rule is determined by using all features $\alpha(j,b,k)$ in $\mathcal{F}$. Let $\alpha_i = [\alpha_i(j,b,k), (j,b,k) \in \mathcal{F}]$ be the vector of smoothed WP periodograms for object i. We estimate the posterior probability p_{ig}, conditioned on α_i, that object i belongs to group g. Under the assumption that the features in the best clustering basis $\mathcal{B}$ are independent, the joint density of these features is:

$$
\begin{aligned}
H_g(\alpha_i | g_i = g) = & \prod_{(j,b,k)\in\mathcal{F}} [\Gamma(\nu/2)]^{-1} \left[\frac{\nu}{2f_g(j,b,k)}\right]^{\nu/2} \alpha_i(j,b,k)^{\nu/2-1} \\
& \times \exp\left[-\frac{\nu\,\alpha_i(j,b,k)}{2f_g(j,b,k)}\right].
\end{aligned} \tag{4.7}
$$

The posterior probability p_{ig} can then be estimated via the EM algorithm similarly to the one given in Appendix 4.1 [simply replacing $h(\alpha_i(j,b,k)|g_i = g)$ in the formulae given in Appendix 4.1 by $H_g(\alpha_i|g_i = g)$] and the object i is assigned to group g^* with the largest posterior probability (i.e., $g^* = \arg\max_g p_{ig}$).

4.5 SIMULATIONS

To demonstrate the validity of our proposed clustering procedures, three sets of simulations were run.

4.5.1 Simulation 1: Two Groups from the AR(1) Process

The first simulation considers time series generated under different time-varying auto-regressive processes. The observations from the first group were generated as follows:

$$X_t = \begin{cases} 0.9X_{t-1} + W_t^{(1)}, & 1 \le t \le T/2, \\ -0.9X_{t-1} + W_t^{(1)}, & T/2 \le t \le T, \end{cases} \tag{4.8}$$

where $W_t^{(1)}$ is normally distributed independent random noise. The observations from group 2 were generated by the same two processes but in reverse temporal order:

$$Y_t = \begin{cases} -0.9Y_{t-1} + W_t^{(2)}, & 1 \le t \le T/2, \\ 0.9Y_{t-1} + W_t^{(2)}, & T/2 \le t \le T, \end{cases} \tag{4.9}$$

where $W_t^{(2)}$ is normally distributed independent random noise.

The length of time series was set to 512, and ten time series were generated for group 1 and five for group 2. Figure 4.5 shows an example of the signals in the two groups from $T = 1$ to $T = 256$. The simulations were repeated 100 times, and the results are summarized in Table 4.2. As shown in the second column of Table 4.2, 70 times out of 100, the data were correctly clustered into two groups based on our proposed procedures.

To examine how the number of signals in each group affected the result, we increased the number of signals in both groups to 30. As shown in the last column of Table 4.2, it is clear that the result for the model-based method has substantially improved; the accuracy rate has increased to 98%.

In the simulation, the best basis that was most frequently chosen was formed by $B(1,0)$ and $B(1,1)$, as it should be, as half of the signals differed in the low-frequency band and the other half differed in the high-frequency band.

4.5.2 Simulation 2: Two Groups from the White Noise Plus AR(2) Process

To further examine the sensitivity of our proposed method, in the second simulation, we considered the signals coming from two groups, but the first

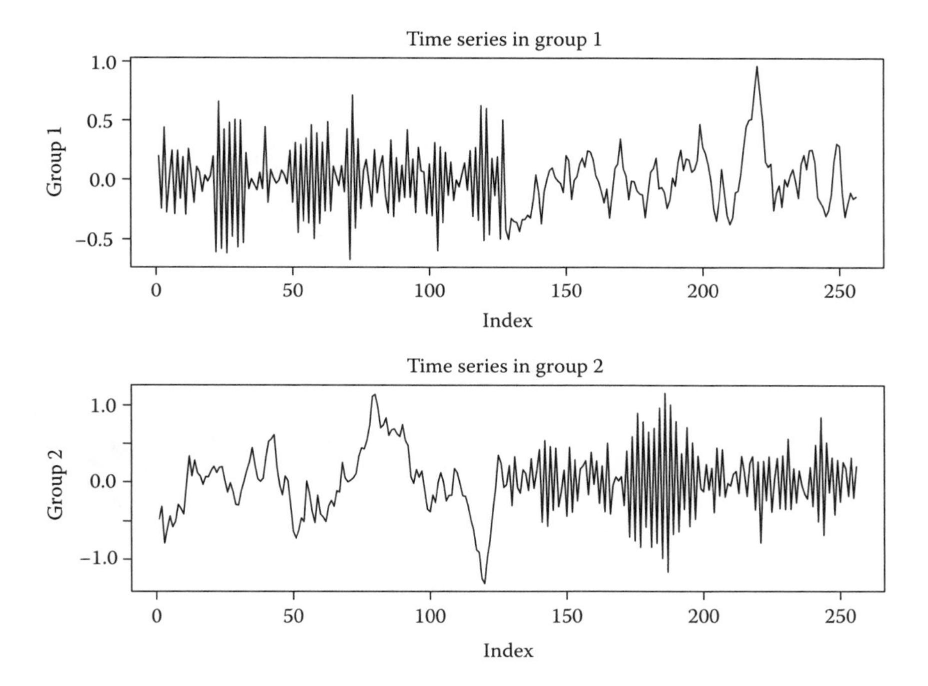

FIGURE 4.5 Signals in two groups.

part of the signals of both groups was random white noise, and the second part was generated from different AR(2) processes. The signals from the first group followed

$$X_t = \begin{cases} W_t^{(1)}, & 1 \leq t \leq 3T/5, \\ Z_t^{(1)}, & 3T/5 \leq t \leq T, \end{cases} \tag{4.10}$$

where $W_t^{(1)}$ is normally distributed random white noise, and $Z_t^{(1)}$ is an AR(2) process: $Z_t^{(1)} = 1.85Z_{t-1}^{(1)} - 0.89Z_{t-2}^{(1)} + W_t$. The signals from the

TABLE 4.2

Number of Clusters for Simulation One when $n_1 = 10$ and $n_2 = 5$

G	$n_1 = 10, n_2 = 5$	$n_1 = 30, n_2 = 30$
2	70	98
3	7	2
4	11	0
5	12	0

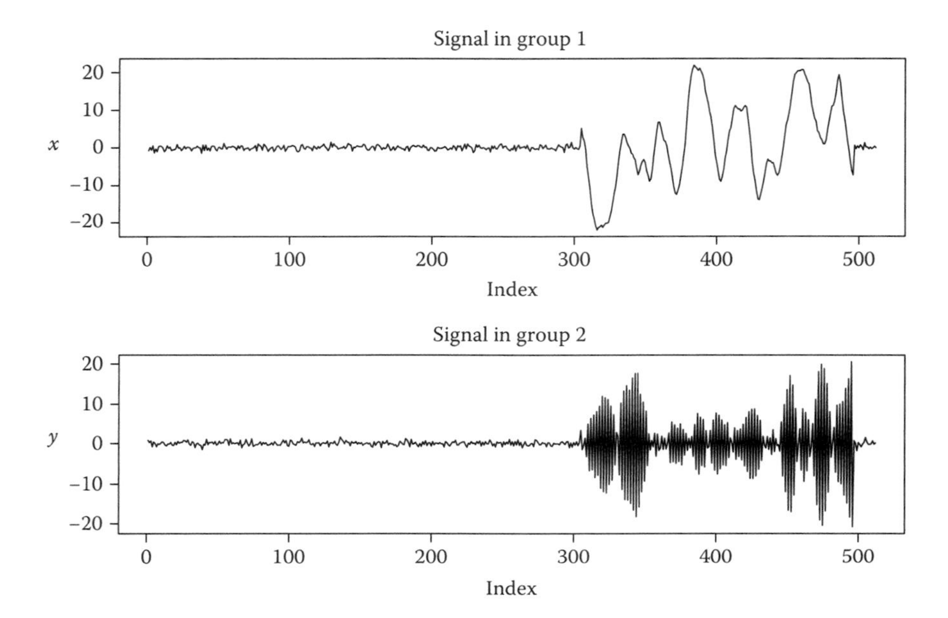

FIGURE 4.6 Two group signals.

second group followed

$$Y_t = \begin{cases} W_t^{(2)}, & 1 \leq t \leq 3T/5, \\ Z_t^{(2)}, & 3T/5 \leq t \leq T, \end{cases} \tag{4.11}$$

where $W_t^{(2)}$ is normally distributed random white noise, and $Z_t^{(2)}$ is an AR(2) process: $Z_t^{(2)} = -1.85Z_{t-1}^{(2)} - 0.89Z_{t-2}^{(2)} + W_t$. An example of the signals from the two groups is shown in Figure 4.6. The spectra of these two AR(2) processes are plotted in Figure 4.7. It can be seen that the spectral power of the signals is localized at the low-frequency range for the first group but is localized at the high-frequency range for the second group. In this simulation, 25 time series were generated for each group, and the length of each time series was 512. Out of 100 simulations, 94 times the signals were correctly classified into two groups and 6 times they were misclassified into three groups. The results demonstrate that our method can still have high sensitivity to distinguish different groups of signals even if 50% of their content were the same.

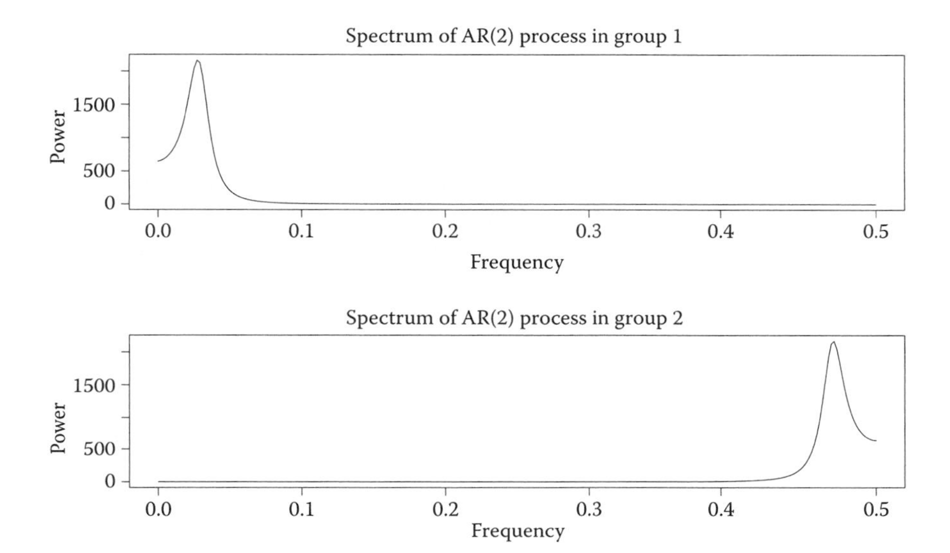

FIGURE 4.7 The spectrum of AR(2) processes.

4.5.3 Simulation 3: Three Groups Generated from WP Coefficients

In the last simulation, classification of signals from three groups was examined. In order to precisely control the spectral power localized at specific time and frequency range, the WP coefficients were explicitly specified which were then converted to time series signals by the inverse WP transform (a "reverse" step of the WP transform). The length of the time series was again set to 512.

For the WP table with $j = 0, \ldots, 3$, at level $j = 3$, there are altogether $2^3 = 8$ blocks and each block has 32 WP coefficients. For group 1, the WP coefficients in block $B(3, 0)$ were generated as follows: the 13th to 28th coefficients in this block were generated from normal distribution with mean 0 and variance 10,000; the rest of coefficients in this block (i.e., 1st to 12th, and 29th to 32nd) and in the remaining seven blocks of level $j = 3$ were generated from normal distribution with mean 0 and variance 1. For group 2, the WP coefficients in block $B(3, 7)$ were generated as follows: the 9th to 24th coefficients in this block were generated from normal distribution with mean 0 and variance 10,000; the rest of the coefficients in this block (i.e., 1st to 7th, and 25th to 32nd) and in the remaining seven blocks of level $j = 3$ were generated from normal distribution with mean

0 and variance 1. For group 3, the WP coefficients in block $B(3, 3)$ were generated as follows: the 5th to 20th coefficients in this block were generated from normal distribution with mean 0 and variance 10,000; the rest of coefficients in this block (i.e., 1st to 4th and 21st to 32nd) and in the remaining seven blocks of level $j = 3$ were generated from normal distribution with mean 0 and variance 1. As a result, the spectral power was localized in the low-frequency band $(0, 1/16)$ in time $t = 192$–448 for group 1, in the high-frequency band $(7/16, 1/2)$ in time $t = 108$–364 for group 2, and in the medium-frequency band $(3/16, 1/4)$ in time $t = 64$–320 for group 3.

The WP coefficients with large spectral power in each of the three groups were highlighted in Figure 4.8 and the corresponding time–frequency plots are shown in Figure 4.9.

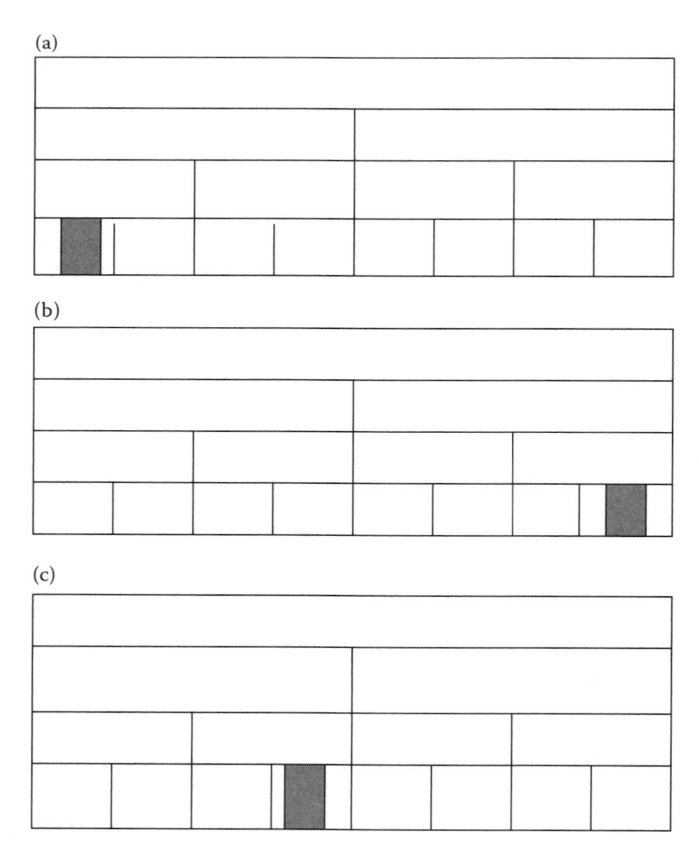

FIGURE 4.8 The WP coefficients selected for each of the three groups.

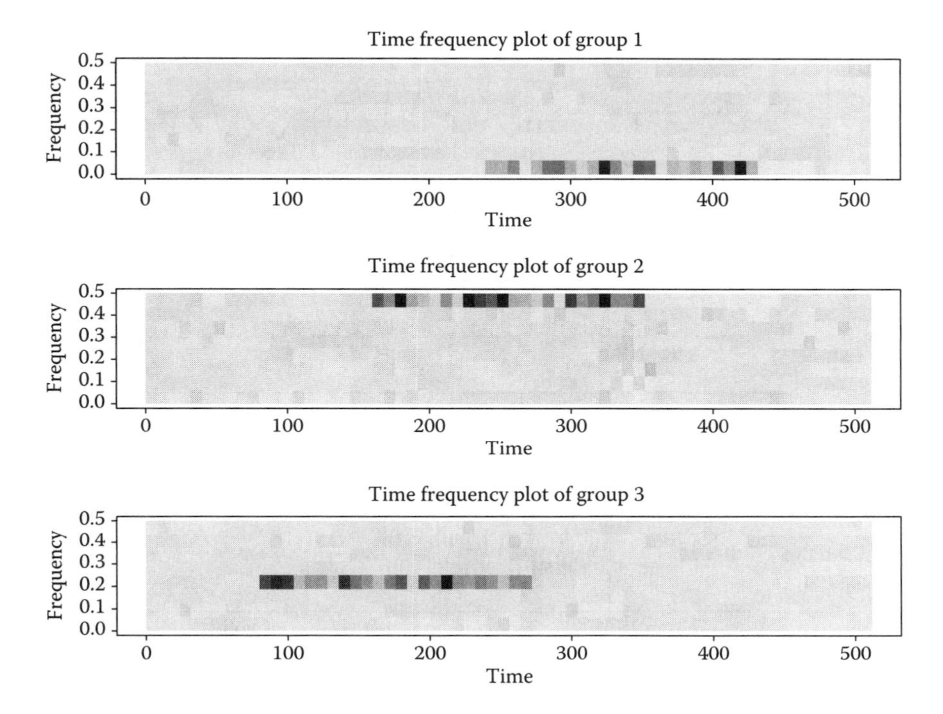

FIGURE 4.9 The true spectra for the three groups in the simulation.

Twenty time series from each of the three groups were generated and the length of each time series was set to 512. Samples of time series from each of the groups are shown in Figure 4.10. Out of 100 simulations, 94 times the signals were correctly classified into three groups corresponding to their true grouping membership in the data generation step, and 5 times to four groups, 1 time to five groups, and 0 times to two groups. The classification results are quite satisfactory.

4.6 ILLUSTRATIVE EXAMPLE

In this section, we demonstrate the validity of our proposed methodology with a dataset that consists of EEGs recorded during two brain states, namely, normal and epileptic seizure states. All the analyses were performed by the software *R* and required the use of two add-on packages, namely, "cluster" and "wavelm."

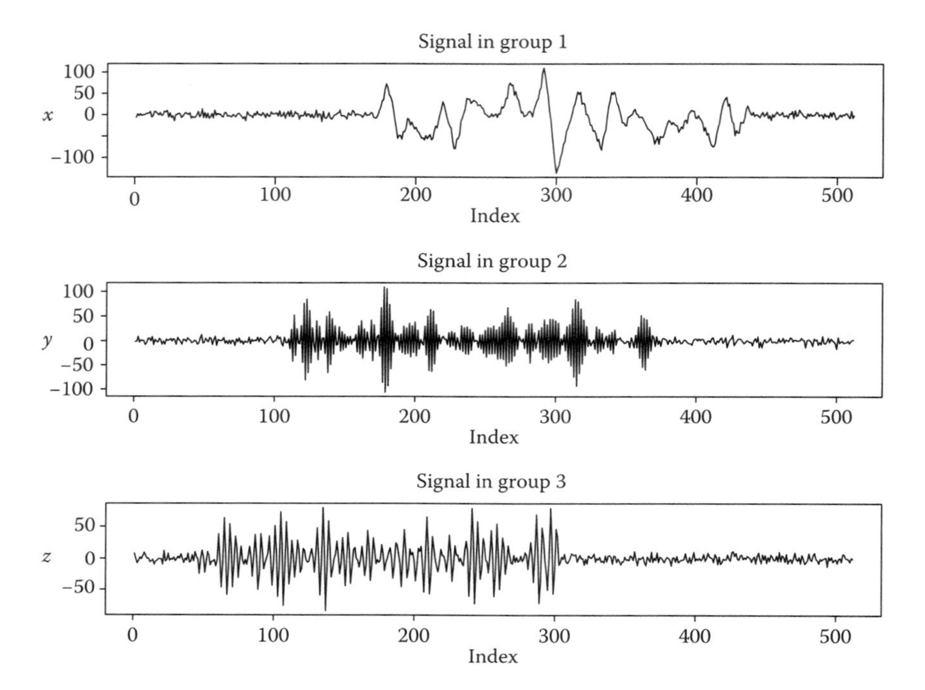

FIGURE 4.10 Samples of time series from the three groups in the simulation.

4.6.1 Electroencephalograms

This data set consists of 34 EEGs recorded during a "normal" brain state and another 34 EEGs recorded at the same channels during the onset of an epileptic seizure. The length of each EEG signal was $T = 512$ and the EEGs were digitized at the rate of 100 Hz (i.e., the duration of the time series was 5.12 s). Figure 4.11 shows an example of the EEG signals prior to and during an epileptic seizure.

The main goal of the analysis is to demonstrate that our proposed clustering method, based on time–frequency features, is able to separate EEGs for the normal state versus EEGs recorded during the epileptic seizure state. In the analysis, we set $J = 5$ for the finest frequency resolution level in the WP table. Instead of fixing the number of clusters *a priori*, we searched for the "optimal" number of clusters based on BIC discussed in Section 4.4.3 from a set of candidate clustering solutions. Our proposed method selected $G = 2$ as the optimal number of clusters,

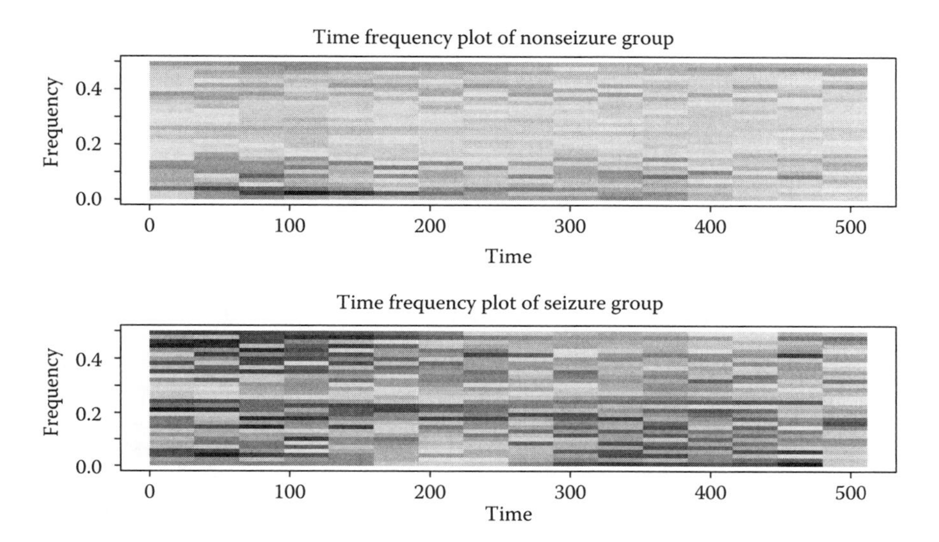

FIGURE 4.11 The time–frequency plots of signals before and during epileptic seizure.

as expected (before vs. during epileptic states). The first cluster contains 33 nonseizure signals, while the second cluster contains the remaining 34 seizure signals and one nonseizure. The best basis being chosen was formed by the 32 frequency blocks at the finest resolution level ($j = 5$) of the WP table. The WP spectra based upon the chosen best basis corresponding to these two clusters are shown Figure 4.11. The plots are a little bit messy and may not be easy to interpret. Using the feature selection procedures delineated in Section 4.4.2, six time–frequency features with largest clustering power were chosen and are shown in Figure 4.12. The detailed time and frequency information is displayed in Table 4.3. These best clustering features primarily consist of frequencies at the beta-band (15–30 Hz) from time $t = 1$ to $t = 300$ (or in the interval $(0, 3]$ seconds). The results are very promising and can be developed for application to seizure detection. This chapter has taken the initial step toward this direction by identifying features that distinguish normal from epileptic seizure states. To be completely useful for clinical applications, an online version of the algorithm will need to be developed so that if technology is available to "normalize" electrical activity, it is able to instantaneously detect abnormal wave patterns and possibly reduce the recurrence of seizure episodes.

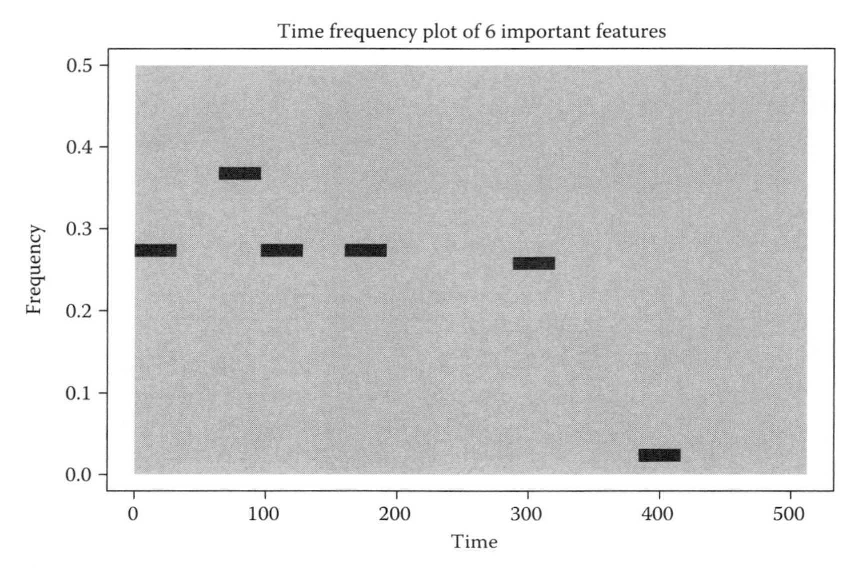

FIGURE 4.12 Important clustering time–frequency features given by the method for clustering the EEG signals data.

TABLE 4.3

Time and Frequency Information of the Six Selected Features of EEG Data

Features ($\alpha(j, b, k)$)	Time (ms)	Frequency (Hz)	f_1	f_2
$\alpha(5, 17, 0)$	0–32	25–26.56	0.22	0.63
$\alpha(5, 23, 2)$	64–96	34.38–35.94	0.34	0.90
$\alpha(5, 17, 3)$	96–128	25–26.56	0.31	0.80
$\alpha(5, 17, 5)$	160–192	25–26.56	0.21	0.60
$\alpha(5, 16, 9)$	288–320	23.44–25	0.20	0.66
$\alpha(5, 1, 12)$	384–416	0–1.56	6.45	2.05

Note: f_1 is the estimated spectrum of nonseizure group (cluster 1), and f_2 is the estimated spectrum of seizure group (cluster 2) at the specific features.

4.7 SUMMARY

Our methodology for clustering nonstationary time series integrates principles of statistical modeling and powerful modern tools for signal processing. We use WP transform to extract a family of time-varying spectral features in the data set and develop an entropy-based criterion to select the basis in the WP table that can best separate clusters in the data set. Our proposed methodology is general. Other localized transforms such as the cosine packet or the Smooth Localized Complex Exponentials (SLEX) transforms (see Ombao et al., 2001 for details) can be used as well. Instead of using the proposed data-driven clustering criterion (see Section 4.4.1), researchers can select the best basis vector depending on some known characteristics of nonstationarity of the time series. One might consider segmenting the time series based on the experimental design directly and search only the best frequency set to distinguish groups, which is less data-dependent than the proposed method.

Not all features contained in the selected basis are relevant for clustering. Thus, we use a model-based feature selection algorithm to select a subset of features in the best basis that are most useful for clustering. The above steps assume that the number of clusters G is known *a priori*. When such information is not known, we include the number of clusters as an unknown parameter in the model and simultaneously select the optimal G and the subset of clustering features using the BIC. Our proposed method gives promising results when applied to an empirical EEG dataset. It can be a useful tool for a variety of practical applications such as predicting seizure onset and for speech recognition.

In the current implementation, the best basis is chosen using a dyadic scheme for simplicity and computational efficiency reasons. However, nondyadic schemes are also feasible, but require more computationally intensive procedures. Other search schemes such as dynamic programming and change-point detection algorithms (see, e.g., Choi, Ombao, & Ray, 2008) are currently being developed to overcome the limitation of dyadic-segmentation-based algorithm.

Our proposed method focuses on univariate analysis of time series, but it can be readily generalized to multivariate application. The periodogram matrix, whose elements contain the auto-periodograms and cross-periodograms, can be used to characterize the relationships between multivariate time series and thus can serve as the building block for clustering.

ACKNOWLEDGMENTS

This research was supported in part by the National Science Foundation DMS 04-05243 (B. Gao & H. Ombao) and the Academic Research Fund (RG30-05), Ministry of Education, Singapore (M.-H. R. Ho).

APPENDIX 4.1: ESTIMATION OF THE POSTERIOR PROBABILITY IN EQUATION 4.4

For feature $\alpha(j, b, k)$, the conditional distribution of the smoothed WP periodogram $\alpha_i(j, b, k)$, given that it belongs to group g ($g = 1, \ldots, G$), is

$$h[\alpha_i(j, b, k)|g_i = g] \\ = [\Gamma(\nu/2)]^{-1} \left[\frac{\nu}{2f_g(j, b, k)}\right]^{\nu/2} \alpha_i(j, b, k)^{\nu/2-1} \exp\left[-\frac{\nu\alpha_i(j, b, k)}{2f_g(j, b, k)}\right], \tag{4.12}$$

where $\{f_g(j, b, k)\}$ is the spectrum for group g. Denote τ_g as the prior probability that $\alpha_i(j, b, k)$ belongs to group g. Then the unconditional probability density function of $\alpha_i(j, b, k)$ is

$$h[\alpha_i(j, b, k)] = \sum_{g=1}^{G} \tau_g \, h[\alpha_i(j, b, k)|g_i = g]. \tag{4.13}$$

This is a finite mixture model with G components; each component has a different spectrum, $f_g(j, b, k)$. The estimators of f_g and $\tau_g, g = 2, \ldots, G$, are obtained by maximizing the observed likelihood:

$$\mathcal{L}^M = \prod_{i=1}^{n} \sum_{g=1}^{G} \tau_g h_g[\alpha_i(j, b, k)|g_i = g]. \tag{4.14}$$

We employ the EM algorithm (Dempster et al., 1977) to maximize the likelihood $\mathcal{L}^M$.

EM algorithm

Denote the unobserved data, z_{ig}, to be the group membership indicator that takes on the value of 1 if the ith object belongs to group g and 0 otherwise. Define $\mathrm{z_i} = [z_{i1}, \ldots, z_{iG}]$, where $\mathrm{z_i} \in \{(1, 0, \ldots, 0), \ldots, (0, \ldots, 0, 1)\}$ and $\tau = [\tau_1, \ldots, \tau_G]$. Under this setup, $\mathrm{z_i}$ is multinomial$(1, \tau)$ so that $p(\mathrm{z_i}|\tau) = \prod_{i=1}^{n} \tau_i^{z_{ig}}$. Consider the "complete" data $w_i = (\alpha_i(j, b, k), \mathrm{z_i})$; the vector $\mathrm{z_i}$ gives us the information on g, so the density of the observation α_i given $\mathrm{z_i}$ is the same as the density of α_i given g_i in Equation 4.14. However, in order to express the log-likelihood of the "complete" data effectively, we express it as $p(\alpha_i(j,b,k)|\mathbf{z_i}) = \prod_{g=1}^{G}[h(\alpha_i(j,b,k)|g_i = g)]^{z_{ig}}$. Because only one element in $\mathbf{z_i}$ is 1, all the others are 0, this product essentially computes the conditional density of group g. The likelihood for the "complete" data $[\alpha_i(j,b,k), \mathbf{z_i}]$ can be formed from $\mathcal{L}^c = \prod_{i=1}^{n}\prod_{g=1}^{G}\{\tau_g\, h_g[\alpha_i(j,b,k)|g_i = g]\}^{z_{ig}}$ and the corresponding log-likelihood of the "complete" data is given by

$$\ell^c = \sum_{i=1}^{n}\sum_{g=1}^{G} z_{ig}\{\log \tau_g + \log h_g[\alpha_i(j,b,k)|g_i = g]\}. \tag{4.15}$$

This complete data log-likelihood is maximized using the EM algorithm. In the E-step, the expectation of log-likelihood is calculated on the basis of previous estimate of the parameter vector $\theta = [(f_g, \tau_g), g = 1, \ldots, G]$. For a given estimate $\widehat{\theta}$, we obtain the posterior probability $p_{ig}(j,b,k) = \tau_g h_g[\alpha_i(j,b,k)|\widehat{\theta}]/\sum_{g=1}^{G}\tau_g h_g[\alpha_i(j,b,k)|\widehat{\theta}]$. In the M-step, the expectation is maximized to obtain the new estimates. To maximize the expectation of complete log-likelihood in Equation 4.15 with respect to θ, first replace the unobserved data z_{ig} by its conditional expectation $\widehat{z}_{ig} = p_{ig}(j,b,k) = E(z_{ig}|\alpha_i(j,b,k), \widehat{\theta})$ and then solve the likelihood equation to get the new estimates $\widehat{\theta}_{\text{new}}$, namely,

$$\widehat{\tau}_g = \sum_{i=1}^{n}\widehat{z}_{ig}/n \quad \text{and} \quad \widehat{f}_g = \frac{\sum_{i=1}^{n}\widehat{z}_{ig}\alpha_i(j,b,k)}{\sum_{i=1}^{n}\widehat{z}_{ig}}.$$

Upon convergence, denote the value of $\widehat{z}_{ig}$ returned from the algorithm as z^*_{ig}, the estimate of conditional probability that observations i belong to group g; and the classification of an observation $\alpha_i(j,b,k)$ is taken to be $g* = \arg\max_g z^*_{ig}$.

APPENDIX 4.2: BBA FOR SELECTING THE BEST CLUSTERING BASIS

In this appendix, we outline the steps in selecting the "best" basis for clustering. The BBA finds an orthogonal basis $\mathcal{B}$ from the WP table to maximize the additive clustering power function:

$$\mathcal{B} = \arg\max_{\mathcal{B}^*} \mathcal{D}(\mathcal{B}^*), \tag{4.16}$$

where $\mathcal{B}^*$ is an orthogonal basis in a WP library. Moreover, $\mathcal{D}(\mathcal{B}^*)$ is an additive function:

$$\mathcal{D}(\mathcal{B}) = \sum_{j,b\in\mathcal{I}} \mathcal{D}(j,b), \tag{4.17}$$

where $\mathcal{I}$ is the set of index pairs (j,b) of the blocks in the basis $\mathcal{B}^*$. The clustering power function for block (j,b) is defined in Equation 4.4.

This algorithm searches for the optimal basis according to the criterion defined in Equation 4.16. The WP tree is explored from the bottom up, and the optimal combination of $\Psi(j,b)$ is kept. Let $B(j,b)$ represent the block in the best basis, and $\Psi(j,b)$ denote a WP block in general. Given a set of n time series $\{\mathbf{X}_\mathrm{i}\}_{i=1}^n$, the search procedure is as follows:

- *Step 0:* Specify the maximum depth of WP decomposition J.
- *Step 1:* For each time series $\mathbf{X}_\mathrm{i}$ $(i = 1, \ldots, n)$, calculate the WP coefficients, then get smoothed wavelet periodograms $\alpha_i(j,b,k)$, which is the estimator of the spectrum.
- *Step 2:* For each object i and WP index (j,b,k), compute the posterior probability $p_{ig}(j,b,k)$, then calculate the clustering power function $\mathcal{D}(j,b,k)$ as defined in Equation 4.3.
- *Step 3:* Sum up the clustering power across the shift for each block in the WP table, get the clustering power for each WP block (j,b), defined by Equation 4.4.
- *Step 4:* At the maximal resolution level J, initialize the best basis with $B(J,b) = \Psi(J,b), b = 0,\ldots,2^J - 1$. For the scales $J-1$ until 0, determine the best block $B(j,b)$ by the following rule:
  If $\mathcal{D}(j,b) \geq \mathcal{D}(j+1,2b) + \mathcal{D}(j+1,2b+1)$, then choose $B(j,b) = \Psi(j,b)$, else choose $B(j,b)$ to be the union of $\Psi(j+1,2b)$ and $\Psi(j+1,2b+1)$, that is,

$$B(j,b) = \Psi(j+1,2b) \cup \Psi(j+1,2b+1), \text{ and set}$$
$$\mathcal{D}(j,b) = \mathcal{D}(j+1,2b) + \mathcal{D}(j+1,2b+1).$$

The above procedure will extract the basis from the library that gives the maximal separation among groups based on the criterion defined

TABLE 4.4

Block Distance in WP Table when $J = 2$

15			
10*		11	
3	5	10*	2*

in Equation 4.16; the output is the best basis $\{B(j, b)\}$. The procedure is computationally efficient because it follows the BBA of Coifman and Wickerhauser (1992).

Table 4.4 presents a simple example when maximum level J is 2. In this table, there are five possible choices of basis (see Section 4.3 for details). The values in the table indicate the clustering power function measure (or any distance measure in general) at each WP block. At $J = 2$, the total clustering power of $B(2, 0)$ and $B(2, 1)$ is $3 + 5 = 8$, which is smaller than their "parent" block $B(1, 0)$. Thus, $B(1, 0)$ is chosen (as it gives a larger clustering power than splitting this block into two "children" blocks). On the contrary, the total clustering power of $B(2, 2)$ and $B(2, 3)$ is $10 + 2 = 12$, which is larger than their "parent" block $B(1, 1)$. Thus, $B(2, 2)$ and $B(2, 3)$ are chosen instead of their parent block. Therefore, the best basis chosen consists of $B(1, 0), B(2, 2)$, and $B(2, 3)$, indicated by $*$ in the table. However, we notice that the clustering power in block $B(2, 3)$ is only 2, the smallest one in level 2; it is chosen only because its sibling block $B(2, 2)$ has large clustering power. Maybe $B(2, 3)$ does not contain critical features and can be removed without affecting the clustering results. The variable selection step discussed in Section 4.4.2 helps us to detect and remove these "unimportant" features from the best basis in an automatic manner.

APPENDIX 4.3: MODEL-BASED FEATURE SELECTION ALGORITHM

Step 1: The first clustering feature is chosen to be the one that gives the greatest difference between the BIC of two models: (i) the first being the model where the feature gives G clusters versus (ii) the second where there is no clustering on this feature (i.e., a single group structure). Note that we do not require that the greatest difference be positive.

For each feature $\alpha(j,b,k) \in \mathcal{B}$, compute

$$\mathrm{BIC_d}[(j,b,k)] = \mathrm{BIC_c}[(j,b,k)] - \mathrm{BIC_{nc}}[(j,b,k)], \tag{4.18}$$

where $\mathrm{BIC_c}(j,b,k)$ is computed from the first model where the feature $\alpha(j,b,k)$ gives G number of clusters,

$$\mathrm{BIC_c}[(j,b,k)] = 2\ell_c[(j,b,k),\widehat{\theta}] - \ m\log n, \tag{4.19}$$

where $\ell_c[(j,b,k)]$ is the maximized log-likelihood for the model (in Equation 4.13); and m is the number of independent parameters to be estimated in the model (in this case $m = 2G - 1$). On the other hand, $\mathrm{BIC_{nc}}$ is the case with only a single group structure. That is, we consider that the smoothed WP periodograms from all objects come from the same group so that $\alpha_1(j,b,k), \ldots, \alpha_n(j,b,k)$ are i.i.d. $f(j,b,k)\chi^2_\nu/\nu$. The maximum likelihood estimator (MLE) of the common spectrum is the sample average of the smoothed WP periodograms $\widehat{f}(j,b,k) = \frac{1}{n}\sum_{i=1}^{n}\alpha_i(j,b,k)$. One then computes $\mathrm{BIC_{nc}}[(j,b,k)]$ to be

$$\mathrm{BIC_{nc}}(j,b,k) = 2\ell_{\mathrm{nc}}(j,b,k) - \log n, \tag{4.20}$$

where the log-likelihood under the single group structure evaluated at the MLE is

$$\ell_{\mathrm{nc}}[\widehat{f}(j,b,k)] = \sum_{i=1}^{n}\log\left\{\frac{\left[\nu/2\widehat{f}(j,b,k)\right]^{\nu/2}\alpha_i(j,b,k)^{\nu/2-1}\exp\left[-[(\nu/2\widehat{f}(j,b,k))\alpha_i(j,b,k)]\right]}{\Gamma(\nu/2)}\right\}.$$

We choose the best feature, $\alpha(j_1,b_1,k_1)$, to be the one that satisfies

$$\alpha(j_1,b_1,k_1) = \arg\max_{\alpha(j,b,k)\in\mathcal{B}} \mathrm{BIC_d}(j,b,k) \tag{4.21}$$

and set $X^{(1)} = \{\alpha(j_1,b_1,k_1)\}$ and $X^{(3)} = \mathcal{B}\setminus\{\alpha(j_1,b_1,k_1)\}$, where $\mathcal{B}\setminus\alpha(j_1,b_1,k_1)$ denotes the set of features in $\mathcal{B}$ excluding the feature $\alpha(j_1,b_1,k_1)$.

Step 2: Next we select that second feature $\alpha(j_2,b_2,k_2)$ from $X^{(3)}$ such that $\alpha(j_2,b_2,k_2)$ maximizes

$$\begin{aligned}\mathrm{BIC_d}[(j,b,k)] = {} & \mathrm{BIC_c}[(j_1,b_1,k_1),(j,b,k)] \\ & - \left\{\mathrm{BIC_c}[(j_1,b_1,k_1)] + \mathrm{BIC_{nc}}[(j,b,k)]\right\}.\end{aligned} \tag{4.22}$$

Note that we do not assume that the greatest difference is positive since the only criterion the variables need to satisfy is being the best initialization variables. We set $X^{(1)} = \{\alpha(j_1, b_1, k_1), \alpha(j_2, b_2, k_2)\}$ and $X^{(3)} = X \setminus \{\alpha(j_1, b_1, k_1), (j_2, b_2, k_2)\}$.

General inclusion step: Suppose that we have already selected $(m-1)$ features in $X^{(1)}$. At this step, consider the set of candidate features for inclusion $C^{(m)} = \{\alpha(j_m, b_m, k_m), \ldots, \alpha(j_T, b_T, k_T)\}$. Compute

$$\text{BIC}_\text{d}[(j,b,k)] = \text{BIC}_\text{c}[X^{(1)}, (j,b,k)] - \left\{\text{BIC}_\text{c}[X^{(1)}] + \text{BIC}_\text{nc}[(j,b,k)]\right\}. \tag{4.23}$$

We choose the best feature $\alpha(j_m, b_m, k_m)$, such that

$$\alpha(j_m, b_m, q_m) = \arg\max_{\alpha(j,b,k)\in C^{(m)}} \text{BIC}_\text{d}[(j,b,k)]. \tag{4.24}$$

If this difference is positive, then it suggests that the proposed variable gives additional information about the clustering, so we will add it to the set of selected clustering variables $X^{(1)}$. If the difference is negative, then we will not add it into the selected clustering variable set $X^{(1)}$, and the set $X^{(1)}$ remains the same. The sets $X^{(1)}$ and $X^{(3)}$ are defined to be

- If $\text{BIC}_\text{d}[(j_m, b_m, k_m)] > 0$, then $X^{(1)} = X^{(1)} \cup (j_m, b_m, k_m)$ and $X^{(3)} = X^{(3)} \setminus (j_m, b_m, k_m)$.
- Otherwise $X^{(1)} = X^{(1)}, X^{(3)} = X^{(3)}$.

General exclusion step: Suppose that we already have selected m features. At this step, we determine whether or not we need to remove any of these m features. Consider the features in $X^{(1)}$, namely, $\alpha(j_1, b_1, k_1), \ldots, \alpha(j_m, b_m, k_m)$. For each of these, compute

$$\text{BIC}_\text{d}[(j,b,k)] = \text{BIC}_\text{c}[X^{(1)}] - \left\{\text{BIC}_\text{c}[X^{(1)} \setminus \alpha(j,b,k)] + \text{BIC}_\text{nc}[(j,b,k)]\right\}. \tag{4.25}$$

If this difference is negative, then it suggests that the proposed feature does not provide enough additional information about the clustering, so we will remove it from the set of selected clustering features $X^{(1)}$. Otherwise, the set $X^{(1)}$ remains the same. We choose the candidate feature $\alpha(j^*, b^*, k^*)$, such that

$$\alpha(j^*, b^*, k^*) = \arg\min_{\alpha(j,b,k)\in X^{(1)}} \mathrm{BIC_d}[(j, b, k)] \qquad (4.26)$$

and thus

- If $\mathrm{BIC_d}(j^*, b^*, k^*) \leq 0$, then $X^{(1)} = X^{(1)} \setminus \alpha(j^*, b^*, k^*)$ and $X^{(3)} = X^{(3)} \cup \alpha(j^*, b^*, k^*)$
- Otherwise $X^{(1)} = X^{(1)}$ and $X^{(3)} = X^{(3)}$.

The general inclusion/exclusion steps are iterated until consecutive inclusion and exclusion proposals are rejected. The algorithm stops at this point because any further proposed feature will be the same ones already rejected. Thus, for a known number of clusters G, we obtain the best subset of features, denoted as $\mathcal{F}_G$. This set maximizes the BIC over the subset of features $\mathcal{F}' \subset \mathcal{B}$, that is,

$$\mathcal{F}_G = \arg\max_{\mathcal{F}'\subset\mathcal{B}} \mathrm{BIC}_G(F'). \qquad (4.27)$$

REFERENCES

Arabie, P., Hubert, L.J., & De Soete, G. (1996). *Clustering and classification*. New Jersey: World Scientific.

Basar, E., Basar-Eroglu, C., Karakas, S. & Schurmann, M. (2001). Gamma, alpha, delta, and theta oscillations govern cognitive processes. *International Journal of Psychophysiology, 39*, 241–248.

Bloomfield, P. (2000). *Fourier analysis of time series: An introduction* (2nd ed.). New York: Wiley.

Brillinger, D. (1981). *Time series: Data analysis and theory*. San Francisco: Hölden Day.

Brockwell, P. & Davis, R. (1991). *Time series: Theory and methods*. New York: Springer.

Brockwell, P. & Davis, R. (2002). *Introduction to time series and forecasting* (2nd ed.). New York: Springer.

Bruce, A. & Gao, H. (1996). *Applied wavelet analysis with S-PLUS*. New York: Springer.

Choi, H., Ombao, H., & Ray, B. (2008). Sequential change-point detection method in time series. *Technometrics, 50*, 40–52.

Coifman, R. & Wickerhauser, M. (1992). Entropy-based algorithms for best basis selection. *IEEE Transactions on Information Theory, 38*, 713–718.

Craigmile, P. & Percival, D. (2005). Asymptotic decorrelation of between scale wavelet coefficients. *IEEE Transactions on Information Theory, 51*, 1039–1048.

Dahlhaus, R. (1997). Fitting time series models to nonstationary processes. *Annals of Statistics, 25*, 1–37.

Dempster, A., Laird, N., & Rubin, D. (1977). Maximum likelihood from incomplete data via the EM algorithm. *Journal of the Royal Statistical Society, Series B, 39*, 1, 1–38.

Fowlkes, B., Gnanadesikan, R., & Kettenring, J. (1988). Variable selection in clustering. *Journal of Classification, 5*, 205–228.

Fraley, C., & Raftery, A. (2002). Model-based clustering, discriminant analysis, and density estimation. *Journal of the American Statistical Association, 97*, 611–631.

Friedman, J., & Meulman, J. (2004). Clustering objects on subsets of attributes. *Journal of the Royal Statistical Society, Series B, 66*, 815–839.

Gray, C.M. & McCormick, D.A. (1996). Chattering cells: superficial pyrmical neurons contributing to the generation of synchronous oscillations in the visual cortex. *Science, 274*, 109–113.

Huang, H-Y., Ombao, H., & Stoffer, D. (2004). Classification and discrimination of nonstationary time series using the SLEX model. *Journal of the American Statistical Association, 99*, 763–774.

Kakizawa, Y., Shumway, R., & Taniguchi, M. (1998). Discrimination and clustering for multivariate time series. *Journal of the American Statistical Association, 93*, 328–340.

Klimesch, W., Schack, B., & Sauseng, P. (2005). The functional significance of theta and upper alpha oscillations. *Experimental Psychology, 52*, 99–108.

Kopell, N., Ermentrout, G.B., Whittington, M.A., & Traub, R.D. (2000). Gamma rhythms and beta rhythms have different synchronization properties. *Proceedings of the National Academy of Science, 97*, 1867–1872.

McQueen, J. (1967). Some methods for classification and analysis of multivariate observations. *Fifth Berkeley Symposium on Mathematics, Statistics and Probability, 1*, 281–298.

McLachlan, G., Bean, R., & Peel, D. (2002). A mixture model-based approach to the clustering of microarray expression data. *Bioinformatics, 18*, 413–422.

Meyer, F. (2003). Analysis of event-related fMRI data using best clustering bases. *IEEE Transactions on Medical Imaging, 22*, 933–939.

Ombao, H., Raz, J., von Sachs, R., & Malow, B. (2001). Automatic statistical analysis of bivariate nonstationary time series. *Journal of the American Statistical Association, 96*, 543–560.

Pantev, C., Markeig, S., Hoke, M., Galambos, R., Hampson, S., & Gallen, C. (1991). Human auditory evoked gamma-band magnetic fields. *Proceedings of the National Academy of Science of the United States of America, 88*, 8986–9000.

Percival, D. (1995). On estimation of the wavelet variance. *Biometrika, 82*, 619–631.

Percival D. & Walden, A. (2000). *Wavelet methods for time series analysis*, New York: Cambridge University Press.

Raftery, A. & Dean, N. (2006). Variable selection for model-based clustering. *Journal of the American Statistical Association, 101*, 168–178.

Shumway, R. & Stoffer, D. (2000). *Time series analysis and its applications*. New York: Springer.

Shumway, R. (2003). Time-frequency clustering and discriminant analysis. *Statistics and Probability Letters, 63*, 307–314.

Tadesse, M., Sha, N., & Vannucci, M. (2005). Bayesian variable selection in clustering high-dimensional data. *Journal of the American Statistical Association, 100*, 602–617.

Traub, R.D., Whittington, M.A., Buhl, E.H., Jeffreys, J.G., & Faulkner, H.J. (1999). On the mechanism of the gamma → beta frequency shift in neuronal oscillations induced in the rat hippocampal slices by titanic stimulation. *Journal of Neuroscience, 19*, 1088–1105.

Vidakovic, B. (1999). *Statistical modelling by wavelets*. New York: Wiley.

Wickerhauser, M. V. (1994). *Applied wavelet analysis: From theory to software.* Boston, MA: AK Peters Ltd.

Whittington, M.A., Traub, R.D., & Jeffreys, J.G. (1995). Synchronized oscillations in interneuron networks driven by metatropic glutamate receptor activation. *Nature, 373*, 612–615.

5

Characterizing Latent Structure in Brain Signals

Raquel Prado

5.1 INTRODUCTION

5.1.1 Quasiperiodic Nature of Electroencephalogram Signals

Electroencephalograms or EEGs are recordings that represent the dynamics of the electrical activity in the brain over time. These types of signals are frequently used by neuroscientists to study the brain behavior in clinical and nonclinical settings. Typically, EEG activity is broken up into four frequency bands, referred to as the *delta* (0–4 Hz), *theta* (4–8 Hz), *alpha* (8–13 Hz), and *beta* (above 13 Hz) bands. Different kinds of activity/behavior may induce brain waves in one or more of these frequency bands. For instance, the normal resting EEG usually consists of brain activity in the alpha and beta bands (Dyro, 1989). In the context of characterizing cognitive fatigue, previous EEG studies have suggested that the fatigue is associated with an increase in the theta band power in mid-frontal locations, accompanied by an increase in the alpha band power in parietal locations (Trejo et al., 2006). Therefore, developing and implementing models and methodology that allow us to infer the latent quasiperiodic structure underlying EEG signals over time are the key to understanding brain activity.

Autoregressive (AR) models, time-varying autoregressive (TVAR) models, and related time series decompositions have proven very useful in characterizing the latent quasiperiodic structure present in EEG signals. In particular, such models have been successfully applied to describe EEGs recorded in patients who received electroconvulsive therapy (ECT), a treatment for major depression (Krystal, Prado, & West, 1999). AR and TVAR models belong to the much broader class of dynamic linear models, or DLMs (West & Harrison, 1997). We now give a brief overview of DLMs and discuss why it is useful to consider DLM representations of AR and TVAR processes in the context of studying EEG signals.

5.1.2 DLM Overview

DLMs constitute a large and very flexible class of models that are particularly useful to study time series whose main characteristics change over time (i.e., nonstationary time series). Time series that display trends, periodic or quasiperiodic components with time-varying amplitudes, or those whose linear relationship with a given explanatory variable changes over time are examples of nonstationary time series. In the case of EEGs, the nature of the nonstationarities displayed by these signals varies with the application. For instance, the EEG signals analyzed in West, Prado, and Krystal (1999) and Krystal et al. (1999) display changes in their quasiperiodic latent components that are well captured by AR models whose parameters change smoothly over time. These models are referred to as time-varying autoregressions or TVARs.

DLMs date back to at least Kalman (1960). The book by West and Harrison (1997) details the structure and theory of several DLMs and discusses Bayesian approaches to inference and forecasting within such a modeling framework. Here, we follow the notation of West and Harrison (1997). More specifically, DLMs are defined by two equations. First, the *observation equation* describes the sampling distribution of the time series y_t conditional on the parameters θ_t, that is,

$$y_t = \mathbf{F}_t'\boldsymbol{\theta}_t + \nu_t. \tag{5.1}$$

In this setting, y_t is a univariate time series [although DLMs for multivariate time series can also be considered, see West and Harrison (1997)], $\mathbf{F}_t$ is a p-dimensional vector, θ_t is a p-dimensional parameter vector, and ν_t is a univariate random quantity for each t. Then, a second equation called the *state* or *system* equation defines the way in which the model parameters $\boldsymbol{\theta}_t$

change over time and is given by

$$\boldsymbol{\theta}_t = \mathbf{G}_t \boldsymbol{\theta}_{t-1} + \mathbf{w}_t. \tag{5.2}$$

The most commonly used DLMs are the so-called normal DLMs or NDLMs. These are models in which the terms v_t and $\mathbf{w}_t$ in Equations 5.1 and 5.2 follow normal distributions, that is $v_t \sim N(0, V_t)$ and $\mathbf{w}_t \sim N(\mathbf{0}, \mathbf{W}_t)$. $\mathbf{G}_t$ is a $p \times p$ matrix, also referred to as the evolution matrix. Extensions to non-Gaussian models are possible and often used in practice, but will not be considered here. Therefore, in NDLMs, the quadruple $\{\mathbf{F}_t, \mathbf{G}_t, V_t, \mathbf{W}_t\}$ defines the model structure at time t.

In order to illustrate the use of the DLM notation, we consider two simple examples. We begin with the simplest DLM, that is, the one defined by the equations $y_t = \mu_t + v_t$ and $\mu_t = \mu_{t-1} + w_t$, or equivalently by the quadruple $\{1, 1, V_t, W_t\}$. This model is used to represent random variation in time series whose level μ_t is relatively steady, but does not remain constant over time and is instead modeled as a random walk. Another simple DLM is the dynamic regression model, defined by taking $y_t = \alpha_t + \beta_t x_t + v_t$, and so $\mu_t = \alpha_t + \beta_t x_t$, and then allowing the intercept and slope parameters α_t and β_t to change over time according to a random walk. That is, $\alpha_t = \alpha_{t-1} + w_{t,1}$ and $\beta_t = \beta_{t-1} + w_{t,2}$. Such a model has a DLM representation specified by Equations 5.1 and 5.2 with $\mathbf{F}'_t = (1, x_t)$, $\boldsymbol{\theta}_t = (\alpha_t, \beta_t)'$, $\mathbf{G}_t - \mathbf{I}$ (where $\mathbf{I}$ is the 2×2 identity matrix), and $\mathbf{W}_t$ a two-dimensional matrix. x_t is a predictor, assumed to be known at each time t. This DLM is suitable for cases in which simple linear models are locally satisfactory, but do not adequately describe the global relationship between y_t and x_t as time evolves.

Bayesian inference in NDLMs is summarized later in this chapter. We now focus on AR and TVAR models given that, as mentioned above, they are helpful in describing some types of EEG signals. DLM representations of AR and TVAR models are useful for posterior inference and for deriving decompositions of the time series y_t in terms of scientifically meaningful latent components.

AR and TVAR models. AR models assume that at time t, the series y_t can be "regressed" on its past values, and hence the term *autoregression*. In other words, an AR model of order p, or AR(p), is a model in which y_t is expressed in terms of its past p values, that is

$$y_t = \phi_1 y_{t-1} + \phi_2 y_{t-2} + \cdots + \phi_p y_{t-p} + v_t. \tag{5.3}$$

Typically, $v_t \sim N(0, V_t)$ with $V_t = V$, but other distributions can be considered. It is possible to write this model in NDLM form by taking $\mathbf{F}_t' = (y_{t-1}, y_{t-2}, \ldots, y_{t-p}), \theta_t = \phi$, with $\phi = (\phi_1, \phi_2, \ldots, \phi_p)'$, and setting $\mathbf{G}_t = \mathbf{I}$ and $\mathbf{W}_t = \mathbf{0}$ for all t, indicating no changes on the AR parameters over time. This DLM representation is useful for inference and forecasting. An alternative DLM representation was proposed by West (1997) and used for characterizing the latent quasiperiodic components in geological time series records, with the purpose of determining if, and how, such components relate to climate change. This later representation is also used here to infer the quasiperiodic components underlying the EEG signals recorded during a cognitive fatigue experiment.

In many applied scenarios, AR models provide a good description of their quasiperiodic structure for relatively short periods of time, but fail to sequentially adapt to the changes observed in the frequency content of such signals. In cases where AR models are locally satisfactory but not globally appropriate, it is possible to consider a single AR model whose parameters change—often smoothly—over time. Such a model is referred to as time-varying autoregression (TVAR), and is defined by the following observation and system equations:

$$y_t = \phi_{t,1} y_{t-1} + \phi_{t,2} y_{t-2} + \cdots + \phi_{t,p} y_{t-p} + v_t, \tag{5.4}$$

$$\boldsymbol{\phi}_t = \boldsymbol{\phi}_{t-1} + \mathbf{w}_t, \tag{5.5}$$

with $\boldsymbol{\phi}_t = (\phi_{t,1}, \ldots, \phi_{t,p})'$, $v_t \sim N(0, V_t)$, and $\mathbf{w}_t \sim N(\mathbf{0}, \mathbf{W}_t)$. Therefore, a DLM representation of this model is obtained by taking $\mathbf{F}_t' = (y_{t-1}, y_{t-2}, \ldots, y_{t-p})$, $\boldsymbol{\theta}_t = (\phi_{1,t}, \ldots, \phi_{p,t})'$, and $\mathbf{G}_t = \mathbf{I}_p$ for all t, where $\mathbf{I}_p$ denotes the $p \times p$ identity matrix. As in the AR case, it is possible to consider alternative DLM representations that lead to TVAR-based time series decompositions. In particular, West et al. (1999) present extensions of the AR decomposition results to TVAR models, and use such results to study EEG signals recorded on patients who received ECT. Further methodological issues and various analyses of these EEG series can be found in Prado (1998), Krystal et al. (1999), Prado, West, and Krystal (2001), and Aguilar, Huerta, Prado, and West (1999). The software `TVAR`, available at http://www.stat.duke.edu/research/software/, provides code for fitting and exploring time series via TVAR models and latent decompositions. Extensions of the methods described above have been considered to handle multivariate time series (Prado, 1998, Molina, Prado, & Huerta,

2006) and TVAR models with model orders that vary over time (Prado & Huerta, 2002).

This chapter presents analyses of electroencephalographic signals recorded on a subject who performed simple arithmetic operations continuously for up to 3 h. The objective of the analyses is to determine whether cognitive fatigue can be detected automatically from the EEG signals. Previous analyses of these data appear in Trejo et al. (2006) and Trejo et al. (2007). More specifically, this chapter has two major aims: (1) to give a didactic introduction to approaches for fitting time series models within a Bayesian DLM setting, focusing on AR and TVAR models, and (2) to illustrate how posterior estimates derived from such models help shed light on human brain dynamics.

5.2 INFERRING LATENT STRUCTURE VIA AR AND TVAR MODELS

In this section, we summarize some general features of AR and TVAR models and briefly comment on some computational issues related to performing Bayesian inference in such models. We then review the time series decomposition results of West et al. (1999) and Prado (1998).

5.2.1 AR and TVAR Models: General Features

We begin by defining the AR characteristic polynomial and describe how the roots of this polynomial determine several features of the process, such as stationarity and quasiperiodic behavior. Let $\boldsymbol{\phi} = (\phi_1, \ldots, \phi_p)'$ be the p-vector of AR oefficients of the process given in Equation 5.3. The characteristic polynomial of this process is given by

$$\Phi(u) = (1 - \phi_1 u - \cdots - \phi_p u^p).$$

The process is stationary if the roots of $\Phi(u)$ lie outside the unit circle. In other words, the process is stationary if $\Phi(u) = 0$ only when $|u| > 1$ (u is complex valued), or equivalently if all the reciprocal roots of $\Phi(u)$ have moduli below unity.

The reciprocal characteristic roots can be real or complex. If complex reciprocal roots are present, they appear in pairs of complex conjugates and so each pair can be represented in terms of its modulus, say r, and its wavelength, say λ (or equivalently, its frequency $2\pi/\lambda$). Each pair of complex roots captures a quasiperiodic component in the series whose amplitude is a function of modulus r.

We now illustrate how the values of r and λ affect the structure of a time series process. The left panels in Figure 5.1 depict data simulated from AR(1) processes with AR coefficients $0.9, -0.9, 0.1, -0.1$, and 0.0. More specifically, these pictures show how the data, simulated from the two AR(1) processes with coefficients 0.9 and $-0.9, y(1)$ and $y(2)$ respectively,

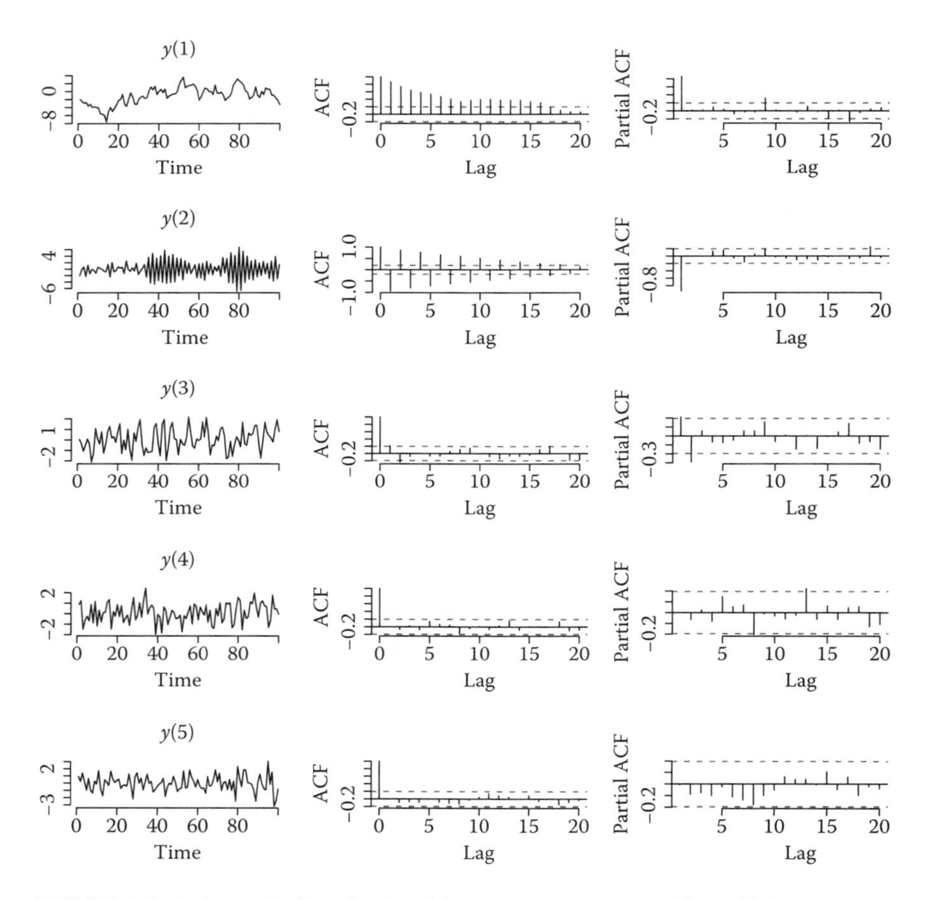

FIGURE 5.1 Left panels: data simulated from AR(1) processes with coefficients $\phi = 0.9$ (series $y(1)$), $\phi = -0.9$ [series $y(2)$], $\phi = 0.1$ (series $y(3)$), $\phi = -0.1$ [series $y(4)$], and $\phi = 0.0$ [white noise, series $y(5)$]. Center panels: sample autocorrelation plots of the series. Right panels: sample partial autocorrelation plots of the series.

do not resemble the data simulated from a white noise process (series $y(5)$ was simulated from a white noise process since $\phi = 0$), while the series $y(3)$ and $y(4)$, simulated from AR processes with coefficients 0.1 and -0.1 respectively, are much closer to white noise. Similarly, the left panels in Figure 5.2 show the data simulated from AR(2) processes with complex characteristic roots. In particular, series $y(1)$ was simulated from a process whose characteristic reciprocal roots had modulus $r = 0.95$ and wavelength $\lambda = 6$, series $y(2)$ was simulated from a process whose characteristic reciprocal roots had modulus $r = 0.95$ and wavelength $\lambda = 12$,

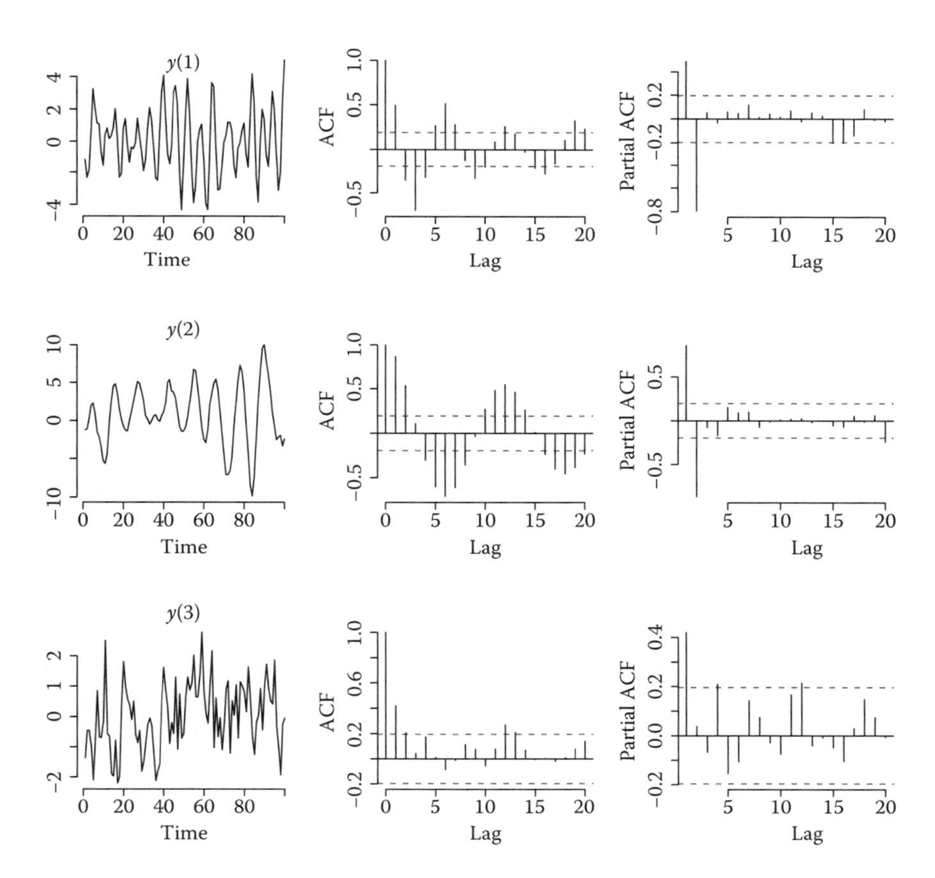

FIGURE 5.2 Left panels: data simulated from AR(2) processes with complex characteristic reciprocal roots with modulus $r = 0.95$ and wavelength $\lambda = 6$ [series $y(1)$], $r = 0.95$ and $\lambda = 12$ [series $y(2)$], and $r = 0.4$ and $\lambda = 6$ [series $y(3)$]. Center panels: sample autocorrelation plots of the series. Right panels: sample partial autocorrelation plots of the series.

and, finally, series $y(3)$ was simulated from a process whose characteristic reciprocal roots had modulus $r = 0.3$ and wavelength $\lambda = 12$. The series $y(1)$ and $y(2)$ show a very persistent quasiperiodic behavior—both were simulated from ARs that had reciprocal roots with modulus 0.95—but $y(1)$ has a much higher frequency. The series $y(3)$ was simulated from a process with the same wavelength as that used to simulate series $y(2)$; however, the quasiperiodicity is less apparent because the modulus of the reciprocal roots of the third process was relatively small [$r = 0.3$ for $y(3)$].

The center and right panels in Figures 5.1 and 5.2 display, respectively, the sample autocorrelation function (ACF) plots and the sample partial autocorrelation function (PACF) plots of the simulated series. For formal definitions of the ACF, the sample ACF, the PACF, and the sample PACF, see for example Shumway and Stoffer (2005). The plots are used to highlight relevant features of the time series. First, there is an important result in AR theory that says that if a process is an AR(p) the PACF will be zero after lag p (again, see Shumway and Stoffer, 2005). Such behavior is clearly illustrated in the sample PACF plots of the series $y(1)$ and $y(2)$ in Figure 5.1, generated from AR(1) processes with $\phi = 0.9$ and $\phi = -0.9$ (see the top two right panels in Figure 5.1), and the sample PACF plots of the series $y(1)$ and $y(2)$ displayed in Figure 5.2 (see the two top right panels in Figure 5.2), both simulated from AR(2) processes whose reciprocal roots had modulus $r = 0.95$. In these cases, it is clear that the sample PACF values at lags greater than $p = 1$ for the AR(1) cases, and those at lags greater than $p = 2$ for the AR(2) cases are not significant (i.e., these values are all inside or very close to the dotted confidence bands). It can also be seen from the PACF plots that the series simulated from processes whose characteristic reciprocal roots had moduli close to zero display no significant PACF values (see PACF plots of series $y(3)$ and $y(4)$ in Figure 5.1), or suggest a model order that is smaller than that used to simulate the series, as in the case of the PACF plot of series $y(3)$ in Figure 5.2. The ACF plots do not provide information about the order of the model in the case of AR processes; however, they also summarize relevant features of the series such as the quasiperiodicity, as it is illustrated in the sample ACF plots of series $y(1)$ and $y(2)$ shown in Figure 5.2.

When TVAR models are considered, a characteristic polynomial is defined at each time t, since the AR coefficients vary with time. Such a polynomial is given by $\Phi_t(u) = 1 - \phi_{t,1}u - \cdots - \phi_{t,p}u^p$. Then, a collection of reciprocal roots and, consequently, a collection of moduli and frequencies are available at each time t, and so it is possible to show traces of such moduli and frequencies over time. These plots are useful to describe changes in the latent components of the series over time, and have been used in applied scenarios to interpret the nature of such components in a scientifically meaningful way. For instance, West et al. (1999) and Krystal et al. (1999) used such plots in the context of assessing the clinical efficacy of a treatment for major depression. An association was found between the rate of decay over time of one of the latent frequencies and the efficacy of the treatment. Here we show frequencies and moduli traces of some of the latent components estimated from a relatively short EEG dataset, with the purpose of offering intuitive insights on how these plots might be useful in time series analyses, particularly in EEG analyses. Such an EEG series with 1664 observations is displayed at the bottom of Figure 5.4. The series corresponds to 13 s of EEG recording from an individual who solved a simple arithmetic equation that appeared on a computer monitor exactly at 5 s, and is part of a much larger dataset that will be described later in this chapter. Figure 5.3 depicts traces of the estimated frequencies and moduli of two of the latent components (corresponding to two pairs of reciprocal complex roots at each time t) of this EEG series. A TVAR model of order $p = 10$ was fitted to the series. Details about the inference process will be given below. To obtain this picture, we computed the posterior mean of the AR coefficients at each time t, denoted by $\hat{\boldsymbol{\phi}}_t = (\hat{\phi}_{t,1}, \ldots, \hat{\phi}_{t,10})'$, and then computed estimates of the moduli and frequencies of the characteristic reciprocal roots at each time t based on $\hat{\phi}_t$. The top panel in Figure 5.3 shows the frequency traces of the complex characteristic roots with the lowest frequencies, while the bottom panel shows the moduli traces of these components (solid and dashed lines), together with the trace of the modulus of the real reciprocal root with the largest modulus (dotted–dashed line). These pictures may be useful in various ways. For example, if the decrease observed in the moduli of these components around 4 s appears consistently in repeated experiments of this sort, that is, each time the individual is asked to solve a similar algebraic equation, it may indicate that the subject is getting ready for solving the arithmetic problem. As will be seen later in this chapter, our interest in this EEG context is to characterize cognitive fatigue in subjects who solved arithmetic problems continuously, and for a long period of time, from a collection of EEG signals similar to that plotted in Figure 5.4. Therefore, we did not properly investigate if there is an association between

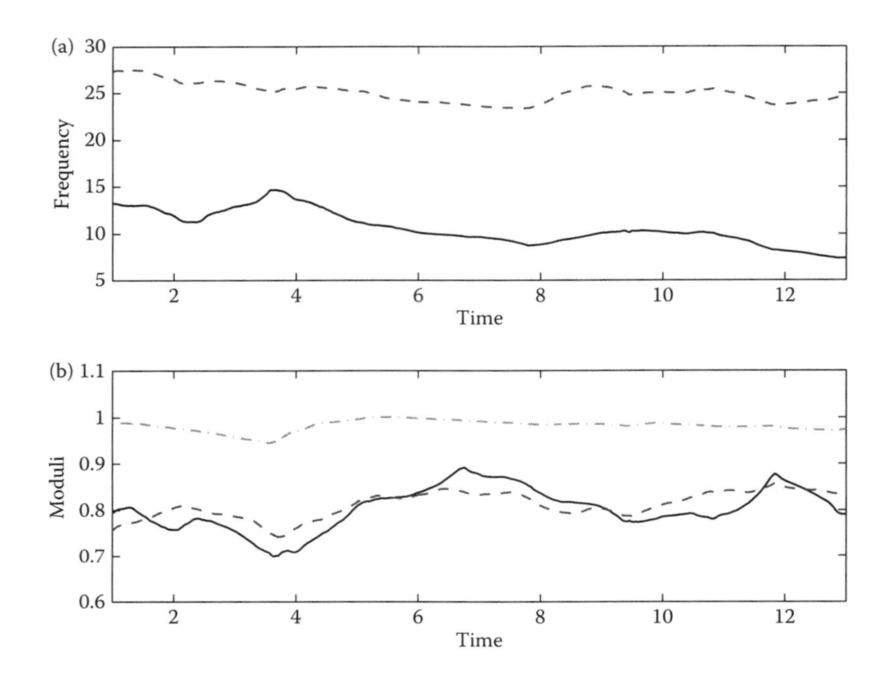

FIGURE 5.3 (a) Traces of the frequencies associated with two of the latent components of an EEG portion from a particular subject recorded at channel *FT8*. (b) Traces of the moduli of latent quasiperiodic process with the lowest frequencies (solid and dashed lines, respectively). The trace of the modulus of the real reciprocal root with the largest modulus at each time t is also shown [dotted–dashed line in plot (b)].

the time-varying behavior of the latent frequencies and moduli underlying these relatively short time series, and the appearance of the stimuli (i.e., the moments when the equations appeared on the computer monitor). However, as mentioned before, TVAR models and related time series decompositions have been useful in other EEG studies and so, in addition to discussing and illustrating various aspects of Bayesian AR inference and AR-based decompositions, we also summarize some key results for TVAR models.

5.2.2 AR and TVAR Models: Bayesian Inference

In order to perform Bayesian inference in an AR(p) framework, prior distributions need to be specified for the model parameters $\boldsymbol{\phi}$ and V. The reference priors $p(\boldsymbol{\phi}) \propto 1$ and $p(V) \propto 1/V$ can be considered. In this

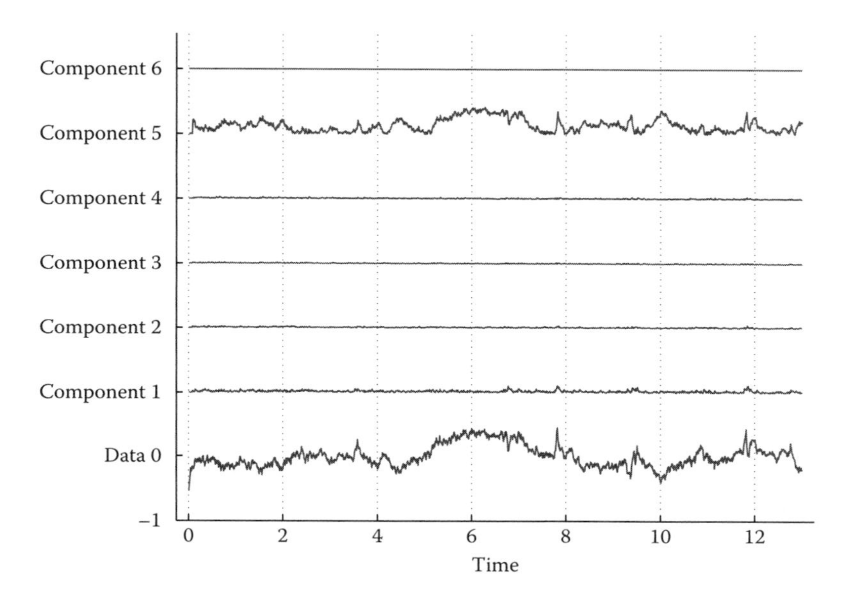

FIGURE 5.4 The series at the bottom corresponds to the first epoch (1664 observations and 13 s of duration) recorded at channel *FT8* in subject **skh**. The remaining components are estimated latent processes based on an AR(10). Components 1–4 are quasiperiodic, while components 5 and 6 are related to real characteristic roots. The quasiperiodic components are ordered by frequency, that is, process 1 is related to the AR reciprocal root with the lowest frequency, while component 4 is related to the AR reciprocal roots with the highest frequency.

case, the conditional posterior distribution of $\boldsymbol{\phi}$ given V, and based on T observations—whose density is denoted as $p(\boldsymbol{\phi}|V, y_{1:T})$—is multivariate Gaussian, while $p(V|y_{1:T})$ is an inverse-gamma density. Note that in spite of the fact that the priors are improper, the posterior distributions are proper if $T > 2p$. Normal-inverse-gamma priors can also be considered, that is, $(\boldsymbol{\phi}|V) \sim N(\mathbf{m}_0, V\mathbf{C}_0^*)$ and $V^{-1} \sim Gamma(n_0/2, n_0 s_0/2)$, resulting in normal-inverse-gamma posteriors. Posterior inference under these priors can be easily achieved via direct simulation. For a review on Bayesian methods, see for example Gelman, Carlin, Stern, and Rubin (2003). More sophisticated prior structures have been developed and used in practice. In particular, Huerta and West (1999) proposed a class of structured prior distributions on the roots of the AR characteristic polynomials. Such an approach offers several interesting features but, due to its complexity, it is not considered here.

As described before, the model in Equation 5.3 can be extended to consider time series that can be well described locally by a single stationary AR model, but that would require several AR models to capture the non-stationarities displayed globally. Such a model is the TVAR(p) defined in Equations 5.4 and 5.5. In the system Equation 5.5, a random walk is used to describe the evolution of the AR coefficients over time. The variation in $\boldsymbol{\phi}_t$ can be controlled by a discount factor $\delta \in (0, 1]$. δ accounts for loss of information over time in the following sense. If we think of $\mathbf{P}_t$ as the variance of $\boldsymbol{\phi}_t$ prior to observing y_t in an ideal scenario in which $\boldsymbol{\phi}_t$ is stable and requires no variation over time, then the actual prior variance of $\boldsymbol{\phi}_t$ at time t, $\mathbf{R}_t \equiv V(\boldsymbol{\phi}_t|y_{1:(t-1)})$, can be set to $\mathbf{R}_t = \mathbf{P}_t/\delta$ for $\delta \in (0, 1]$, and so the prior variance at time t is that of a model with no stochastic variation in the parameters, times a correction factor that inflates such variance to account for loss of information when evolving from $t - 1$ to t. Computational details appear in the Appendix. Low values of δ are consistent with a high variation in $\boldsymbol{\phi}_t$ over time, while large values, in the range of 0.85–0.999, are typically relevant in practice. In particular, if $\delta = 1$ we obtain the standard AR model in Equation 5.3. An optimal discount factor value can be found by maximizing a log-likelihood function defined in terms of the observed predictive density (see Appendix). For a general discussion about discount factors, see West and Harrison (1997). For a further discussion about discount factors in the TVAR model setting, see Prado (1998).

Our TVAR(p) posterior inference is conditional on the first p observations of the time series. Following West and Harrison (1997), we use $\mathcal{D}_t$ to denote all the information available at time t. Typically, $\mathcal{D}_t = \{\mathcal{D}_{t-1}, y_t\}$ and so $\mathcal{D}_t = \{y_{1:t}, \mathcal{D}_0\}$, with $\mathcal{D}_0$ the information available initially. Then, we assume that $(\boldsymbol{\phi}_{p+1}|\mathcal{D}_p, V)$ follows a p-dimensional Gaussian distribution, and that $(V|\mathcal{D}_p)$ follows an inverse-gamma distribution. The distributions of $(\boldsymbol{\phi}_t|\mathcal{D}_t)$, $(V|\mathcal{D}_t)$, and $(\boldsymbol{\phi}_{t-k}|\mathcal{D}_t)$ for $k < t$ can be obtained using the DLM filtering and smoothing equations of West and Harrison (1997). These equations are summarized in the Appendix. The software `TVAR`, available at http://www.stat.duke.edu/research/software, implements these models and also estimates the time series decompositions summarized below. For instance, the frequencies and moduli trajectories displayed in Figure 5.3 were computed after fitting a TVAR(10) with a discount factor of $\delta = 0.9$ to an EEG portion of 1664 observations. The priors used for the AR coefficients and the variance V were normal-inverse-gamma, that is, a Gaussian prior $N(\mathbf{0}, V\mathbf{I}_p)$ was set on ϕ_{p+1}, and an inverse-gamma prior was used for V, or equivalently a gamma prior was set on V^{-1} with parameters $n_0/2$ and $n_0 s_0/2$. The values of n_0 and s_0 were set at $n_0 = 1$ and $s_0 = 10$. Changes in these prior values did not result in major changes on the posterior distributions of the model parameters. The trajectories shown in Figure 5.3 were obtained by computing the characteristic reciprocal roots at the posterior means of $\boldsymbol{\phi}_t$, $\hat{\boldsymbol{\phi}}_t$, for $t = 11{:}1664$. In some applications it is clear that TVAR models should be used instead of static AR models. When long time series with clear changes in their quasiperiodic patterns are considered, TVARs are typically appropriate (e.g., see West et al., 1999). However, in the case of the single epoch EEG data analyzed here it can be shown that, if the purpose of the analysis is characterizing cognitive fatigue, AR models are preferred over TVAR models for most epochs, since ARs are able to capture relevant features of the data that can be associated with cognitive fatigue, and are more parsimonious than TVAR models. In other EEG applications (e.g., Krystal et al., 1999; Prado et al., 2001), using TVAR over AR models is crucial to appropriately describe the latent structure underlying the data.

5.2.3 Time Series Decompositions

West (1997), West et al. (1999), Prado (1998), and Prado et al. (2001) show how AR and TVAR processes can be decomposed into latent processes that are interpretable in many practical scenarios.

Assume that y_t follows an AR(p) process with R real and distinct characteristic reciprocal roots, denoted by r_j for $j = 1{:}R$, and C pairs of distinct complex reciprocal characteristic roots (and so $p = R + 2C$), represented in terms of their modulus and frequency, that is, $r_j \exp(\pm i\omega_j)$, for $j = (R+1){:}(R+C)$. Then, it can be shown that

$$y_t = \sum_{j=1}^{R} x_{t,j} + \sum_{j=R+1}^{R+C} z_{t,j}, \tag{5.6}$$

where each $x_{t,j}$ is a real AR(1) process with AR coefficient r_j, for $j = 1{:}R$, and each $z_{t,j}$ is a real ARMA(2, 1) process with AR coefficients given by $2r_j \cos(\omega_j)$ and $-r_j^2$, for $j = (R+1){:}(R+C)$. The AR(2) component in $z_{t,j}$ is quasiperiodic, with modulus r_j and frequency ω_j, both constant over time.

These decomposition results can be extended to include the TVAR(p) case. If y_t follows a TVAR(p), then, at each time t, the process will have an instantaneous characteristic polynomial given by $\Phi_t(u) = (1 - \phi_{t,1} u - \cdots - \phi_{t,p}u^p)$. If we assume that the numbers of real and complex characteristic reciprocal roots of $\Phi_t(u)$ do not vary over time, or in other words, if at each time t we have R real and distinct reciprocal roots and C pairs of distinct complex roots, then we can decompose y_t as in Equation 5.6. This assumption holds in many practical scenarios where AR parameters change smoothly over time. In particular, it holds in the TVAR analysis of a single EEG epoch considered above. What changes in the TVAR(p) case with respect to the AR(p) case is the nature of the $x_{t,j}$ and $z_{t,j}$ processes. Let $\alpha_{t,j} = r_{t,j}$ denote the R real reciprocal roots for $j = 1{:}R$, and $\alpha_{t,j} = (r_{t,j}, \omega_{t,j})$ be the C pairs of complex roots for $j = (R + 1){:}C$. Then, it can be shown that each $x_{t,j}$ behaves *approximately* as a TVAR(1) with time-varying AR coefficient $r_{t,j}$. Similarly, each $z_{t,j}$ behaves *approximately* as a TVARMA(2, 1) whose TVAR(2) component has time-varying characteristic modulus and frequency $r_{t,j}$ and $\omega_{t,j}$, respectively. Such decomposition has an interpretation in the frequency domain. The spectrum of y_t is time varying: at each time t is the product of the instantaneous spectra of $x_{t,j}$ and $z_{t,j}$. If the TVAR characteristic polynomial has complex reciprocal roots, its spectral density will be peaked around the frequencies $\omega_{t,j}$ and the sharpness of the peaks will be proportional to the moduli $r_{t,j}$. Note also that the $x_{t,j}$ and $z_{t,j}$ processes behave *approximately* as TVAR(1) and TVARMA(2, 1), respectively. How close are the $x_{t,j}$ and $z_{t,j}$ processes to TVAR(1) and TVARMA(2, 1) depends on how similar are the reciprocal roots at time $t - 1$ to those at time t. In general, if ϕ_t changes very slowly over time, the latent processes will be basically dominated by the TVAR(1) and TVARMA(2, 1) structures described above. For a detailed discussion on this, see Prado (1998). If the number of real and complex roots varies with time, the interpretation of the latent structure in the decomposition in Equation 5.6 becomes more complicated. For instance, suppose that you have a TVAR(3) process, y_t, that shows one real root $r_{t,1}$ and a pair of complex roots $(r_{t,2}, \omega_{t,2})$ for $t = 1{:}100$, and then has three real roots $r_{t,j}$, for $j = 1{:}3$, at times $t = 101{:}200$. This means that y_t can be decomposed as $x_{t,1} + z_{t,1}$, with $x_{t,1} \approx$ TVAR(1) and $z_{t,1} \approx$ TVARMA(2, 1) for $t = 1{:}100$, and as $y_t = x_{t,1} + x_{t,2} + x_{t,3}$, with $x_{t,j} \approx$ TVAR(1) for $t = 101{:}200$, and so no quasiperiodic components are present in y_t for $t = 101{:}200$.

The following section illustrates the decomposition results summarized here in the context of characterizing cognitive fatigue from EEG signals.

5.3 DETECTING FATIGUE FROM EEGS: EXPERIMENTAL SETTING AND DATA ANALYSIS

5.3.1 Data Description and Experimental Setting

The EEG data analyzed here were recorded at the NASA Ames Research Center in Moffett Field, California. We now summarize the most important aspects of the experimental setting. For a detailed description of the experiment and preliminary analyses of the data, see Trejo et al. (2006, 2007).

We study EEG recordings of a subject who performed continuous simple arithmetic operations for a period of 3 h. We refer to this subject as **skh**. The complete dataset includes recordings of 15 additional individuals. During the experiment, the participants sat in front of a computer with their right hand resting on a keypad, and were asked to solve summation problems that appeared on the computer monitor. The summations consisted of four randomly generated single digits, three operators (only $+$ and $-$ were considered) and a target sum (e.g., $2 + 3 - 1 + 7 = 11$). The subjects had to solve each problem and decide whether their calculated sums were less than ($<$), equal to ($=$), or greater than ($>$) the target sums provided by pressing the appropriate button on the keypad. Participants were told to answer as quickly as possible without sacrificing accuracy. Once a response was received, the monitor was blank for 1 s and after this a new summation appeared on the screen. The 16 participants performed the task until they quit from exhaustion or 180 min had elapsed. All subjects performed the task for at least 90 min. Subject **skh** completed the maximum period of 180 min.

Subjective moods for the participants were indexed by the Activation Deactivation Adjective Checklist (AD-ACL, see Trejo et al., 2006 and references therein). Observed behavior included ratings of activity and alertness from videotape recordings of each participant's performance. The performance measures were response time and response accuracy. From self-report analyses, it was found that average self-reported energy and calmness were higher prior to the experiment than after the experiment ended, while average self-reported tiredness was lower before the experiment than after the experiment. Observed activity increased over time, while observed alertness decreased over time. Similarly, there was an increase in the average response time as the experiment progressed, but no significant differences were found in the pre- and postexperiment levels of response accuracy. These results indicate that, on average, the subjects experienced mental fatigue, but did not sacrifice accuracy. Further details and discussion about the implications of these results in terms of assessing cognitive fatigue appear in Trejo et al. (2006).

EEGs were recorded from the participants using 32 Ag/AgCl electrodes. Vertical and horizontal electrooculograms were also recorded. The EEGs were amplified, digitized, and stored on hard disk drives and were then submitted to algorithms for the detection and elimination of eye-movement artifacts, as well as visually inspected to reject blocks of data containing artifacts (see details in Trejo et al., 2006). In addition, the signals were epoched around the times of the stimuli, which were marked as the times at which the summation problems appeared on the screen. More specifically, an *epoch* corresponds to the EEG recording that goes from 5 s prior to a given stimulus, to 8 s after that stimulus. The EEG data of subject **skh** analyzed here consist of 864 consecutive epochs per channel. The epochs were decimated at a sampling rate of 128 Hz, resulting in a total of 1664 observations per epoch. For instance, the series displayed at the bottom in Figure 5.4 is the EEG time series of the first epoch recorded at channel *FT8* for subject **skh**. A total of 1664 observations are displayed, corresponding to 13 s of recording.

5.3.2 Data Analysis

5.3.2.1 AR-Based Decompositions of Single-Epoch Data

In order to illustrate the use of AR models and related decompositions, we analyze single-epoch EEG data obtained from subject **skh**. Figure 5.4 displays the data and the estimated time series decomposition of the first 13 s of EEG recording (first epoch) for subject **skh** at channel *FT8*. The decomposition was computed assuming that the epoch follows an AR(10) model. An AR(10) was fitted to the data under reference priors for $\boldsymbol{\phi}$ and V. Other priors were considered. In particular, we repeated the analyses using normal-inverse-gamma priors with $(\boldsymbol{\phi}|V) \sim N(\mathbf{0}, V\mathbf{C}_0^*)$, $\mathbf{C}_0^* = c_0\mathbf{I}_p$, and values of $c_0 = 1$, $c_0 = 10$, and $c_0 = 100$. These analyses produced very similar results in terms of parameter inference and estimated AR-based decompositions.

The processes $x_{t,j}$ and $z_{t,j}$ in Equation 5.6 were estimated using the posterior mean values of $\boldsymbol{\phi}$, denoted as $\hat{\boldsymbol{\phi}}$. Component 1 in Figure 5.4 is quasiperiodic, with an estimated wavelength of 13.10, or equivalently a frequency of 9.77 Hz, and modulus 0.81. Components 2, 3, and 4 are also quasiperiodic, with estimated wavelengths of 5.18 (24.71 Hz), 3.09 (41.42 Hz), and 2.16 (59.26 Hz), and moduli 0.81, 0.80, and 0.82, respectively. Finally, components 5 and 6 are not quasiperiodic, since they are associated with real reciprocal roots with moduli 0.99 and 0.20, respectively. Clearly, the real component 5 is the most persistent in terms of its modulus, and it is also the one that has the largest contribution to the observed series in terms of its amplitude. Components 2–4 and component 6 have negligible amplitude contributions to the series.

Similarly, Figure 5.5 displays the estimated decomposition for the last 13 s of EEG recorded at channel *FT8* for subject **skh**. Once again, the decomposition was computed based on the posterior mean of the AR coefficients of an AR(10). As in the previous case, the first four components are quasiperiodic, with wavelengths (frequencies) of 11.64 (10.99 Hz), 4.85 (26.39 Hz), 3.08 (41.55 Hz), and 2.16 (59.26 Hz), and corresponding moduli 0.87, 0.79, 0.80, and 0.86. Components 5 and 6 are AR(1) processes with AR coefficients 0.97 and 0.38, respectively. It can be seen that the estimated frequency and modulus of the first quasiperiodic component (component 1 in Figure 5.5) are higher for the last epoch than the estimated frequency and modulus of the same component (component 1 in Figure 5.4) for the first epoch. The amplitude of component 1 is also larger for the last epoch than for the first epoch, and component 5 in the decomposition of the last epoch showed a smaller estimated modulus than that of component 5 in the first epoch. Once again components 2–4 have negligible amplitude contributions to the series.

Many of the latent features found in the first and last epochs were also found in the AR-based analyses of the 864 epochs recorded in subject **skh**. In particular, components 1 and 5 appeared in all epochs for all the channels recorded. The remaining components were not as persistent. For example, some epochs showed three quasiperiodic components in addition to component 1, while some epochs showed only two.

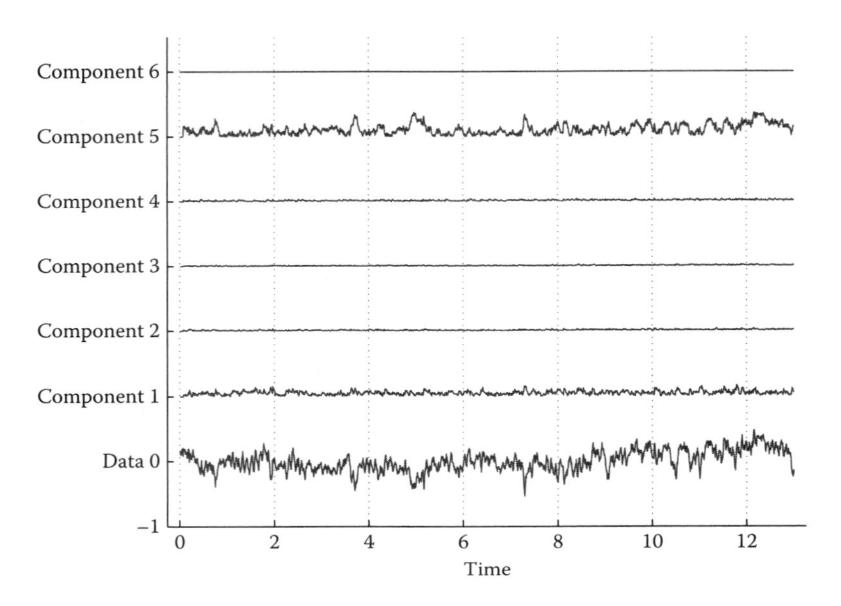

FIGURE 5.5 The series at the bottom corresponds to the last epoch (1664 observations and a duration of 13 s) recorded at channel *FT8* in subject **skh**. The remaining components are estimated latent processes based on an AR(10). Components 1–4 are quasiperiodic, while components 5 and 6 are related to real characteristic roots. The quasiperiodic components are ordered by frequency, that is, process 1 is related to the AR reciprocal root with the lowest frequency, while component 4 is related to the AR reciprocal roots with the highest frequency.

After fitting the AR(10) models to the two epochs considered above, samples from the posterior distributions of the AR parameters can be obtained in each case. Each of those samples can then be used to obtain samples from the posterior distribution of the characteristic reciprocal roots. Figure 5.6 displays 5000 samples of the frequency associated with the quasiperiodic component 1 in the decomposition of the first epoch, namely $\omega_{t,1}^{\text{first}}$, and 5000 samples of the frequency associated with the quasiperiodic component 1 in the decomposition of the last epoch, denoted as $\omega_{t,1}^{\text{last}}$. Density estimates are also displayed to summarize the posterior distribution of $\omega_{t,1}^{\text{first}}$ (solid line) and that of $\omega_{1,t}^{\text{last}}$ (dotted–dashed line). These pictures summarize the uncertainty around the estimated frequencies (in the 8–14 Hz range) of component 1 in the first and last epochs, indicating that there are differences in the alpha band frequency characteristics of the two epochs.

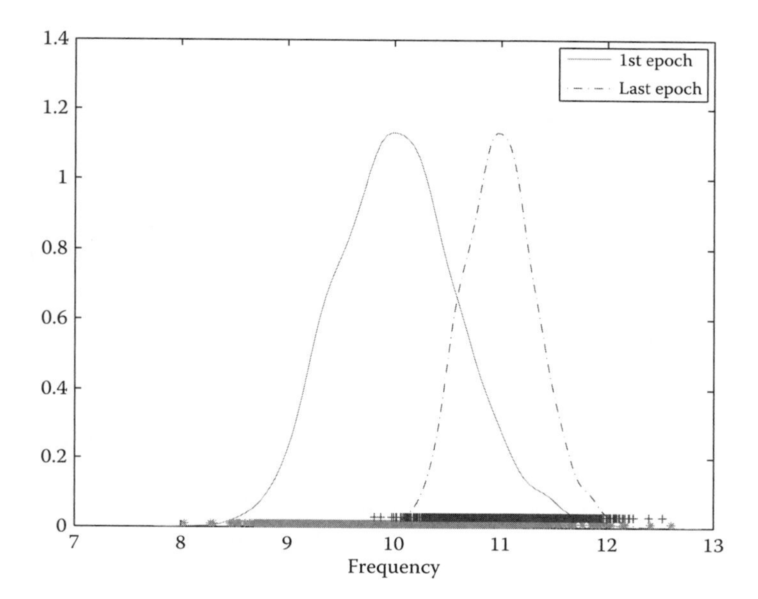

FIGURE 5.6 Solid line: density estimate of $\omega_{t,1}^{\text{first}}$, the frequency of the quasiperiodic component 1 in the decomposition of the first epoch for channel *FT8*. The 5000 samples used to estimate the density appear at the bottom. Dotted–dashed line: density estimate of $\omega_{t,1}^{\text{last}}$, the frequency of the quasiperiodic component 1 in the decomposition of the last epoch for channel *FT8*. Again, the 5000 samples used for density estimation are also displayed.

5.3.2.2 Full Analysis and Classification

Following Trejo et al. (2006), we divide the entire EEG recording of 3 h into 12 intervals, each corresponding to 15 min of recording. Each interval has a variable number of epochs, depending on how fast the subject solved the summation problems that appeared on the screen and also depending on the portions of EEG recording that were excluded from the analysis due to artifacts. We treat the time series from two consecutive epochs as consecutive time series. This assumption was also made by Trejo et al. (2006) and Trejo et al. (2007) and so the results obtained here can be directly compared to those appearing in these references.

Let $y_{1:1664}^{(i,j,k)}$ denote the time series of 1664 observations—corresponding to 13 s of recording—recorded at interval i, epoch j, and channel k. We then have that $i = 1{:}12$, $j = 1{:}n_i$, where n_i is the total number of epochs available during interval i, and $k = 1{:}30$. We begin our analysis by fitting AR(p) models to all the epochs of the first 15 min of recording, that is, those in interval 1, and all the epochs of the last 15 min of recording, that is, those in interval 12. We assume that the subject was *alert* during the first 15 min of the experiment and was *fatigued* during the last 15 min. We also assume that $p = 10$ for all the epochs. Later, we give a justification for choosing this AR model order.

Figure 5.7 displays plots of the estimated frequencies in the alpha band (above 8 Hz and below 14 Hz) and their corresponding moduli for 16 of the 30 EEG channels recorded in subject **skh**. The light dots correspond to values of the frequencies and moduli for epochs of the first interval, while the dark triangles correspond to epochs of the last interval. These are obtained by computing the reciprocal AR characteristic roots at the posterior means of the AR coefficients for each epoch and then extracting the reciprocal roots with frequencies in the alpha band. The channels displayed in the plot are those showing the largest discrepancies between the epochs recorded during the first 15 min (alert) and those recorded during the last 15 min (fatigue). For some of the channels the fatigued epochs display higher frequencies than those shown by the alert epochs, and can also have higher moduli (e.g., channel *FT8*). Some of the channels show discrepancies in the alert and fatigued frequencies, but not in the moduli (e.g., see channel *C4* in the picture) and vice versa (e.g., channel *FC3*).

Based on these results we hypothesize that two cognitive states can be discriminated in terms of the alpha frequency and/or its corresponding modulus at some channel locations. We can use the estimated alpha frequencies and moduli of the epochs of the first and the last 15 min of recording to build a simple classifier that will then allow us to estimate the probability that an epoch recorded during the course of the experiment is an epoch from one of the two cognitive states. We explain how we build such a classifier below.

We begin by choosing the channels that are best at discriminating epochs from the first 15 and last 15 min, as not all the channels are equally informative. In order to do this, for each channel, we fit a bivariate Gaussian mixture model with two components to the estimated alpha frequencies and moduli for the epochs in the first and last intervals (i.e., intervals 1 and 12 or, equivalently, alert and fatigue), leaving one epoch out, and then use such a model to predict if the point that corresponds to the epoch that was left out is a point from the first interval (alert) or the last interval (fatigue). We then compute how many points were correctly classified in this way for each channel, and choose only those channels that lead to good

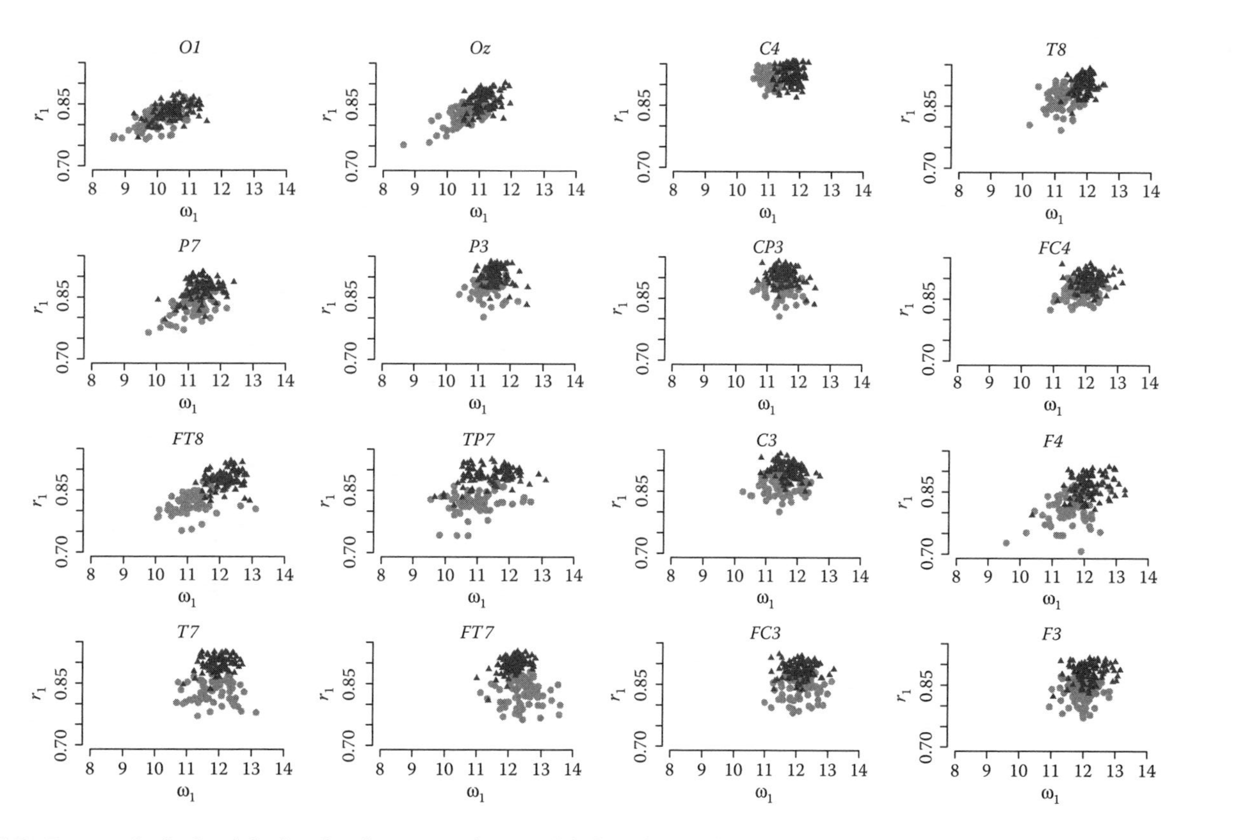

FIGURE 5.7 Frequencies in the alpha band and corresponding moduli for subject **skh** at selected channels. The light dots correspond to the alert state while the dark triangles correspond to the fatigue state. The labels r_1 and ω_1 denote the modulus and frequency, respectively.

predictions. More specifically, let $\boldsymbol{\alpha}^k_{(1,12)}$ denote the estimated frequencies in the alpha band and their corresponding moduli for all the epochs of intervals 1 and 12 at channel k, and let $\boldsymbol{\alpha}^{(k)}_{(1,12)}\{-(i,j,k)\}$ denote all the estimated alpha frequencies and moduli for intervals 1 and 12, except for the estimated frequency and modulus in the alpha band of epoch j at interval i (with $i = 1$ and $i = 12$ in this case), and for the same channel k, denoted by $\alpha(i,j,k)$. Similarly, let $\mathbf{m}_a\{-(i,j,k)\}$ and $\mathbf{m}_f\{-(i,j,k)\}$ be the two-dimensional vectors of means and let $\mathrm{C}_a\{-(i,j,k)\}$ and $\mathrm{C}_f\{-(i,j,k)\}$ be the 2×2 covariance matrices of the two-component Gaussian mixture model fitted using all the epochs at channel k except for epoch j from interval i. Then, the probability that epoch (i,j,k) is from the alert period is defined by $P_a(i,j,k) \equiv Pr[\boldsymbol{\alpha}(i,j,k) \in \mathcal{I}_a|\boldsymbol{\alpha}^{(k)}_{(1,12)}\{-(i,j,k)\}]$, with

$$Pr[\boldsymbol{\alpha}(i,j,k) \in \mathcal{I}_a|\boldsymbol{\alpha}^{(k)}_{(1,12)}\{-(i,j,k)\}]$$

$$\times \propto \frac{\pi_a(i,j,k) \times K_a(i,j,k)}{\pi_a(i,j,k) \times K_a(i,j,k) + \pi_f(i,j,k) \times K_f(i,j,k)}, \qquad (5.7)$$

where

$$K_a(i,j,k) = N[\boldsymbol{\alpha}(i,j,k)|\mathbf{m}_a\{-(i,j,k)\}, \mathrm{C}_a\{-(i,j,k)\}],$$

$$K_f(i,j,k) = N[\boldsymbol{\alpha}(i,j,k)|\mathbf{m}_f\{-(i,j,k)\}, \mathrm{C}_f\{-(i,j,k)\}],$$

and $\pi_a(i,j,k)$ and $\pi_f(i,j,k)$ are prior probabilities that $\alpha(i,j,k)$ is in $\mathcal{I}_a$ and $\mathcal{I}_f$, respectively. For these calculations we set $\pi_a(i,j,k) = \pi_f(i,j,k) = \pi_a = \pi_f = 0.5$ for all the epochs. We normalize the probabilities so that $P_a(i,j,k) + P_b(i,j,k) = 1$ for each epoch (i,j,k).

In order to fit a mixture of two Gaussians to the alpha frequencies and their corresponding moduli of the epochs recorded during the first and last intervals of the experiment, we first used `kmeans` to partition the points into two clusters. This is one of the simplest unsupervised clustering algorithms. We used the MATLAB® implementation of the method. The algorithm is iterative, and aims to minimize the sum over the number of clusters (two in this case) of the within cluster sum of the distances between the observed points and the centers of the clusters. The algorithm starts with initial locations for the centers of the two clusters and then recalculates such locations at each step, stopping when the positions are the same in two consecutive iterations. The function `kmeans` in MATLAB® returns a vector of indicator values whose size is the number of data points. Each value in this vector corresponds to the cluster index for each point. The algorithm can use any distance, and so we use the Euclidean distance which is the default distance implemented in MATLAB®. We then fitted two Gaussian distributions, one to the points that were assigned to one of the two indexes by the `kmeans` function, and another Gaussian to the remaining points. We used the function `normfit` in MATLAB® to obtain estimates for the moments of such Gaussian distributions. This function returns the minimum variance unbiased estimators of the means and the variances of the Gaussian distributions. Clearly, there are better and more sophisticated methods of clustering, but the algorithm presented here is simple and has provided reasonable results when analyzing EEG epochs from different subjects who participated in the experiment.

Figure 5.8 quantifies the performance of the different channels in discriminating between epochs of the first and last intervals, referred to as the alert and fatigue states, respectively, using only the information at the alpha frequency band. For each epoch, we computed Equation 5.7 and assigned the epoch to the alert state if such probability was above 0.5. Otherwise, we assigned the epoch to the fatigued state. We then computed the accuracy of the prediction for each channel based on all the epochs. The figure shows the accuracy at each channel location, computed as the percentage

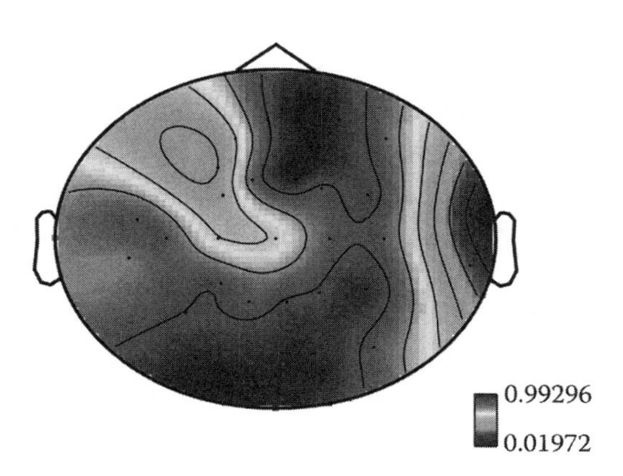

FIGURE 5.8 Predictive performance of the 30 channels in terms of classifying epochs from intervals 1 and 12 for subject **skh**. The predictive performance was measured in terms of the accuracy in the classification for each channel.

of epochs correctly identified as epochs from interval 1 or from interval 12. An image created by linearly interpolating those values over a grid defined by the approximate electrode locations is also displayed. It can be seen that channels located at right frontal locations and those at parietal locations are the best channels for discriminating the two types of epochs for this subject, while channels located at the very right of the scalp, near the right ear, are the worst.

Figure 5.8 shows results based on fitting AR(10) models to each epoch for each of the channels. We repeated the same type of analysis using model orders $p = 8, \dots, 15$, and chose $p = 10$ as the optimal model order since it gave the best predictive performance in terms of accuracy. Using the maximum accuracy among all the channels, and the average accuracy for the 30 channels as measures of performance, we found that the model order $p = 10$ maximized both measures.

We now proceed to discuss the results of the analysis for all the epochs recorded after the first 15 min and prior to the last 15 min of the experiment. As mentioned before, our criterion for choosing how many channels are going to be used in the final analysis is based on the predictive accuracy of the "leave-one-epoch-out" procedure described above. We complete the analysis using only those channels that had accuracies of at least $\kappa \times 100\%$ and let the user specify $\kappa \in (0, 1)$. For instance, if $\kappa = 0.75$, only channels *Oz*, *C4*, *T8*, *FT8*, and *F4* are selected for subject **skh**, since those are the ones that have a predictive accuracy of at least 75%. For each of these channels, we fit a two-component Gaussian mixture model to the estimated frequencies and moduli of all epochs in the first and last intervals (intervals 1 and 12). We use $\mathbf{m}_a(k), \mathbf{C}_a(k), \mathbf{m}_f(k)$, and $\mathbf{C}_f(k)$ to denote the means and covariance matrices for the two Gaussians for channel k, corresponding to the alert and fatigue periods. We then consider the remaining epochs from intervals 2 to 11, in addition to those from intervals 1 and 12. We begin by fitting AR(10) models to all the EEG epochs and compute the estimated alpha frequencies and corresponding moduli using the posterior means of the AR coefficients in each case. Then, we proceed to estimate the probabilities that each epoch is an epoch from one of the two states, alert or fatigue, as follows. We first rearrange the estimated frequencies and moduli for the epochs from intervals 1 to 12 consecutively and so, instead of using (i, j, k) to denote the jth epoch from interval i, and channel k, with $i = 1{:}12$ and $j = 1{:}n_i$, we now switch to the notation (l, k) for epoch l of channel k, with

$l = 1 : \sum_{i=1}^{12} n_i$. Then, the probability that the lth epoch is in the alert state is estimated via

$$P_{\beta,a}(l,k) = \beta P_{\beta,a}(l-1,k) + (1-\beta)P_a(l,k), \text{ with } \beta \in [0,1], \quad (5.8)$$

where

$$P_a(l,k) \propto \frac{K_a(l,k)}{K_a(l,k) + K_f(l,k)}, \quad (5.9)$$

normalized such that $P_a(l,k) + P_f(l,k) = 1$, and with $K_a(l,k) = N(\alpha(l,k)|\mathbf{m}_a(k), \mathbf{C}_a(k)), K_f(l,k) = N(\alpha(l,k)|\mathbf{m}_f(k), \mathbf{C}_f(k))$, and $P_{\beta,a}(1,k) = P_a(1,k)$. Once again, $\mathbf{m}_a(k), \mathbf{C}_a(k)$, $\mathbf{m}_f(k)$, and $\mathbf{C}_a(k)$ are the means and covariance matrices that define the mixture of Gaussians for channel k computed using only epochs from the first and last intervals. In Equation 5.8, β acts as a smoothing parameter to balance the weight given to the probability of alert computed using Equation 5.9—that only uses information from epochs in the first and last interval, but not from any other epochs—and the probability of alert of the previous epoch, computed by evaluating Equation 5.8 at $l-1$. When $\beta = 0$ we use Equation 5.9 to compute the probability of alert for epoch l. When β is close to one, most of the weight is given to the probability of alert of the previous epoch. Therefore, Equation 5.8 allows us to introduce a Markovian structure in the calculation of the alert and fatigue probabilities.

Figure 5.9 shows the estimated probabilities $P_{\beta,a}(l,k)$ and $P_{\beta,f}(l,k)$ for all the epochs and each of the channels that have a predictive accuracy of at least 75%. These results were obtained using $\beta = 0.9$. The right panel in the figure displays the average of those probabilities computed using the channels shown at the left. As seen in the picture, the probability of alert at the beginning of the experiment is relatively high and decreases towards the end when the subject enters the fatigue state.

Figure 5.10 shows the average probabilities of alert and fatigue based on channels *Oz, C4, T8, FT8*, and *F4*. The only difference with respect to the results displayed in Figure 5.9 is that the smoothing factor is $\beta = 0.7$, and so less weight is now given to the probability of alert estimated in the past. Consequently, the weight given to the probability that is computed using solely the data from the current epoch in Equation 5.8 is increased. Note that, regardless of the value of β, the pictures show an increase of the probability of fatigue towards the end of the experiment.

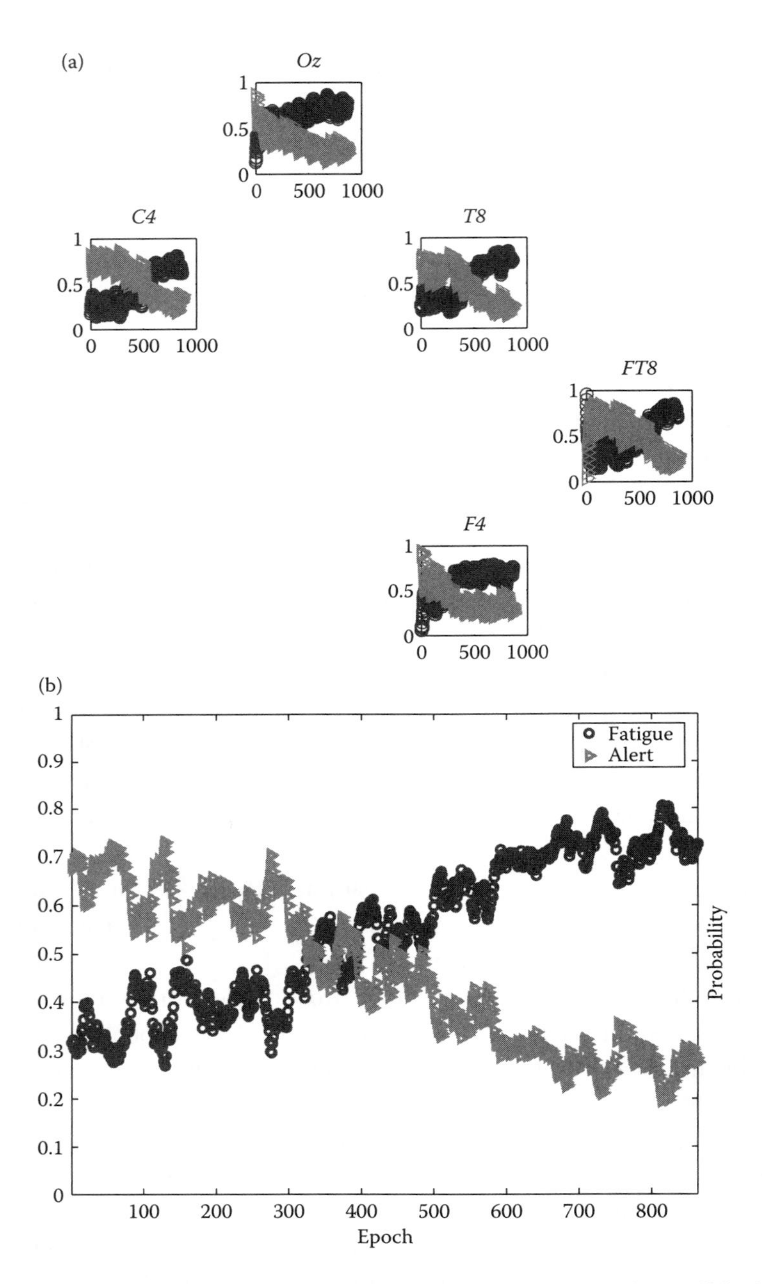

FIGURE 5.9 (a) Probabilities of being in the alert state (light triangles) and the fatigue state (dark circles) for channels *Oz, C4, T8, FT8,* and *F4*. These channels were the only ones with a predictive accuracy of at least 75%. (b) Average (computed using only the channels listed before) alert probabilities (light triangles) and average fatigue probabilities (dark circles). A smoothing factor of $\beta = 0.9$ was used to update the probabilities over time.

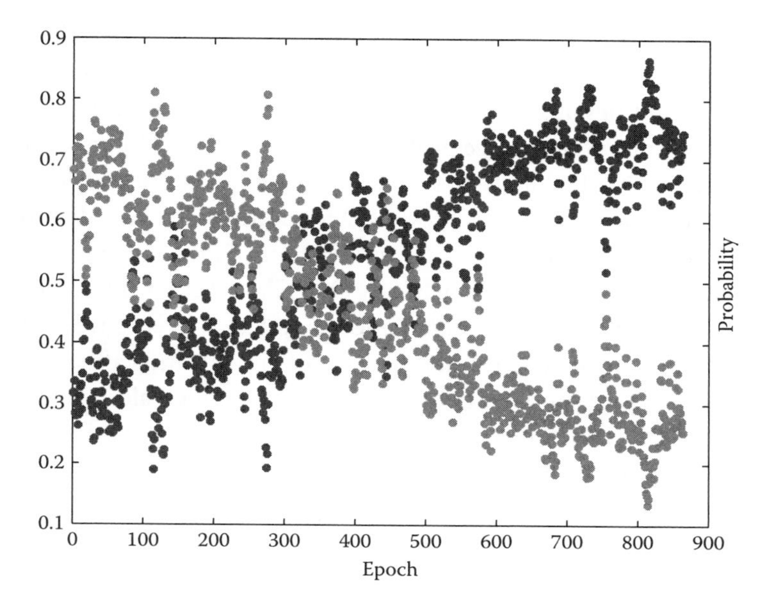

FIGURE 5.10 Average probabilities of being in the alert and fatigued states (light dots and dark dots, respectively) using channels with a predictive accuracy of at least 75% and a smoothing factor of $\beta = 0.7$.

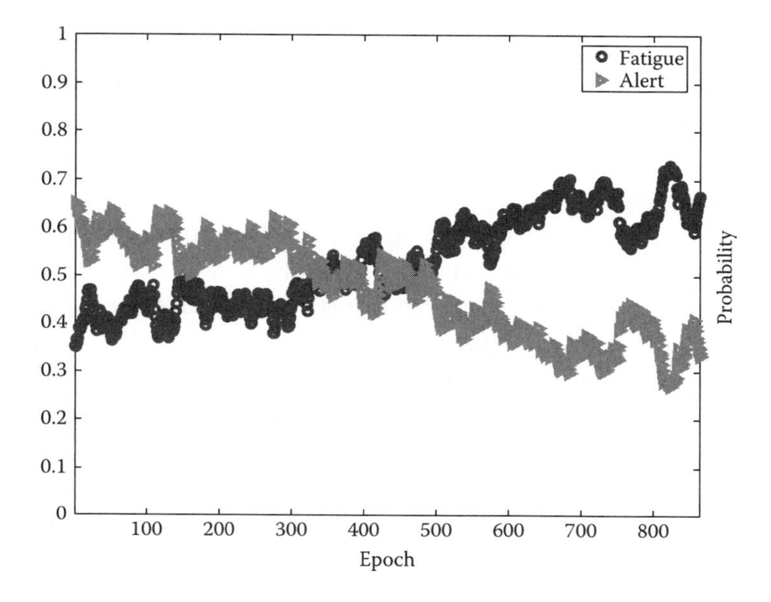

FIGURE 5.11 Average probabilities of being in the alert state (light triangles) and the fatigue state (dark circles) computed using channels *O2, O1, Oz, C4, TP8, T8, CPz, Cz, FC4, FT8, TP7,C3, F4, F8, FT7*, and *F3*. These channels were the only ones with a predictive accuracy of at least 60%. A smoothing factor of $\beta = 0.9$ was used to update the probabilities over time.

Finally, it is worth comparing the plot on the right panel of Figure 5.9 with Figure 5.11 to assess the effect of using more channels to compute the average probabilities of alert and fatigue over the course of the experiment. Figure 5.11 displays the average probabilities of alert and fatigue computed using channels that had a predictive performance of at least 60%, instead of 75%. The value of β was set at $\beta = 0.9$ for comparison with Figure 5.9. Then, in addition to channels *Oz*, *C4*, *T8*, *FT8*, and *F4* that have a predictive accuracy of at least 75%, channels *O2*, *O1*, *TP8*, *CPz*, *Cz*, *FC4*, *TP7*, *C3*, *FT7*, and *F3* were also considered, since they had a predictive accuracy in the 60–75% range. The estimates are very similar, indicating that the subject has a higher probability of being in the so-called alert state at the beginning of the experiment and this probability decays toward the end as the subject enters the fatigue state, with an estimated probability of fatigue in the 0.6–0.75 range.

5.4 CONCLUSIONS AND FUTURE DIRECTIONS

We summarize general features of AR and TVAR models and related decomposition results and illustrate how these models can be used to characterize latent processes in EEG signals that can be associated with two cognitive states, namely alert and fatigue. These models are easy to use and the decompositions provide interpretable results in terms of processes that are scientifically meaningful.

Various models are fitted to the data to provide descriptive analyses. These analyses do not take into account the uncertainty in the estimated frequencies for each epoch, as the estimated probabilities of alert and fatigue are based on point estimates of the AR parameters. Analyses that allow us to take into account such uncertainty are possible but very computationally intensive, and so they are not feasible for online detection of cognitive fatigue.

Here we present the complete analysis for a single subject, **skh**, assuming that there are only two cognitive states, and using a single frequency band to characterize these states. We analyzed data from other subjects (see Trejo et al., 2007) using an approach similar to the one presented here, but assuming that there is a third intermediate state between the alert and fatigue states. The analyses in Trejo et al. (2007) indicate that, at least for some of the subjects who participated in the experiment, there is evidence that such an intermediate state is present. Furthermore, we believe that a reasonable representation of the process that leads to cognitive fatigue is the one in which the individual is assumed to enter such a state gradually in a smooth way. In technical terms this implies considering models in which the number of mental states is not discrete. We did not consider such modeling approaches since the EEG data analyzed are segmented into epochs that are consecutive but not necessarily contiguous, and hence considering models in which we have a discrete number of states seems appropriate here. We also performed spectral analyses of the signals of some of the subjects (not shown) that suggest that other frequency bands should be considered in the analysis, as they may also be useful in discriminating epochs from different cognitive states.

Future extensions will consider modeling the signals using mixtures of autoregressions, where each process—or each cognitive state—in the mixture is characterized by model parameters for which informative priors, such as those proposed in Huerta and West (1999), are used to define specific features that characterize a given cognitive state in terms of various frequency bands. Such models typically require methods for online parameter estimation that are based on sequential Monte Carlo algorithms.

Further research also needs to be done exploring different ways of summarizing and combining the information provided by the 30 channels. Some of the questions related to how to automatically detect fatigue from EEG signals that still remain unanswered include, among others: how many channels should be used to detect fatigue? If more than one channel is used, should they all have the same weight in estimating the probability of a given state? Is the number and location of the channels the same for different subjects? Should the information from different channels be combined using a principal component analysis or a factor model approach? Several paths can be taken in terms of choosing models that can combine the information from the 30 channels. One possibility is to consider factor models and dynamic factor models, in which the EEG series recorded at the 30-channel locations can be expressed in terms of a small number of series or "factors" that characterize the different cognitive states as well as the main spatial features of the multichannel data. Another alternative is to use mixtures of vector autoregressions as proposed by Molina et al. (2006) in the context of modeling and classification of EEG signals.

ACKNOWLEDGMENTS

We are grateful to the referees and the editors for their valuable advice and review of this Chapter. We thank Yuzheng Zhang for preparing Figure 5.8 and L. J. Trejo for providing access to the data.

APPENDIX 5.1: POSTERIOR ESTIMATION IN NDLMS

1. Filtering equations: We summarize the filtering and smoothing equations presented in West and Harrison (1997) for posterior inference in DLMs of the form

$$\begin{aligned} y_t &= \mathbf{F}_t'\boldsymbol{\theta}_t + v_t, \quad v_t \sim N(0, V_t), \\ \boldsymbol{\theta}_t &= \mathbf{G}_t\boldsymbol{\theta}_{t-1} + \mathbf{w}_t, \quad \mathbf{w}_t \sim N(\mathbf{0}, \mathbf{W}_t). \end{aligned}$$

We assume that $V_t = V$ for all t and use a discount factor $\delta \in (0, 1]$ to specify $\mathbf{W}_t$. For other more general cases see West and Harrison (1997).

The marginal posterior distributions for $\boldsymbol{\theta}_t$ and V are given by $(\boldsymbol{\theta}_t|\mathcal{D}_t) \sim T_{n_t}(\mathbf{m}_t, \mathbf{C}_t)$, a multivariate Student-t distribution with n_t degrees of freedom, mean $\mathbf{m}_t$ and scale matrix $\mathbf{C}_t$, and $(V^{-1}|\mathcal{D}_t) \sim \text{Gamma}(n_t/2, n_t s_t/2)$. The updating equations are

$$\begin{aligned} \mathbf{m}_t &= \mathbf{G}_t\mathbf{m}_{t-1} + \mathbf{A}_t e_t, \\ \mathbf{C}_t &= (\mathbf{R}_t - \mathbf{A}_t\mathbf{A}_t' q_t)(s_t/s_{t-1}), \\ n_t &= n_{t-1} + 1, \\ s_t &= s_{t-1} + \frac{s_{t-1}}{n_t}\left(\frac{e_t^2}{q_t} - 1\right), \end{aligned}$$

where

$$\begin{aligned} e_t &= y_t - f_t, \\ f_t &= \mathbf{F}_t'\mathbf{G}_t\mathbf{m}_{t-1}, \end{aligned}$$

$$q_t = \mathbf{F}_t'\mathbf{R}_t\mathbf{F}_t + s_{t-1},$$
$$\mathbf{A}_t = \mathbf{R}_t\mathbf{F}_t/q_t,$$
$$\mathbf{R}_t = \mathbf{C}_{t-1} + \mathbf{W}_t,$$
$$\mathbf{W}_t = \frac{1-\delta}{\delta}\mathbf{G}_t\mathbf{C}_{t-1}\mathbf{G}_t'.$$

The analysis requires an initial conjugate normal inverse gamma prior $(\boldsymbol{\theta}_0|V,\mathcal{D}_0) \sim N(\mathbf{m}_0, V\mathbf{C}_0^*)$ and $(V^{-1}|\mathcal{D}_0) \sim$ Gamma $(n_0/2, n_0 s_0/2)$.

2. Smoothing equations: The marginal posterior distribution of $(\boldsymbol{\theta}_{t-k}|\mathcal{D}_t)$ for $1 \leq k \leq t$ is a multivariate Student-t distribution, $T_{n_t}(\mathbf{a}_t(-k), (s_t/s_{t-k})\mathbf{R}_t(-k))$, where

$$\mathbf{a}_t(-k) = \mathbf{m}_{t-k} + \mathbf{B}_{t-k}[\mathbf{a}_t(-k+1) - \mathbf{a}_{t-k+1}],$$
$$\mathbf{R}_t(-k) = \mathbf{C}_{t-k} + \mathbf{B}_{t-k}[\mathbf{R}_t(-k+1) - \mathbf{R}_{t-k+1}]\mathbf{B}_{t-k}',$$

with $\mathbf{B}_t = \mathbf{C}_t\mathbf{G}_{t+1}'\mathbf{R}_{t+1}^{-1}$, starting values $\mathbf{a}_t(0) = \mathbf{m}_t, \mathbf{R}_t(0) = \mathbf{C}_t$, and with $\mathbf{a}_{t-k}(1) = \mathbf{a}_{t-k+1}$, $\mathbf{R}_{t-k}(0) = \mathbf{R}_{t-k+1}$. If a discount factor is considered then $\mathbf{B}_{t-k} = \delta\mathbf{G}_{t-k+1}^{-1}$ and so

$$\mathbf{a}_t(-k) = (1-\delta)\mathbf{m}_{t-k} + \delta\mathbf{G}_{t-k+1}^{-1}\mathbf{a}_t(-k+1),$$
$$\mathbf{R}_t(-k) = (1-\delta)\mathbf{C}_{t-k} + \delta^2\mathbf{G}_{t-k+1}^{-1}\mathbf{R}_t(-k+1)\mathbf{G}_{t-k+1}^{-1}.$$

3. Choosing the discount factor: The discount factor $\delta \in (0, 1]$ can be chosen to maximize the function

$$l(\delta) \equiv p(y_T, \ldots, y_{p+1}|\mathcal{D}_p, \delta) = \prod_{t=p+1}^{T} p(y_t|\mathcal{D}_{t-1}),$$

where $p(y_t|\mathcal{D}_{t-1})$ is a univariate Student-t distribution with n_t degrees of freedom, mean f_t, and scale matrix q_t.

REFERENCES

Aguilar, O., Huerta, G., Prado, R., & West, M. (1999). Bayesian inference on latent structure in time series (with discussion). In J. Bernardo, J. Berger, A. Dawid, & A. Smith (Eds.), *Bayesian statistics* 6 (pp. 3–26). Oxford: Oxford University Press.

Dyro, F. (1989). The EEG handbook. Boston, MA: Little, Brown and Company.

Gelman, A., Carlin, J., Stern, H., & Rubin, D. (2003). *Bayesian data analysis* (2nd ed.). New York: Chapman & Hall/CRC.

Huerta, G., & West, M. (1999). Priors and component structures in autoregressive time series models. *Journal of the Royal Statistical Society, Series D* 61, 881–899.

Kalman, R. (1960). A new approach to linear filtering theory and prediction problems. *Transactions of the ASME, Series D, Journal of Basic Engineering*, 82, 35–45.

Krystal, A. D., Prado, R., & West, M. (1999). New methods of time series analysis of non-stationary EEG data: Eigenstructure decompositions of time-varying autoregressions. *Clinical Neurophysiology*, 110, 2197–2206.

Molina, F., Prado, R., & Huerta, G. (2006). Multivariate time series modelling and classification via hierarchical VAR mixtures. *Computational Statistics and Data Analysis*, 51(3), 1445–1462.

Prado, R. (1998). *Latent structure in non-stationary time series*. Unpublished doctoral dissertation, Duke University, Durham, NC.

Prado, R., & Huerta, G. (2002). Time-varying autoregressions with model order uncertainty. *Journal of Time Series Analysis*, 23, 599–618.

Prado, R., West, M., & Krystal, A. (2001). Multi-channel EEG analyses via dynamic regression models with time-varying lag/lead structure. *Journal of the Royal Statistical Society, Series C (Applied Statistics)*, 50, 95–109.

Shumway, R., & Stoffer, D. (2005). *Time series analysis and its applications*. New York: Springer.

Trejo, L., Knuth, K., Prado, R., Rosipal, R., Kubitz, K., Kochavi, R., et al. (2007). EEG-based estimation of mental fatigue: Convergent evidence for a three-state model. In D. Schmorrow & L. Reeves (Eds.), *Foundation of augmented cognition, LNCS 4565* (pp. 201–211). Berlin/Heidelberg: Springer.

Trejo, L., Kochavi, R., Kubitz, K., Montgomery, L., Rosipal, R., & Matthews, B. (2006). *EEG-based estimation of mental fatigue* (Technical Report). Available at http://publications.neurodia.com/Trejo-et-al-EEG-Fatigue2006-Manuscript.pdf.

West, M. (1997). Time series decomposition. *Biometrika*, 84, 489–494.

West, M., & Harrison, J. (1997). *Bayesian forecasting and dynamic models* (2nd ed.). New York: Springer.

West, M., Prado, R., & Krystal, A. (1999). Evaluation and comparison of EEG traces: Latent structure in nonstationary time series. *Journal of the American Statistical Association*, 94, 1083–1095.

6

A Closer Look at Two Approaches for Analysis and Classification of Nonstationary Time Series

Hernando Ombao and Raquel Prado

We summarize the relevant aspects of the two approaches for the analysis and classification of several nonstationary time series presented in this book. In Gao et al. (2009), the interest lies in grouping several time series into clusters according to their time-scale characteristics. In Prado (2009), the goal is to estimate the probability that a given time series, from a large collection of them, is a realization from one of multiple processes that can be characterized in terms of their quasi-periodic structure. The methodology of Gao et al. (2009) assumes that there is a known number of clusters G and so, at the end of the analysis, each time series is assigned to one of these clusters. Moreover, the method assumes that there is no training data available (i.e., the group membership of all time series in the data is not known). Prado (2009) assumes that there is a known number of states K and estimates the probability that each time series is a realization from the process that underlines each of the k states for $k = 1{:}K$. Both methodologies take into account the spectral characteristics of the time series.

The methods presented in both chapters are model-based and hence offer many advantages with respect to other non-model-based approaches commonly used in classification, such as support vector machines (SVM) (see Table 6.1 for a comparison of model-based versus SVM methods). Relevant features of model-based approaches include, for example: (a) their ability

TABLE 6.1

Comparison Between Model-Based and SVM Methods for Classification

Model-Based	SVM
Highly structured	Highly flexible, few constraints
Can incorporate information across trials	Not easily generalizable to multiple trials
Can incorporate common information across subjects	Not easily generalizable to multiple subjects
Can provide estimates of uncertainty in predictions	Do not account for uncertainty in prediction
Can model and test for covariate effects	Covariate effects cannot be incorporated

to incorporate scientifically meaningful information collected during previous trials of a given experiment; this can be done by using informative prior distributions on the model parameters; (b) their ability to model and estimate uncertainty in predictions; and (c) the fact that covariates can be easily handled. It is not obvious how these can (if at all possible) be incorporated in SVM methods.

There are several possible approaches that can be considered when analyzing time-series data. These methods can be broadly classified as either frequency domain or spectral domain. Table 6.2 summarizes some of the differences between time-domain and frequency-domain methods. In general, time-domain models are parametric—they model the conditional mean explicitly as a function of its own past values as well as those of the other time series. They allow us to incorporate information across trials and subjects in experimental settings. Often, their parameters cannot be easily interpreted. In contrast, frequency-domain methods are typically nonparametric, providing intuitive interpretation of the result through estimates of the spectral power (variance decomposition of time series across frequency

TABLE 6.2

Comparison Between Time-Domain and Frequency-Domain Approaches

Time Domain	Spectral Domain
Typically parametric	Often nonparametric
Massive data summarized via model parameters	Require more data
Parameters may not be easily interpreted	Power and coherence offer intuitive interpretation
Incorporate information across trials and subjects	Not easily done; work still in its infancy stage

bands) and coherence (frequency-specific cross-correlation between two filtered time series).

The methodology of Gao et al. (2009) is a frequency-domain approach that uses the WP transform which is localized in time and can generate time-varying spectra, capturing the relevant features that describe the variance (or energy) of the time series over time. This makes the methodology suitable for analyzing nonstationary time series. The method in Prado (2009) also employs spectral features for classification. However, it differs from the Gao et al. method because it extracts spectral quantities via AR and TVAR models. AR models are appropriate for stationary time series, whereas TVARs are appropriate to describe changes in the series over time. Note also that the spectrum of a stationary time series can be estimated parametrically by fitting an AR (or ARMA) model to the time series. The spectrum of an AR (or ARMA) process can be expressed in terms of the ARMA coefficients and the spectrum is indirectly estimated via the AR (or ARMA) coefficients. Like the WP-based approach of Gao et al. (2009), it produces time-varying spectra in the following sense. At each time t, a TVAR(p) model is described by a set of p parameters that are related nonlinearly to a set of reciprocal characteristic roots as described in Prado (2009). These roots can be represented in terms of their moduli and frequencies. Therefore, when a series y_t is modeled by a TVAR process, its spectrum is time varying, with peaks around the characteristic frequencies. The sharpnesses of these peaks are proportional to the corresponding characteristic moduli. These two approaches of modeling time-varying spectra (WP versus TVAR) have both advantages and disadvantages as outlined in Table 6.2.

REFERENCES

Prado, R. (2009). Characterizing latent structure in brain signals. In S. Chow, E. Ferrer and F. Hsieh (Eds.), *Statistical methods for modeling human dynamics.* New York: Psychology Press, Taylor and Francis Group.

Gao, B., Ombao, H., & Ho, M. R. (2009). Cluster analysis for nonstationary time series. In S. Chow, E. Ferrer and F. Hsieh (Eds.), *Statistical methods for modeling human dynamics*, pp. 85–122. New York: Psychology Press, Taylor and Francis Group.

Part II

Representing and Extracting Intraindividual Change

7

Generalized Local Linear Approximation of Derivatives from Time Series

Steven M. Boker, Pascal R. Deboeck, Crystal Edler, and Pamela K. Keel

7.1 INTRODUCTION

Recent developments in dynamical systems modeling of repeated observations data have led to first- and second-order differential equations being fit to psychological data using local linear approximation (LLA) of derivatives (Boker & Graham, 1998; Boker, 2001; Butner, Amazeen, & Mulvey, 2005). The LLA method provides simplified explicit estimation of derivatives from repeated observations using a three-dimensional time-delay embedding (Abarbanel, Carroll, Pecora, Sidorowich, & Tsimring, 1994; Noakes, 1991; Sauer, Yorke, & Casdagli, 1991; Takens, 1981; Whitney, 1936) in a manner similar to Savitzky–Golay filtering (Savitzky & Golay, 1964), but has several weaknesses. Three-dimensional embedding is sensitive to time-independent noise, which can bias estimates of the differential equations parameters unless the delay time, τ, used to create the time-delay embedded matrix is chosen correctly (Boker & Nesselroade, 2002; Deboeck, Boker, & Bergeman, submitted). In addition, as it is currently used, LLA is only able to estimate first and second derivatives. Some differential equation models may require higher-order derivatives.

One method that has been proposed as an alternative to LLA is the latent differential equations (LDE) method (Boker, Neale, & Rausch, 2004; Boker, 2007). This method uses a fixed loading measurement model to estimate latent derivatives and their covariances. The covariances between the derivatives in the structural part of the model are used to estimate regression coefficients relating the derivatives and thus estimating a differential equation or system of differential equations. The LDE method is much less sensitive to time-independent noise and is somewhat more lenient with respect to the choice of time delay than is LLA. However, sometimes the explicit calculation of approximate derivatives by LLA can still be the preferred method, particularly when the system is composed of data that are nested in a multilevel framework (Boker & Ghisletta, 2001; Butner et al., 2005; Maxwell & Boker, 2007).

The LLA and LDE methods are two methods that are currently in use for the estimation of differential equations models in the social sciences. Other methods include the exact discrete (Singer, 1993) and approximate discrete (Oud & Jansen, 2000) methods for estimating stochastic differential equations and Kalman filtering techniques (e.g., Chow, Hamaker, Fujita, & Boker, in press). These three methods have the advantage of explicitly modeling stochastic innovation, exogenous influences that may be time varying and thus nonstationary. However, these methods require that the user have an analytic integral of the differential equation model prior to being able to begin modeling. An advantage of the LLA and LDE methods is that the differential equation can be specified and fit directly, rather than fitting the integral of the differential equation to the data. Functional data analysis (Ramsay, Hooker, Campbell, & Cao, 2007) is another candidate for fitting differential equations directly, which bypasses the need for an integral solution of the differential equation. The functional data analysis approaches share some similarity with LLA and LDE in that they estimate derivatives from data and use the covariances between the derivatives to estimate parameters of the target differential equation. The strength of this family of methods is that it is flexible and can deal with nonstationarity. One weakness is that the method is relatively complicated, requires relatively long time series, and requires the researcher to make informed choices about the algorithm that can influence the estimates.

This chapter presents a method that generalizes LLA so that it is less sensitive to time-independent noise and so that the choice of time delay becomes independent of the choice of coverage of cycles in the data while still explicitly calculating approximate derivatives. In order to unpack the previous statement, let us start by examining time-delay embedding and then show how a generalization of LLA can be formed from the fixed loading matrices of LDE.

7.2 TIME-DELAY EMBEDDING

Consider a time series X where individuals $i = 1, \ldots, N$ are observed on occasions $j = 1, \ldots, P$ separated by a fixed time interval Δt. As a first step, each individual's data are centered around either an estimated or a known equilibrium value. The equilibrium value (or equilibrium set) are values such that if no external perturbation to the system were to occur, the system would remain at equilibrium. One type of equilibrium is a homeostatic set point. If a fixed equilibrium value is known, it is subtracted from each individual's data to create deviations about the equilibrium. If the equilibrium value is not known, one common simple method is to use residuals from linear trends fit individually through each participant's time series. In this case, each individual has a separate estimated equilibrium that may be changing linearly over time. More complex methods for estimating changing equilibria can also be used when theory provides a reasonable functional form to the equilibrium change (Boker & Bisconti, 2006).

Once the time series has been centered around the equilibrium values, we can calculate approximate derivatives from a time-delay embedded matrix created from the time series. For instance, consider that d is a three-dimensional embedded matrix such that the time delay between embedded columns is $\tau\Delta t$, where $\tau = 2$, so that the embedding delay is twice the interval between occasions of measurement. If the original time series X is ordered by occasion $j = \{1, \ldots, P)$ within individual $i = \{1, \ldots, N)$, then the series of all observations $x_{(i,j)}$ can be written as a vector of scores

$$X = \{x_{(1,1)}, x_{(1,2)}, \ldots, x_{(1,P)}, x_{(2,1)}, x_{(2,2)}, \ldots, x_{(2,P)}, \ldots,$$
$$x_{(N,1)}, x_{(N,2)}, \ldots, x_{(N,P)}\}. \quad (7.1)$$

A three-dimensional time-delay embedded matrix $\mathbf{X}^{(3)}$ of order $M \times 3$ where $\tau = 2$ can then be written as a matrix with three columns such that

$$\mathbf{X}^{(3)} = \begin{bmatrix} x_{(1,1)} & x_{(1,3)} & x_{(1,5)} \\ x_{(1,2)} & x_{(1,4)} & x_{(1,6)} \\ \vdots & \vdots & \vdots \\ x_{(1,P-8)} & x_{(1,P-6)} & x_{(1,P-4)} \\ x_{(2,1)} & x_{(2,3)} & x_{(2,5)} \\ x_{(2,2)} & x_{(2,4)} & x_{(2,6)} \\ \vdots & \vdots & \vdots \\ x_{(2,P-8)} & x_{(2,P-6)} & x_{(2,P-4)} \\ \vdots & \vdots & \vdots \\ x_{(N,1)} & x_{(N,3)} & x_{(N,5)} \\ x_{(N,2)} & x_{(N,4)} & x_{(N,6)} \\ \vdots & \vdots & \vdots \\ x_{(N,P-8)} & x_{(N,P-6)} & x_{(N,P-4)} \end{bmatrix}. \tag{7.2}$$

This time-delay embedded matrix is referred to as being a "three-dimensional embedding" because each row can be thought of as a point in a three-dimensional space. This is why time delay is commonly referred to as embedding. What we are doing is taking the time dependency of a univariate (one-dimensional) time series and converting it into a geometric shape in a higher-dimensional space. Thus, we are capturing the time dependency in the time series into the rows of the time-delay embedded matrix. We then perform local smoothing in this higher dimensional space so that points that are near each other in the embedding space help give an estimate of the tangent slope and curvature along the geometric shape. Covariances between estimates of derivatives of this geometric shape are used in the estimation procedure to give parameter estimates for the differential equation. This is sometimes referred to as "trading time for geometry." All of that may seem complicated, but in practice it turns out to be quite simple.

Let us look more carefully at the matrix in Equation 7.2. Each row of $\mathbf{X}^{(3)}$ is composed of an ordered triplet from the time series X where there is an interval of length $\tau = 2$ occasions of measurement separating each column. Note that data from individual i never appear on the same row with individual $i + 1$.

7.3 LLA ESTIMATES OF DERIVATIVES

LLAs of derivatives (Boker, 2001) can now be calculated from $\mathbf{X}^{(3)}$ and stored in matrix $\mathbf{Y}$ of the same $M \times 3$ order as $\mathbf{X}^{(3)}$ where the kth row of $\mathbf{Y}$ is

$$y_{k1} = x_{k2}, \tag{7.3}$$

$$y_{k2} = \frac{x_{k3} - x_{k1}}{2\tau\Delta t}, \tag{7.4}$$

$$y_{k3} = \frac{x_{k1} - 2x_{k2} + x_{k3}}{(\tau\Delta t)^2}. \tag{7.5}$$

Thus, the first column of $\mathbf{Y}$ is the value of x for person i at the occasion of measurement indexed in the second column of $\mathbf{X}^{(3)}$, and the second and third columns of $\mathbf{Y}$ are the approximated first and second derivatives, respectively, at that same occasion of measurement.

7.4 LDE ESTIMATES OF DERIVATIVES

Another method for estimating and modeling the covariance between derivatives of a time series is LDE, which uses a form of a latent growth curve model with fixed loadings (Boker et al., 2004). The fixed loading matrix for an LDE model is constructed so that the covariances between the latent variables will be those that best account for the time series such that the latent variables are derivatives of the time series. When a first- or second-order linear LDE model is specified, it is often fit to a five-dimensional time-delay embedded matrix. Consider the LDE model in Figure 7.1. The latent variables' relationship with the indicators is established by setting the loadings of the first latent variable to be equal to 1, the loadings of the second latent variable to be increasing linearly with a step of $\tau\Delta t$, and the loadings of the third latent variable to be the indefinite integral of the loadings for the second latent variable. These fixed loadings can be specified in a matrix $\mathbf{L}$ so that

$$\mathbf{L} = \begin{bmatrix} 1 & -2\tau\Delta t & (-2\tau\Delta t)^2/2 \\ 1 & -1\tau\Delta t & (-1\tau\Delta t)^2/2 \\ 1 & 0 & 0 \\ 1 & 1\tau\Delta t & (1\tau\Delta t)^2/2 \\ 1 & 2\tau\Delta t & (2\tau\Delta t)^2/2 \end{bmatrix}. \tag{7.6}$$

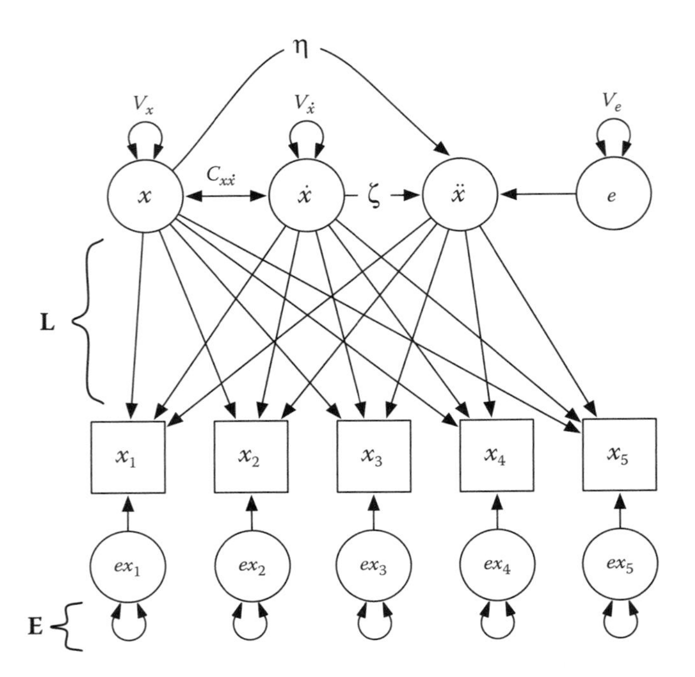

FIGURE 7.1 Path diagram of a second-order LDE model using a five-dimensional time-delay embedding.

Since Δt and τ are fixed, no coefficients are estimated in **L**. In the model in Figure 7.1, covariances between the latent variables, the displacement x, first derivative $\dot{x}$, and second deriviative $\ddot{x}$ estimate the coefficients of the second-order differential equation

$$\ddot{x}(t) = \eta x(t) + \zeta \dot{x}(t) + e(t), \tag{7.7}$$

where η is related to the frequency of oscillation and ζ is the damping or amplification. Now if we define two 3×3 matrices **A** and **S** such that

$$\mathbf{A} = \begin{bmatrix} 0 & 0 & 0 \\ 0 & 0 & 0 \\ \eta & \zeta & 0 \end{bmatrix}, \tag{7.8}$$

$$\mathbf{S} = \begin{bmatrix} V_x & C_{x\dot{x}} & 0 \\ C_{x\dot{x}} & V_{\dot{x}} & 0 \\ 0 & 0 & V_{e\ddot{x}} \end{bmatrix}, \tag{7.9}$$

and a 5×5 diagonal matrix **E** to contain the five residual variances for the five indicators $(x_1, x_2, x_3, x_4, x_5)$, we can calculate the expected covariance matrix **R** for this model as

$$\mathbf{R} = \mathbf{L}(\mathbf{I} - \mathbf{A})^{-1}\mathbf{S}(\mathbf{I} - \mathbf{A})^{-1'}\mathbf{L}' + \mathbf{E}. \tag{7.10}$$

The five columns of $\mathbf{X}^{(5)}$ give us 15 degrees of freedom in the data covariances. There are five degrees of freedom used by **E**, two degrees of freedom used by **A**, and five degrees of freedom used by **S**, leaving four degrees of freedom with which to test the fit of the model.

7.5 RELATIONSHIP BETWEEN LLA AND THE LDE LOADING MATRIX

Consider a second-order LDE model with only three indicators, in other words an LDE model to be fit to a three-dimensional time-delay embedded matrix $\mathbf{X}^{(3)}$. This model would not be identified due to negative degrees of freedom. However, for our purposes, we will construct the 3×3 loading matrix **L** for this LDE model according to the same restrictions used in the LDE model fit to the five-dimensional embedded matrix above:

$$\mathbf{L} = \begin{bmatrix} 1 & -1\tau\Delta t & (-1\tau\Delta t)^2/2 \\ 1 & 0 & 0 \\ 1 & 1\tau\Delta t & (1\tau\Delta t)^2/2 \end{bmatrix}. \tag{7.11}$$

Let us assume that $\mathbf{E} = 0$, so that the previously latent scores become identified as linear combinations of the three columns of indicators in the time-delay embedded matrix $\mathbf{X}^{(3)}$. Now, let **Y** be the $M \times 3$ matrix of latent derivatives x, $\dot{x}$, and $\ddot{x}$. Thus, each row i of **Y** will consist of three columns containing the latent derivatives x, $\dot{x}$, and $\ddot{x}$ corresponding to the data for row i of $\mathbf{X}^{(3)}$. We can now construct an equation that relates the latent derivatives **Y** to the data $\mathbf{X}^{(3)}$ by postmultiplying **Y** by the transpose of the loading matrix **L**:

$$\mathbf{X}^{(3)} = \mathbf{Y}\mathbf{L}'. \tag{7.12}$$

Now, if $\mathbf{L}'\mathbf{L}$ is nonsingular, we can solve for $\mathbf{Y}$ while accounting for the possibility that $\mathbf{L}$ might not be square by the following:

$$\mathbf{X}^{(3)}\mathbf{L} = \mathbf{Y}\mathbf{L}'\mathbf{L}, \tag{7.13}$$

$$\mathbf{X}^{(3)}\mathbf{L}(\mathbf{L}'\mathbf{L})^{-1} = \mathbf{Y}(\mathbf{L}'\mathbf{L})(\mathbf{L}'\mathbf{L})^{-1}, \tag{7.14}$$

$$\mathbf{X}^{(3)}\mathbf{L}(\mathbf{L}'\mathbf{L})^{-1} = \mathbf{Y}. \tag{7.15}$$

Substituting the values from Equation 7.11 into $\mathbf{L}$, we can calculate matrix $\mathbf{W}$ as

$$\mathbf{W} = \mathbf{L}(\mathbf{L}'\mathbf{L})^{-1} \tag{7.16}$$

$$= \begin{bmatrix} 0 & -1/2\tau\Delta t & 1/(\tau\Delta t)^2 \\ 1 & 0 & -2/(\tau\Delta t)^2 \\ 0 & 1/2\tau\Delta t & 1/(\tau\Delta t)^2 \end{bmatrix}. \tag{7.17}$$

Now it becomes obvious that the matrix $\mathbf{W}$ contains coefficients from Equations 7.3 through 7.5 that LLA uses to transform the embedded matrix $\mathbf{X}^{(3)}$ into the approximate derivatives $\mathbf{Y}$, such that

$$\mathbf{Y} = \mathbf{X}\mathbf{W}. \tag{7.18}$$

An equivalent transformation matrix $\mathbf{W}$ can be calculated for any number of columns in a time-delay embedding. For instance, the five-dimensional embedding $\mathbf{X}^{(5)}$ has a loading matrix $\mathbf{L}$ defined in Equation 7.6. If we choose $\tau = 1$ and $\Delta t = 1$, we can apply Equation 7.16 to find that

$$\mathbf{W} = \begin{bmatrix} -0.0857 & -0.2 & 0.2857 \\ 0.3429 & -0.1 & -0.1429 \\ 0.4857 & 0.0 & -0.2857 \\ 0.3429 & 0.1 & -0.1429 \\ -0.0857 & 0.2 & 0.2857 \end{bmatrix}. \tag{7.19}$$

In the enclosed CDROM, R code for a function gllaWMatrix to calculate the $\mathbf{W}$ matrix for approximating derivatives can be found, given a selected embedding dimension D, a time interval between successive observations Δt, a number of observations delay τ between columns of the embedded matrix, and the highest order of derivatives you wish to calculate. The requested embedding dimension should be greater than or equal to the requested order plus one.

By adding columns to the time-delay embedding matrix (i.e., increasing the embedding dimension) and using a generalized local linear approximation (GLLA) transformation to estimate derivatives, one increases the amount of smoothing applied to the geometric shape in the embedded space. This has the effect of removing noise at the cost of attenuating rapid changes in the signal. If the target signal is changing relatively slowly in comparison to the sampling rate, increasing the embedding dimension can improve point estimates of differential equation parameters by reducing the effect of time-independent noise on the parameters.

7.6 SIMULATION

A simulation was conducted comparing GLLA with LDE for a series of noisy stationary time series generated by a second-order linear differential equation

$$\ddot{x}_t = \eta x_t + \zeta \dot{x}_t + e_t \tag{7.20}$$

in a $3 \times 3 \times 3 \times 3$ design, where $\eta = \{-0.01, -0.02, -0.03\}$, $\zeta = \{-0.01, 0.00, 0.01\}$, the order of the derivatives estimated was $o = \{2, 3, 4\}$, and the dimension of the embedding matrix was $d = \{3, 5, 9\}$. The case where $o = 2$ and $d = 3$ corresponds to LLA and the other values of o and/or d correspond to GLLA. Two hundred replications of a time series with length $N = 300$ were simulated for each cell, GLLA was used to estimate derivatives, and then the parameters of the differential equation were estimated with ordinary least squares regression.

The results of the simulation were predicted by the manipulated parameters d and o so as to better understand the effects of increased smoothing due to increasing the embedding dimension and/or increasing the order of the maximum derivative that was used in the smoothing. The results of predicting the R^2 and mean parameter bias in the simulation as a standardized multiple regression are presented in Tables 7.1 and 7.2.

It can be seen that increasing the number of columns in the time-delay embedding matrix (increasing the embedding dimension) provides a large

TABLE 7.1

R^2 and Parameter Bias Predicted as Multiple Regressions with Standardized Predictors Embedding Dimension d and Derivative Order o

	Value	SE	t	p
R^2				
Intercept	0.285	0.0194	14.742	<0.0001
Dimension	0.230	0.0199	11.548	<0.0001
Order	−0.123	0.0195	−6.327	<0.0001
Dimension × order	−0.064	0.0200	−3.222	0.0020
Multiple R^2: 0.7516; adjusted R^2: 0.739				
η bias				
Intercept	−0.0096	0.00094	−10.198	<0.0001
Dimension	0.0097	0.00097	9.974	<0.0001
Order	−0.0050	0.00095	−5.240	<0.0001
Dimension × order	0.0019	0.00098	1.941	0.0571
Multiple R^2: 0.6451; adjusted R^2: 0.627				
ζ bias				
Intercept	0.0014	0.00027	5.140	<0.0001
Dimension	−0.0014	0.00028	−4.876	<0.0001
Order	0.0005	0.00028	1.854	0.0687
Dimension × order	−0.0001	0.00028	−0.491	0.6251
Multiple R^2: 0.2931; adjusted R^2: 0.2572				

TABLE 7.2

Variability of Parameters (Standard Deviations of the Estimates within Simulation Cells) Predicted as Multiple Regressions with Standardized Predictors Embedding Dimension d and Derivative Order o

	Value	SE	t	p
$\sigma(\eta)$				
Intercept	0.00112	0.00001	11.422	<0.0001
Dimension	−0.00099	0.00010	−9.819	<0.0001
Order	0.00053	0.00001	5.406	<0.0001
Dimension × order	−0.00021	0.00010	−2.082	0.0416
Multiple R^2: 0.6411; adjusted R^2: 0.6228				
$\sigma(\zeta)$				
Intercept	0.00295	0.00024	12.389	<0.0001
Dimension	−0.00200	0.00025	−8.123	<0.0001
Order	0.00104	0.00024	4.341	<0.0001
Dimension × order	−0.00021	0.00025	−0.850	0.399
Multiple R^2: 0.5503; adjusted R^2: 0.5274				

and statistically significant improvement in the R^2 of the differential equation model, whereas increasing the order of the maximum derivative to be estimated has a significant negative impact on R^2. Thus, we can conclude that increasing the area of the local smoothing tends to help separate signal from noise, but increasing the flexibility of that filter by increasing the order of the derivatives to be estimated tends to allow more noise into the estimates of the derivatives.

The bias of the η parameter estimates is larger when the dimension of the embedding matrix is increased, but is lower when the order of the estimates is increased. The bias in the ζ parameter is decreased slightly when the dimension of the embedding matrix is increased. The variabilities of the estimates of ζ and η are both decreased when the embedding dimension is increased, but the variabilities of both parameters increase when order is increased.

Overall, using the order of the differential equation (in our case a second-order equation) is recommended when using GLLA, since increasing the order of the derivative estimates allows more noise to contaminate the signal and thus the parameter estimates have more variability. However, bias of η is increased when the embedding dimension is increased, so one must take care to not increase the embedding dimension more than necessary. How much is necessary will depend on the signal-to-noise ratio in the target data set. If the data are relatively precise, then small embedding dimensions will provide for lower bias while still having acceptable variability of the parameter estimates. But when there is a noisy signal, it may be useful to increase the embedding dimension. One method for determining how to choose the embedding dimension is to choose a range of d in order to see how the parameter estimates behave. This method is illustrated in the example application provided in the next section.

7.7 EXAMPLE APPLICATION

The example data come from four subjects from a study of binge eating and ovarian hormones (Edler, Lipson, & Keel, 2007). Daily data were collected over the course of one menstrual cycle in nine women with Diagnostic and Statistical Manual IV, Bulimia Nervosa (DSM-IV BN) (American Psychiatric Association, 1994). Participants were excluded for (1) body mass index less than $19\,\text{kg/m}^2$ or greater than $25\,\text{kg/m}^2$,

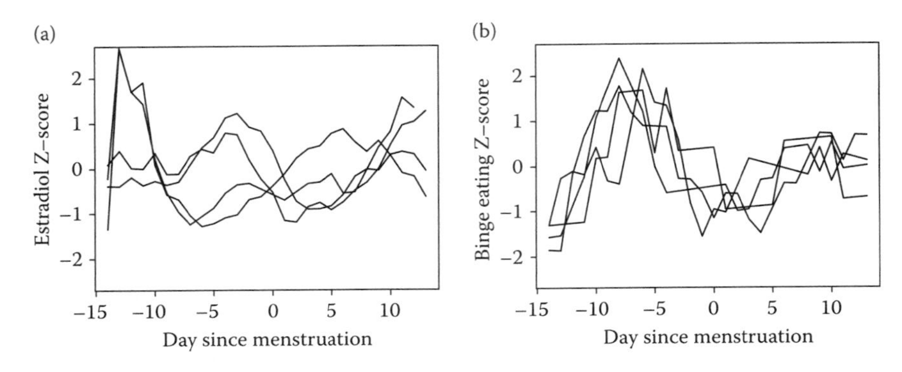

FIGURE 7.2 Daily (a) assays of estradiol and (b) self-reported binge eating scores for four participants aligned to their day of menstruation.

(2) irregular menses, or (3) psychotropic medications or oral contraceptive use. Women recorded daily binge episodes, and daily salivary samples were collected and assayed for estradiol and progesterone (Edler et al., 2007). The detrended and standardized daily values for these data are plotted in Figures 7.2a and b where each line is an individual participant.

It is clear from inspection that there are cyclic patterns in these data, something that would be expected *a priori* from a marker for estrogen, but might not be so readily expected for daily fluctuations in binge eating. The binge eating cycles appear to align themselves with the day of menstruation such that each subject is at a peak during a similar phase offset from menstruation. However, the daily fluctuations in estradiol do not coincide so easily across subjects. If one were to calculate an unrestricted growth curve as a mean of all subjects at each day, the result would obscure the within-subject fluctuations due to the phase offset in estradiol curves between subjects. A differential equations model of these data allows the aggregation of relationships between derivatives; relationships that can still hold when phase offsets such as we see in the estradiol data are present.

Since these data are hypothesized to be cyclic, we will use the GLLA method to calculate derivatives and fit a multilevel second-order differential equation model first to the estradiol data and then to the binge eating data such that

$$\ddot{x}_{it} = \eta_i x_{it} + \zeta_i \dot{x}_{it} + e_{it}, \tag{7.21}$$

$$\eta_i = m_\eta + u_{\eta i}, \tag{7.22}$$

$$\zeta_i = m_\zeta + u_{\zeta i}, \tag{7.23}$$

where x_{it}, $\dot{x}_{it}$, and $\ddot{x}_{it}$ are the displacement, first derivative, and second derivative of the variable of interest (binge eating or estradiol) for person i on day t; η_i and ζ_i can vary across individuals such that they each have means (m_η and m_ζ) and unique contributions from each individual ($u_{\eta i}$ and $u_{\zeta i}$). We will refrain from fitting more complicated coupled oscillator models at this time, since we wish to demonstrate the use of the GLLA estimation method rather than focussing on the details of the relationship between ovarian functioning and disordered eating.

Since the cycle period of menstruation is likely to be near 28 days, we will choose time delays so that the total interval covered across all columns of our time-delay embedding matrix is about one half of the period: 14 days. Previous simulations have shown that the minimum bias in the frequency parameter is found when the coverage of the embedding matrix is near one half the period (see Boker & Nesselroade, 2002, for the case of a three-dimensional embedding). When the period of fluctuations is not known, this coverage must be estimated (Deboeck, 2005; Deboeck et al., submitted).

We will present the results of GLLA estimation for using four different choices of embedding dimension: (1) $d = 3$ and $\tau = 7$ results in a coverage of 14 observations and replicates what would be found using LLA; (2) $d = 6$ and $\tau = 3$ results in a coverage of 15 observations; (3) $d = 9$ and $\tau = 2$ results in a coverage of 16 observations; and (4) $d = 14$ and $\tau = 1$ results in a coverage of 14 observations and is the largest embedding dimension we can use, given that these data were sampled daily.

7.8 EXAMPLE PROGRAM

For the purposes of the example program included in the enclosed CD, data from the four subjects were organized as a three-column data file, with the first column being ID number, the second column being estradiol, and the third column being binge eating. Thus, each row comprised a single occasion of measurement for a single individual. It is important to note that the rows are time ordered and of equal interval so that the jth row for the ith individual is the jth occasion of measurement for that individual. If data are missing for individual i for occasion j, then the jth row for person i must have that person's ID number in the ID column and missing data indicators in the other columns.

The example program uses the two R functions from the enclosed CDROM. The function gllaWMatrix calculates a GLLA transformation matrix **W** according to the methods described in the previous section. The function gllaEmbed takes a vector of time ordered equal interval data and an optional matching vector of IDs and returns a time-delay embedded matrix according to the supplied time delay parameter τ and embedding dimension d. If a participant ID vector is supplied, rows are never time delayed such that multiple individuals appear on the same row of the matrix. If too few rows exist to create an embedding with the supplied embedding dimension and time delay, then the function returns a missing value, NA. These functions and the example program are available electronically from the corresponding author's website http://people.virginia.edu/˜smb3u and as part of this book. An example data file may also be downloaded from the same site. The example data file is the simulated data provided in order to allow the reader to test the functions.

7.9 MODELING RESULTS

The results from the example program run on the example subjects using the four different combinations of embedding dimension d and time delay τ are presented in Tables 7.3 and 7.4. Note that each combination of parameters has a similar total delay from the first to the last column in the embedded matrix that is used to approximate derivatives. Further note that there are small differences in the total N that result from these embeddings. This is due to the interaction of each of these combinations with the pattern of missingness in the data. Since row-wise deletion is performed in this case, larger embedding dimensions can lead to substantially fewer rows available for estimation.

Parameter estimation is relatively stable across the different columns in the estradiol model results in Table 7.3. Recall that the estradiol data plotted in Figure 7.2a were relatively smooth and appeared similar to a damped linear oscillator. Thus, we can see that when the data are relatively low noise, several equivalent choices of derivative approximation may exist. Simulations of LLA estimation with $d = 3$ have shown that estimates of frequency are biased towards the optimum frequency for the

TABLE 7.3

Multilevel Second-Order Differential Equations Model of Estradiol Regulation

	$d = 3$, $\tau = 7$	$d = 6$, $\tau = 3$	$d = 9$, $\tau = 2$	$d = 14$, $\tau = 1$
Total delay	14	15	16	14
N	55	51	47	59
m_η	−0.054	−0.056	−0.058	−0.073
SE	±0.0057	±0.0064	±0.0070	±0.0082
m_ζ	−0.046	−0.033	−0.032	−0.040
SE	±0.0673	±0.0568	±0.0635	±0.0559
Mean r^2	0.915	0.936	0.952	0.906
λ_1	26.57	25.17	25.56	23.59
λ_2	30.50	29.59	31.14	26.63
λ_3	26.50	25.44	25.57	22.65
λ_4	24.93	23.52	23.58	21.09

chosen time delay, thus attenuating individual differences in frequency (Boker & Nesselroade, 2002). Note that the choice of $d = 9$ and $\tau = 2$ not only has the maximum mean r^2 (calculated as the mean of the individual r^2s), but also reduces the attenuation in the between-persons differences in the period of oscillation, λ_i, in days. When ζ is small, the period (or peak-to-peak wavelength), λ_i, can be estimated from η_i for individual i such that $\lambda_i = 2\pi\sqrt{-1/\eta_i}$. Only when η_i is negative does λ_i have a real value.

The data for Binge eating plotted in Figure 7.2b are, by inspection, considerably noisier than those of estradiol. Thus, we might expect that the smoothing that is accomplished by a higher-dimension embedding might

TABLE 7.4

Multilevel Second-Order Differential Equations Model of Binge Eating Regulation

	$d = 3$, $\tau = 7$	$d = 6$, $\tau = 3$	$d = 9$, $\tau = 2$	$d = 14$, $\tau = 1$
Total delay	14	15	16	14
N	55	51	47	59
m_η	−0.055	−0.069	−0.067	−0.091
SE	±0.0040	±0.0028	±0.0024	±0.0059
m_ζ	−0.160	−0.114	−0.119	−0.111
SE	±0.0512	±0.0366	±0.0469	±0.0266
Mean r^2	0.893	0.947	0.957	0.971
λ_1	27.51	23.89	24.23	20.44
λ_2	26.73	23.70	24.36	20.99
λ_3	25.76	24.41	24.19	22.40
λ_4	27.49	23.82	24.24	19.57

help in estimating the parameters of the second-order differential equation. The largest embedding dimension $d = 14$ does have the largest mean r^2. Note that the model results for $d = 14$ also have the smallest standard error for the damping parameter ζ and the largest individual differences in estimated periods for binge eating.

7.10 DISCUSSION

Choosing a combination of embedding dimension and time delay that maximizes the mean proportion of explained variance in the second derivative appears to reduce standard errors in fixed-effects parameters and increase individual differences in periods when fitting a multilevel damped linear oscillator model. These two effects are particularly interesting because they have been the weaknesses of the LLA approach to approximating derivatives from time series.

If many individuals are missing observations, then the high embedding dimensions with small time delays may result in far fewer total usable observed rows than the smaller embedding dimension data. However, if the data are largely complete and there is a fairly large amount of time-independent noise in the data, high embedding dimensions can help reject high-frequency noise. GLLA gives an increased degree of flexibility in the estimation of derivatives from a selected data set.

Several weaknesses remain in the GLLA method. There still remains a built-in dependency between the displacement and second derivative that inflates the apparent r^2. An approximation method that reduces or eliminates this dependency would be a significant advance. Simulations for power analysis of GLLA and combinations of embedding dimension and time delay would also further improve our understanding of the consequences of the choices of these parameters and might lead to an empirically derived optimal embedding algorithm that could automatically choose optimal embeddings for a given data set.

7.11 CONCLUSIONS

The correspondence between LDE estimation and GLLA helps unify two extant methods for the estimation of parameters of differential equations models from time series. In addition, the simplicity of the GLLA estimation method means that approximated derivatives may be quickly and easily calculated for a variety of time series where linear models may not hold and thus analytic derivatives may not be available. GLLA derivative estimation can be added to the list of transformations that may be useful in many areas of physiological and behavioral time series from sources such as EEG, EMG, heart rate, and motion capture data.

ACKNOWLEDGMENTS

Funding for this work was provided in part by NSF Grant BCS–0527485 and NIH Grant 1R21DA024304–01. Any opinions, findings, and conclusions or recommendations expressed in this material are those of the authors and do not necessarily reflect the views of the National Science Foundation or the National Institutes of Health.

REFERENCES

Abarbanel, H. D. I., Carroll, T., Pecora, L. M., Sidorowich, J. J., & Tsimring, L. S. (1994). Predicting physical variables in time-delay embedding. *Physical Review E, 49*(3), 1840–1853.

American Psychiatric Association (Ed.). (1994). *Diagnostic and statistical manual of mental disorders* (4th ed.) Washington, DC: American Psychiatric Association.

Boker, S. M. (2001). Differential structural modeling of intraindividual variability. In L. Collins & A. Sayer (Eds.), *New methods for the analysis of change* (pp. 3–28). Washington, DC: APA.

Boker, S. M. (2007). Specifying latent differential equations models. In S. M. Boker & M. J. Wenger (Eds.), *Data analytic techniques for dynamical systems in the social and behavioral sciences* (pp. 131–159). Mahwah, NJ: Lawrence Erlbaum Associates.

Boker, S. M., & Bisconti, T. L. (2006). Dynamical systems modeling in aging research. In C. S. Bergeman & S. M. Boker (Eds.), *Quantitative methodology in aging research* (pp. 185–229). Mahwah, NJ: Lawrence Erlbaum Associates.

Boker, S. M., & Ghisletta, P. (2001). Random coefficients models for control parameters in dynamical systems. *Multilevel Modelling Newsletter, 13*(1), 10–17.

Boker, S. M., & Graham, J. (1998). A dynamical systems analysis of adolescent substance abuse. *Multivariate Behavioral Research, 33*(4), 479–507.

Boker, S. M. Neale, M. C., & Rausch, J. (2004). Latent differential equation modeling with multivariate multi-occasion indicators. In K. van Montfort, H. Oud, & A. Satorra (Eds.), *Recent developments on structural equation models: Theory and applications* (pp. 151–174). Dordrecht, the Netherlands: Kluwer Academic Publishers.

Boker, S. M., & Nesselroade, J. R. (2002). A method for modeling the intrinsic dynamics of intraindividual variability: Recovering the parameters of simulated oscillators in multi-wave panel data. *Multivariate Behavioral Research, 37*(1), 127–160.

Butner, J., Amazeen, P. G., & Mulvey, G. M. (2005). Multilevel modeling to two cyclical processes: Extending differential structural equation modeling to nonlinear coupled systems. *Psychological Methods, 10*(2), 159–177.

Chow, S.-M., Hamaker, E. L., Fujita, F., & Boker, S. M. (2009). Representing time-varying cyclic dynamics using multiple-subject state-space models. *British Journal of Mathematical and Statistical Psychology, 62*, 683–712.

Deboeck, P. R. (2005). *Using surrogate data analysis to estimate τ for local linear approximation of damped linear oscillators.* Unpublished master's thesis, University of Notre Dame.

Deboeck, P. R., Boker, S. M., & Bergeman, C. S. (2009). Modeling individual damped linear oscillator processes with differential equations: Using surrogate data analysis to estimate the smoothing parameter. *Multivariate Behavioral Research, 43*(4), 497–521.

Edler, C., Lipson, S. F., & Keel, P. K. (2007). Ovarian hormones and binge eating in bulimia nervosa. *Psychological Medicine, 37*, 131–141.

Maxwell, S. E., & Boker, S. M. (2007). Multilevel models of dynamical systems. In S. M. Boker & M. J. Wenger (Eds.), *Data analytic techniques for dynamical systems* (pp. 161–188). Mahwah, NJ: Lawrence Erlbaum Associates.

Noakes, L. (1991). The Takens embedding theorem. *International Journal of Bifurcation and Chaos, 4*(1), 867–872.

Oud, J. H. L., & Jansen, R. A. R. G. (2000). Continuous time state space modeling of panel data by means of SEM. *Psychometrica, 65*(2), 199–215.

Ramsay, J. O., Hooker, G., Campbell, D., & Cao, J. (2007). Parameter estimation for differential equations: A generalized smoothing approach. *Journal of the Royal Statistical Society B, 69*(5), 774–796.

Sauer, T., Yorke, J. & Casdagli, M. (1991). Embedology. *Journal of Statistical Physics, 65*(3,4), 95–116.

Savitzky, A., & Golay, M. J. E. (1964). Smoothing and differentiation of data by simplified least squares. *Analytical Chemistry, 36*, 1627–1639.

Singer, H. (1993). Continuous-time dynamical systems with sampled data, errors of measurement and unobserved components. *Journal of Time Series Analysis, 14*, 527–545.

Takens, F. (1981). Detecting strange attractors in turbulence. In D. Rand & L.-S. Young (Eds.), *Dynamical systems and turbulence. Warwick 1980: Proceedings of a symposium held at the University of Warwick* (pp. 366–381). Berlin: Springer.

Whitney, H. (1936). Differentiable manifolds. *Annals of Mathematics, 37*, 645–680.

8

Unbiased, Smoothing-Corrected Estimation of Oscillators in Psychology

Pascal R. Deboeck and Steven M. Boker

8.1 HOW DO INDIVIDUALS CHANGE OVER TIME? WHEN? WHY?

These loaded questions are becoming more common to a range of psychological contexts and ones that address fundamental psychological issues (Nesselroade, 1991; Nesselroade & Ram, 2004). Examination of individuals through intensive, longitudinal measurement is one way in which researchers will begin to address questions regarding individual change over time. Historically the examination of change over time has been successfully addressed through techniques such as differential equation models and concepts such as those of dynamical systems.

Application of differential equation modeling and dynamical systems to psychological science has proved to be difficult. The difficulty can be attributed to at least two sources. The first is due to the fact that the underlying processes in psychology are likely to be more intricate than those for which these methodologies were developed, that is, the physical and natural sciences (Boker, 2002). This problem will only be remedied as research in psychology becomes more adept at describing change over time. The second source of difficulty are the data common to psychology, which are not measured with the precision and accuracy available in classical physics (Boker, 2002). This creates a host of problems, one of which is the presence of significant amounts of error. These errors may consist of measurement error but may also be due to unknown internal or external sources that perturb a system; this is called *dynamic* or *process error*.

The collection of intense, longitudinal data is particularly difficult in psychology, due to participant load constraints. While the common solution is to collect panel data, these data are not likely to provide the same information that will be provided through repeated, intraindividual measurements (Molenaar, 2004). When time series on individuals are collected, these data typically contain only univariate measures of constructs, as collecting several measures to assess a construct would only further exacerbate the demands on the participant. This practice is problematic for the current derivative estimation techniques available. Methods such as local linear approximation (LLA, Boker & Graham, 1998; Boker & Nesselroade, 2002), latent differential equations (LDE, Boker, Neale, & Rausch, 2004), and generalized local linear approximation (GLLA, Boker, Deboeck, Edler, & Keel, submitted) can produce derivative estimates that are approximately unbiased,* but the parameters of differential equation models produced by univariate time series can be very biased (Boker & Nesselroade, 2002; Boker et al., submitted). And while some methods try to eliminate bias in parameter estimates (e.g., Boker & Nesselroade, 2002; Deboeck, 2005; Deboeck, Boker, & Bergeman, in press), these methods do not address fundamental problems with the estimation of derivatives.

This chapter proposes a method for modeling univariate time series using a differential equation model, the resulting parameter estimates of which do not depend on researcher-selected values during the modeling process. This method is based on a formula that relates the model parameter estimates produced by LLA, which are conditional on a researcher-specified parameter τ, to a model parameter estimate that is not conditional on τ. We begin by presenting some background on dynamical systems and differential equation modeling. We then review some of the methods currently available for fitting differential equation models to time series with noisy observations; we then show that these methods can frequently produce biased estimates of parameters when applied to univariate time

* The estimates produced by LLA are based on the estimation of the tangent of curves, $f'(x) = \lim_{h \to 0}[f(x+h) - f(x)]/h$. Therefore, as the distance between observations is reduced, LLA will produce derivative estimates that are unbiased. GLLA and LDE are based on similar principles. For many applications of LLA, GLLA, and LDE, the error variance due to derivative estimates not truly approximating $\lim_{h \to 0}$ is likely to be very small relative to other sources of variance, such as measurement and process error.

series. The formulas of the new method presented in this chapter, which related the τ-conditional and τ-corrected estimates of model parameters, are then described. Finally, the results from simulation work are presented, including time series with and without oscillating components.

8.1.1 Dynamical Systems

Dynamical systems methodology is one promising methodological route that may allow psychologists to describe intraindividual variability. Dynamical systems are systems, that is, sets of related variables, where the observed characteristics of the the systems are in some way dependent on the characteristics of the said systems at some previous time (Abarbanel, Brown, Sidorowich, & Tsimring, 1993; Boker & Laurenceau, 2005). Systems can be relatively simple, such as the relationships among position, velocity, and acceleration in the case of a simple pendulum, or can be more complicated, such as the three coupled differential equations of the Lorenz attractor (Lorenz, 1963).

The latter example, the Lorenz attractor, demonstrates one reason why dynamical systems methodology may be promising for the study of intraindividual change. One characteristic of dynamical systems is the ability to produce complex and even unexpected behavior using relatively few variables and simple, often linear, relationships. The Lorenz attractor is a classical example that consists of three differential equations:

$$\begin{aligned} \frac{\mathrm{d}x}{\mathrm{d}t} &= c_1(x - y), \\ \frac{\mathrm{d}y}{\mathrm{d}t} &= x(c_2 - z) - y, \\ \frac{\mathrm{d}z}{\mathrm{d}t} &= xy - c_3 z, \end{aligned} \tag{8.1}$$

where x, y, and z are some system of variables and c_1, c_2, and c_3 are constants.* Figures 8.1a through c plot the trajectories of x, y, and z for a

* E. N. Lorenz was a meteorologist interested in weather predictions and the difficulties surrounding making accurate predictions. The equations for the Lorenz attractor arose from his attempts to simplify the problem of weather prediction by considering fluid flow and thermal gradients.

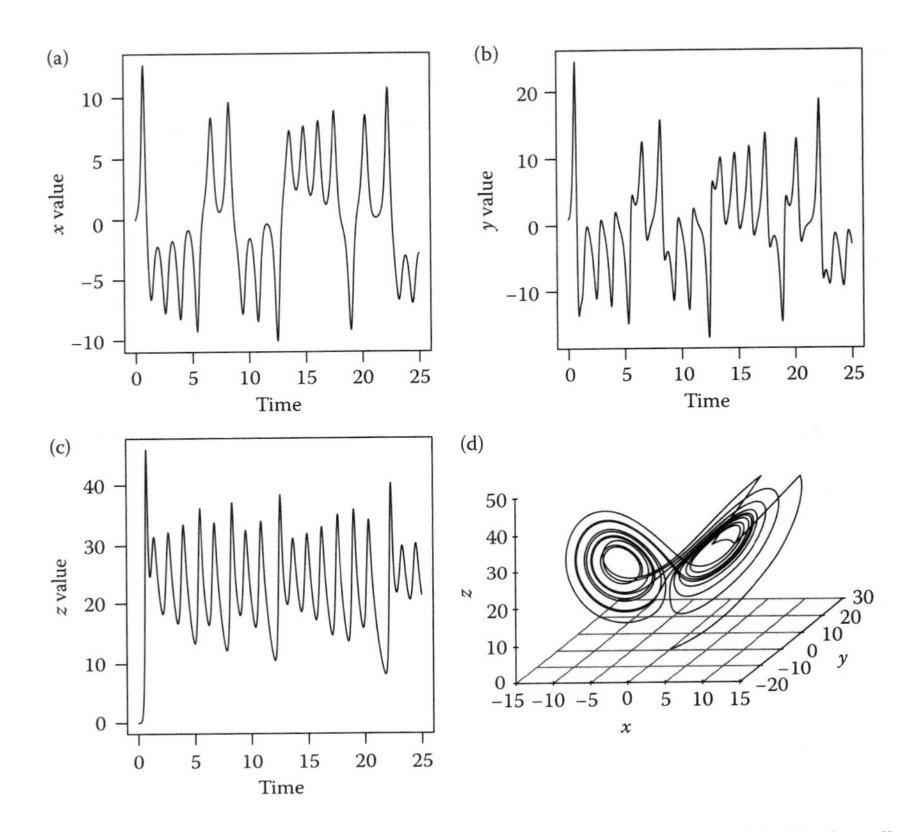

FIGURE 8.1 Trajectories of Lorenz attractor variables x (a), y (b), and z (c). (d) plots all three trajectories simultaneously in three-dimensions. In all figures, $x_0 = 0, y_0 = 1, z_0 = 0$, $c_1 = -3, c_2 = 26.5$, and $c_3 = 1$.

specific set of constants and initial conditions.* Despite the apparent complexity of these observed variables, Figure 1d and Equation set 8.1 betray the underlying simplicity of the Lorenz attractor. The ability to simply express complicated changes over time is likely to be important to the study of intraindividual variability.

The Lorenz attractor also demonstrates a dynamical systems concept called self-regulation. Initially, one might consider modeling the complexity observed in the Lorenz attractor variables as the sum of many different exogenous influences. However, even in the absence of exogenous effects,

* Systems such as the Lorenz attractor demonstrate sensitivity to initial conditions. Plots of x, y, and z can differ greatly depending on the exact set of constants and initial conditions selected.

there is an orderly relationship between the variables of the Lorenz attractor that allows it to remain in a stable, bounded range over time: that is, self-regulation. Many forms of intraindividual variability in psychology seem likely to be due to self-regulating processes (Boker et al. 2004; Carver & Scheier, 1998).

Dynamical systems allow for the representation of some complex, multiple-variable, high-dimensional behavioral models as simpler models with fewer variables. As mentioned previously, the characteristics of dynamical systems are in some way dependent on the characteristics of the system at some previous time (Abarbanel et al., 1993). Changes of variables over time are frequently expressed as derivatives.

8.1.2 Differential Equation Modeling

Derivatives express the change in a variable with respect to change in a second variable. Given the measurement of some variable x, one can examine changes in x with respect to a second variable such as time. The change in x with respect to time, that is the first derivative, is often written as $\mathrm{d}x/\mathrm{d}t$. An alternative notation, primarily used to denote variables that change with respect to time, expresses the first derivative as $\dot{x}$. In physics the variable x often represents position, in which case $\dot{x}$ would represent velocity; that is, a change in position with respect to a change in time. The second derivative of x has a similar notation, $\ddot{x}$, and expresses the change in the first derivative with respect to time. If x represents position, $\ddot{x}$ represents the change in velocity over time, also called acceleration.*

A differential equation is any equation with a variable that is a derivative (Kaplan & Glass, 1995). Rather than defining a meaningful initial time point from which changes occur over time, as with growth curve modeling, one can model the relationship between the current value of the variable, how that variable is changing over time, and other variables of interest (Arminger, 1986; Boker et al. 2004; Oud & Jansen, 2000). Differential equation models assume that there are relationships between the observed variables and how those variables are changing, but do not assume that a specific trajectory over time occurs. Consequently, individuals described

* As all derivatives in this chapter involve changes with respect to time, Newtonian notation, where the order of the derivative is indicated by placing dots above a variable name, will be adopted for all subsequent matter.

by the same model can have very different change over time trajectories, and furthermore a common time scale to align individuals is not required.

8.1.3 Linear Oscillator

One dynamical system that has a simple expression as a differential equation model, and which may have applications in the behavioral sciences, is that of a linear oscillator (e.g., Boker & Graham, 1998; Boker & Nesselroade, 2002). Variables that are well described by this type of model are ones where fluctuations in a variable are expected over time to move back and forth between some set of extreme values around some "typical" or equilibrium value. The prototypical example of a linear oscillator is a pendulum, which oscillates at a particular frequency if displaced from equilibrium. In cases where the maximum displacement (amplitude) is not constant over time, the linear oscillator is called a damped linear oscillator.

In differential equation form, the linear oscillator is expressed as

$$\ddot{x} = \eta x, \tag{8.2}$$

where x is the value of some variable, $\ddot{x}$ is the second derivative of x with respect to time, and η is a parameter that describes the frequency of oscillation. For the damped linear oscillator a second term $\zeta\dot{x}$ is added to Equation 8.2, where $\dot{x}$ is the first derivative of x with respect to time and ζ is a parameter that describes the rate of damping. Naturally, when $\zeta = 0$ one is left with Equation 8.2, an undamped linear oscillator.

One solution for Equation 8.2 is

$$x_t = A\cos(\omega t + \delta), \tag{8.3}$$

where x_t is the position of the oscillator at some time t, A is the amplitude, ω indicates the frequency of oscillation,* and δ corresponds to the phase (Tipler, 1998). Equation 8.3 is an alternative to differential equation modeling for fitting a linear oscillator model to observed data. This raises the question: Given the difficulties associated with estimating differential equations such as Equation 8.2, why shouldn't one use Equation 8.3 to model linear oscillators?†

* The frequency parameters ω and η can be shown to be related by the equation $\omega = \sqrt{-\eta}$.

† That is, leaving aside the issues that arise from the estimation of a nonlinear function like Equation 8.3 compared to the estimation of a linear function like Equation 8.2.

Modeling a linear oscillator with Equation 8.2 versus Equation 8.3 approaches the modeling of time series from very different conceptual frameworks; both will be considered in the case of modeling a single individual's time series. Equation 8.3 focuses on modeling a single trajectory that is assumed to follow a perfect linear oscillation, such as in Figure 8.2a. The disadvantage is that one is trying to model a specific trajectory, that is, the observed scores on some variable. Consequently, if one had the case of a variable that oscillated, but with occasional disturbances (e.g., perturbations to the phase, that is, phase resetting) as in Figure 8.2b, Equation 8.3 would not be a wise choice to model this type of data.

Instead of modeling the observed time-series trajectory, Equation 8.2 models the relationship between the observed variable and its derivatives. From Equation 8.2 it is known that an undamped linear oscillator can be

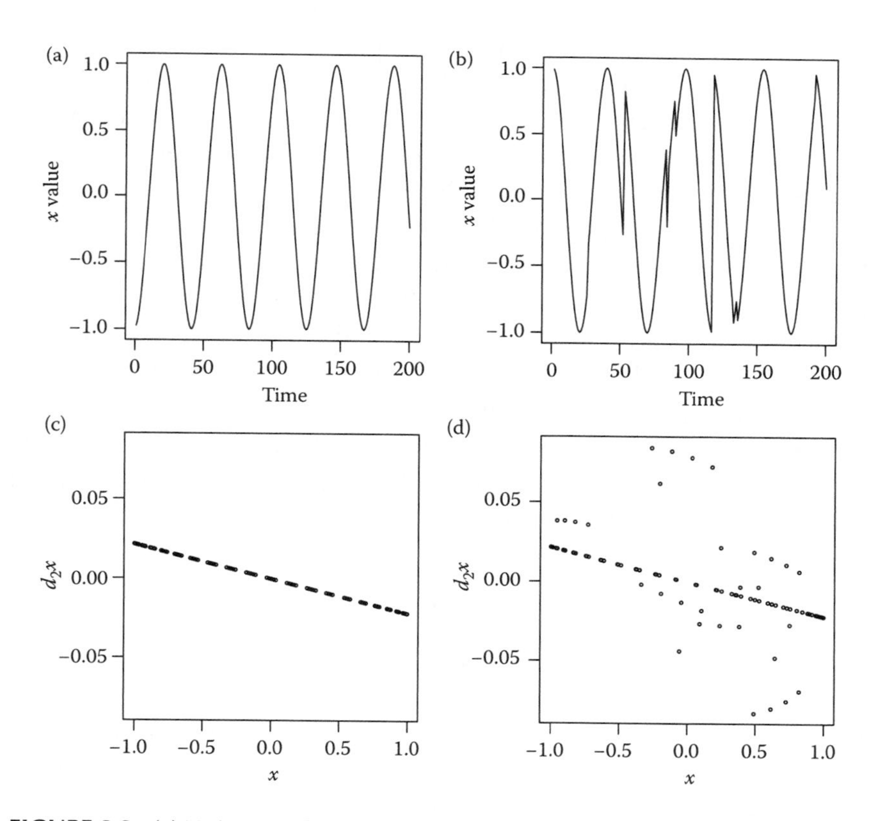

FIGURE 8.2 (a) Trajectory of a linear oscillator. (b) Trajectory of a linear oscillator with random phase resets. (c) State space of the trajectory shown in (a). (d) State space of the trajectory shown in (b).

fully described by a single relationship between x and the second derivative of $\ddot{x}$. If one plots $\ddot{x}$ versus x one can visualize the entire space describing the system, often called the *state space*. Figure 8.2c plots estimates of $\ddot{x}$ versus x for the linear oscillator in Figure 8.2a. Similarly, Figure 8.2d plots estimates of $\ddot{x}$ versus x for the linear oscillator in Figure 8.2b. Comparing Figure 8.2c and d, the similarity of the state space is apparent, despite large differences in the trajectories of Figure 8.2a and b. In these state space examples, the slope of the line apparent in both examples has intrinsic meaning, in this case corresponding to how quickly the time series observations move toward and away from equilibrium (related to frequency).

8.1.4 Estimation Methods for Noisy Observations

Application of differential equation models to data collected with significant proportions of measurement and process error, as is the case in psychology, is difficult. Several available methods for estimating derivatives prior to differential equation modeling are LLA, LDE modeling, and GLLA. Each of these estimation methods is briefly described before we address the problems associated with these methods.

LLA. LLA is a computationally simple method that uses a variable's observed values x to produce estimates of the derivatives associated with a particular x_t (Boker & Graham, 1998; Boker & Nesselroade, 2002). Given a particular observed value x_t, for which the associated first and second derivatives will be estimated, a triplet of values centered on x_t are selected (e.g., $x_{t-\tau}$, x_t, $x_{t+\tau}$). Parameter τ is an integer value selected by the researcher that defines the observations that are to be used to estimate derivatives at x_t. Using LLA, given a triplet of observed values, the first and second derivatives can be estimated:

$$\dot{x}_t \approx \frac{x_{t+\tau} - x_{t-\tau}}{2\tau\Delta t},$$

$$\ddot{x}_t \approx \frac{x_{t+\tau} + x_{t-\tau} - 2x_t}{\tau^2\Delta t^2}.$$

In these equations, Δt is equal to the elapsed time between the equally spaced observations of a time series. Currently there are several advantages to using LLA over other derivative estimation techniques. For instance, work has been done to allow for the automated selection of τ for LLA (Deboeck, 2005), which allows for nearly unbiased parameter estimation for univariate time series; equivalent work has not been done with other derivative-based estimation techniques. The observed derivatives also make it easier to plot and visualize the state space, which is advantageous when applying these techniques to new areas of study where novel models may be required. Observed derivatives also allow one to estimate multilevel derivative models where the derivative model parameters may be predicted by other variables (Bisconti, Bergeman, & Boker, 2006; Maxwell & Boker, 2007).

LDE. LDE modeling is a technique for modeling differential equations using latent variables through structural equation modeling (Boker et al. 2004). With LDE modeling, latent derivatives are estimated from observed data using a method similar to latent growth curve modeling. In latent growth curve modeling, a latent intercept and latent slope are differentiated by how loadings to observed data have been constrained (Duncan, Duncan, Strycket, Li, & Alpert, 1999). Similarly one can constrain loadings to produce latent estimates of x, $\dot{x}$, and $\ddot{x}$.

Boker et al. (2004) have shown that x, $\dot{x}$, and $\ddot{x}$ can be estimated by using loadings matrix $\mathbf{L}$,

$$\mathbf{L} = \begin{bmatrix} 1 & -1.5\tau\Delta t & (-1.5\tau\Delta t)^2/2 \\ 1 & -0.5\tau\Delta t & (-0.5\tau\Delta t)^2/2 \\ 1 & 0.5\tau\Delta t & (0.5\tau\Delta t)^2/2 \\ 1 & 1.5\tau\Delta t & (1.5\tau\Delta t)^2/2 \end{bmatrix}, \tag{8.4}$$

where the first, second, and third columns correspond to the loadings on observed data to identify x, $\dot{x}$, and $\ddot{x}$, respectively. As with LLA, Δt is the elapsed time between equally spaced observations and τ represents an integer that defines which set of four observations will be used to identify a particular derivative.

LDE modeling can be used with either short time series (e.g., four observations) with multiple individuals or with long time series on one or more individuals. In the case of longer time series the data for each individual's time series are usually embedded (Boker et al. 2004; Takens, 1985; Sauer, Yorke, & Casdagli, 1991). In the above example the $\mathbf{L}$ matrix is appropriate for a four-dimensional embedding. To embed the time series of a single individual x, where $x = 1, 2, \ldots, N$, using $\tau = 2$ and four embedded dimensions ($D = 4$), one would create an $(N - \tau(D - 1)) \times D$ matrix $\mathbf{X}$

consisting of offset columns of observed time series x. For this example,

$$\mathrm{X} = \begin{bmatrix} x_1 & x_{1+\tau} & x_{1+2\tau} & x_{1+3\tau} \\ x_2 & x_{2+\tau} & x_{2+2\tau} & x_{2+3\tau} \\ \vdots & \vdots & \vdots & \vdots \\ x_{N-3\tau} & x_{N-2\tau} & x_{N-\tau} & x_N \end{bmatrix}.$$

In principle any number of embeddings can be used, although the number will vary depending on identification of the model.

LDE modeling has several advantages over LLA, primarily related to the flexibility of structural equation modeling. When presented with multivariate time series representing the same construct, for instance, LDE modeling is preferable due to its ability to estimate a single set of latent derivatives (Boker et al. 2004); the estimates from multivariate time series have been shown to have low bias that appears to be independent of τ, within a reasonable range of τ's. LDE can also be used to estimate several equations simultaneously. This can be useful when two or more differential equations have related parameters; an example is the coupled oscillators model (Boker & Laurenceau, 2005; Boker et al., 2004).

GLLA. GLLA is a technique that bridges the direct estimation of derivatives from LLA and the ability to use any number of embedded dimensions from LDE. A complete description of GLLA can be found in Chapter 7 of this book (Boker et al., submitted). GLLA allows for increased flexibility in the application of LLA. The predominant consequence is that calculation of the coefficients in order to explicitly estimate derivatives can be easily performed for any number of embedding dimensions, any τ value, and any order of derivatives. One advantage of GLLA, despite its similarities to LLA, is that one can use additional observations to estimate a particular derivative. By using more than three observations GLLA can provide more precise estimates of the derivative, although this does not necessarily dramatically improve the estimates of the differential equation parameters.

8.1.5 Univariate-Measurement Time Series

Importance of τ selection. Despite their different approaches and unique advantages, LLA, LDE, and GLLA have a common element when applied in practice. All three methods can be used to estimate derivatives from

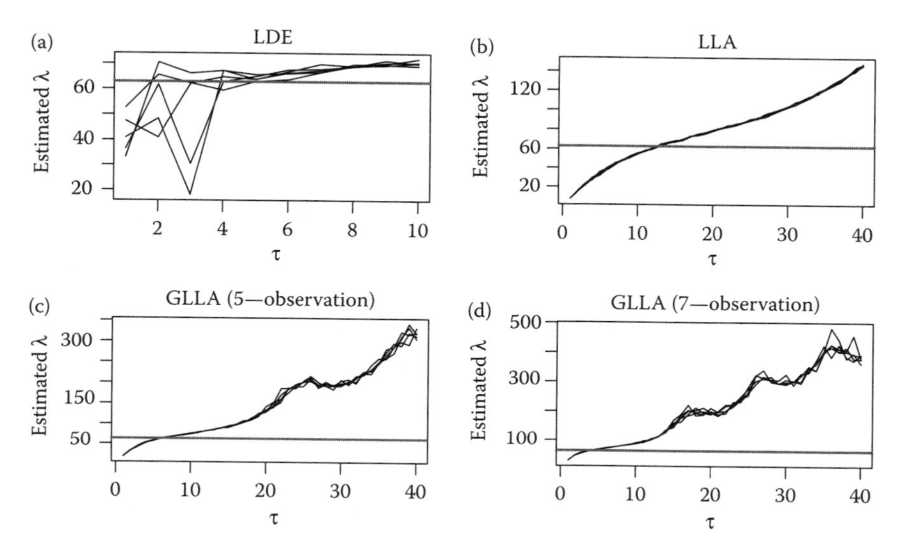

FIGURE 8.3 Estimated values of η (transformed to λ, right) versus τ for LDE, LLA, a five-observation GLLA, and a seven-observation GLLA. The horizonal gray line in all figures is equal to the true parameter value.

observed data such that differential equation models such as the linear oscillator can be fit. However, when all three estimation procedures are applied to univariate time series to estimate an oscillator model, estimates of the frequency parameter η are dependent on selection of τ, even though the extent of bias is reduced in the case of LDE. This is particularly problematic given that multivariate time series of the same construct are not commonly available in psychology due to the difficulties of collecting such data.

For example, consider a linear oscillator with $\lambda = 62.8$, that is 62.8 observations collected per cycle.* Assume this oscillator is measured with a signal-to-noise ratio of 2:1 and observed for five individuals. Figure 8.3 demonstrates the results that might be observed if linear oscillator parameters were estimated for each individual's time series using several values of τ. In all methods the estimates for λ tend to be both biased and dependent on the value of τ used for analysis. The bias in the frequency parameter demonstrates a problem with the current methods for estimating derivatives, the

* The parameter λ is used to indicate wavelength. When the elapsed time between observations is 1, as is the case here, λ is equal to the number of observations measured within on oscillation. With $\Delta t = 1, \lambda = (2 * \pi)/\sqrt{-\eta}$.

implications of which in practice depend on the differential equation model being fit, and the relationships being examined.

8.1.6 τ-Corrected Parameter Estimates

It would be preferable if parameter estimates could be generated that correct for the value of τ used in the analysis. There is evidence that suggests that τ-corrected parameter estimates are possible for differential equation models. This possibility follows from the observation that given a specific model for analysis and one's data, the parameter estimates are expected to change in predictable ways as τ is varied. The equations presented below show a relationship between the τ-conditional estimates of η_τ and the true τ-corrected value of ω.

The differential equation for an undamped linear oscillator can be expressed as

$$\ddot{x} = \eta x,$$

which can be rewritten using the approximate value of $\ddot{x}$ (described by LLA)* and simplified to

$$\eta_\tau \tau_\Delta^2 \approx \frac{x_{(t+\tau_\Delta)} + x_{(t-\tau_\Delta)}}{x_t} - 2. \tag{8.5}$$

In this equation τ_Δ is equal to $\tau \Delta t$, t is the time at which the observation occurred, and η_τ is equal to the τ-conditional estimates of η. Combining one solution for a linear oscillator with error, it is assumed that

$$x_t = A_0 \cos(\omega t) + e_t. \tag{8.6}$$

Substituting Equation 8.6 into Equation 8.5,

$$\eta_\tau \tau_\Delta^2 \approx \frac{A_0 \cos(\omega t + \omega \tau_\Delta) + e_{(t+\tau_\Delta)} + A_0 \cos(\omega t - \omega \tau_\Delta) + e_{(t-\tau_\Delta)}}{A_0 \cos(\omega t) + e_t} - 2.$$

* The equations that follow could be rewritten such that $\ddot{x} + B_2(t|\tau) = (x_{t+\tau} + x_{t-\tau} - 2x_t)/\tau^2 \Delta t^2$ rather than using the approximation stated earlier. However, if one calculates the difference between the approximate solution and an integrated solution, for a linear oscillator it can be shown that $B_2(t|\tau) = A_0 \cos(\omega t)[-\omega^2 + (2/\tau^2)(1 - \cos(\omega\tau))]$. $B_2(t|\tau)$, therefore, has an expected value of zero and should not bias the estimates.

Using the relationship $\cos(\theta_1 \pm \theta_2) = \cos(\theta_1)\cos(\theta_2) \mp \sin(\theta_1)\sin(\theta_2)$, the previous equation can be simplified such that

$$\eta_\tau \tau_\Delta^2 \approx 2\cos(\omega\tau_\Delta)\frac{A_0\cos(\omega t)}{A_0\cos(\omega t) + e_t} + \frac{e_{(t+\tau_\Delta)} + e_{(t-\tau_\Delta)}}{A_0\cos(\omega t) + e_t} - 2. \quad (8.7)$$

The expression of the terms on the right-hand side can be simplified using the relationship $x_t = A_0\cos(\omega t) + e_t$, such that

$$\eta_\tau \tau_\Delta^2 \approx 2\cos(\omega\tau_\Delta)\frac{x_{t(signal)}}{x_{t(signal+noise)}} + \frac{e_{(t+\tau_\Delta)} + e_{(t-\tau_\Delta)}}{x_{t(signal+noise)}} - 2. \quad (8.8)$$

While the parameter δ, which describes the phase of oscillation, is left out of Equation 8.6 to simplify the presentation, it can be shown that this parameter will drop out of the equations and the same conclusion will be reached.

Making common assumptions that errors are uncorrelated with each other, uncorrelated with the true signal, and come from a distribution with a mean of zero, the expected value of the middle term on the right is zero. Expressing the ratio of $x_{t(\text{signal})}/x_{t(\text{signal+noise})}$ as ρ, it is expected that

$$\eta_\tau \tau_\Delta^2 \approx 2\rho\cos(\omega\tau_\Delta) - 2. \quad (8.9)$$

It can be shown that the parameter ρ is an estimate of reliability (see Appendix 8.1), that is, true variance divided by total variance, given the assumption that the equilibrium of the oscillator has been set equal to zero. Furthermore, it can be shown that as $\rho \rightarrow 1$, Equation 8.9 becomes equal to the solution for an undamped linear oscillator measured without error. In addition, as $\rho \rightarrow 0$, Equation 8.9 becomes equal to the solution for a time series consisting of white noise (independent, normally distributed observations) modeled as a linear oscillator. These results suggest that ρ will be related to the amount of true variance of the undamped linear oscillator divided by the total observed variance which could be considered to be the reliability of the univariate measure given a damped linear oscillation model.

8.1.7 Modeling τ-Dependent Characteristics

The equations in the previous section show that there is a relationship between the LLA τ-conditional estimates of frequency and a τ-corrected frequency ω. The previous equations suggest that by varying the parameter τ, which will produce variations in the estimated parameter η_τ (τ-conditional estimates), it is possible to estimate the true frequency of an oscillating system (i.e., a τ-corrected estimate). The equation also suggests two additional properties of interest. First, the relationship is independent of time t, suggesting that this relationship can be used to model the state space of a linear oscillator rather than just a linear oscillator trajectory. Second, the equations produce a parameter ρ, which expresses the ratio of the true signal variance divided by the total signal variance.

The following sections explore the relationship expressed in Equation 8.9 using simulations. The first set of simulations will examine the estimates for the ω and ρ parameters over a wide range of simulated conditions. True linear oscillators and linear oscillators with process error (phase resets) will be examined, as these types of data will provide information regarding estimation when the state space both matches and deviates from the model; however, in both cases the underlying dynamics are similar to those specified by the model. Next, the fitting of Equation 8.9 to time series with no true linear oscillator signal is considered. The models considered consist of two random processes: time series consisting of white noise and time series consisting of a random walk. We first present the method used to estimate parameters for all simulations.

8.2 METHOD FOR τ-CORRECTED ESTIMATION OF PARAMETERS

For the simulations presented in this document, a two-step procedure is used. In the first step, τ-conditional estimates of frequency are produced. Using LLA (Boker & Graham, 1998; Boker & Nesselroade, 2002), η_τ was estimated for a particular time series using a specific value of τ. Recall that LLA estimates values for derivatives such that linear differential equation models can be solved as linear regressions. In the case of the undamped linear oscillator model ($\ddot{x} = \eta_\tau x$), LLA is used to estimate the second derivative $\ddot{x}$ of an observed time series x. The regression of x on the LLA estimates of $\ddot{x}$, which produces an estimate for the parameter η_τ, is repeated for a range of τ values. The result is a vector containing the τ-conditional estimates of η_τ.

In the second step, the τ-conditional estimates of frequency were used to produce a τ-corrected estimate of frequency. This is accomplished using Equation 8.9, which shows the relationship between the τ-conditional η_τ estimates and a τ-corrected ω estimate. As Equation 8.9 is nonlinear, a function that can be minimized or maximized is required for estimation. Minimization of the sum of squared residuals was selected due to its prevalence in statistics and to minimize the assumptions that had to be made. The nonlinear least squares estimate was made using the Broyden, Fletcher, Goldarb, and Shanno method (BFGS; Broyden, 1970; Fletcher, 1970; Goldfarb, 1970; Shanno, 19770), which is a quasi-Newton procedure for the estimation of unconstrained, non-linear problems. The BFGS method as formulated by Broyden, Fletcher, Goldfarb, and Shanno does not include bounds on the parameters. Therefore a modified version of the BFGS method was used, which allows for bounds on the parameters (Byrd, Lu, Nocedal, & Zhu, 1995). The statistical program R (2006), which is used for all the analyses described in this document, includes a function `optim()` that can optimize functions using the BFGS method both with or without bounds.

Like many gradient descent techniques, the BFGS method approximates and minimizes a hessian matrix. In some cases, the parameter space may include local minima, which can be mistaken for a global minimum by gradient descent techniques. In order to achieve the solution corresponding to a global minimum, the optimization procedure was repeated 30 times for each time series. The solution producing the minimum estimate was retained as the best solution. A script using the statistical program R (2006) for this analysis is provided with the software CD accompanying this book.

Bounds were placed on the estimated parameters. The ρ parameter was bounded between 0 and 1, the theoretical limits of this parameter. The same procedure was to be applied to the ω parameter, but early simulations with bounds of 0 and π resulted in a large number of estimates occurring at the bounds; therefore, the bounds on ω were selected to be large (i.e., 10^{-5} and 10^5) such that the ω parameter was essentially unbounded. Using the relationships $\cos(x) = \cos(x + 2\pi)$ and $\cos(x) = \cos(-x)$, the estimated values of ω were transformed into equivalent values bounded* by 0 and π.

* It should be noted that an upper bound of π, when the time between measurements equals 1, corresponds to the measurement of two observations per cycle. This is the minimum number of samples that can be collected without aliasing. This is called the Nyquist limit (Gasquet & Witomski, 1999).

8.3 ESTIMATION OF ω AND ρ

8.3.1 Methods

The primary simulation consisted of applying the method just described to several time series to examine the estimation of ω and ρ. True undamped linear oscillator time series were generated with the statistical program R (2006) using the equation $x_t = A_0 \cos(\omega t + \delta)$, where the initial amplitude A_0 was fixed to a value of 1 and the phase δ was randomly generated number from a uniform distribution bounded by 0 and 2π. The true frequency ω was varied to take five values: 1.50, 0.75, 0.375, 0.1875, and 0.09375; this corresponds to wavelengths of about 4.19, 8.38, 16.76, 33.51, and 67.02 observations per cycle, given that the time between observations was fixed to 1. Time series lengths of 50, 100, and 200 observations were generated. The time between observations and the time series length determined the values of t. The range of τ's was varied to examine the effects of using a larger or smaller number of estimated η_τ values. All time series were examined with τ values beginning with $\tau = 1$ and continuing to a maximum τ of 3, 6, 10, or 20. Independent, normally distributed observations were then added to each time series. Signal-to-noise ratios were varied to have values of 5:1, 3:1, 1:1, 1:3, and 1:5, and a condition with 0 noise variance was also examined.

For this method to retain the advantages of differential equation modeling compared to other methodologies, this method must be able to model systems that have the dynamics of a linear oscillator but not necessarily the trajectory of a linear oscillator. That is, it must be able to model systems that have relationships between the observed scores and derivatives, but these systems should not be required to follow a sine or cosine trajectory over time as they are likely to be subject to unknown sources of noisy internal and external perturbations. Many methodologies are available for the modeling of observed trajectories, but the strengths of differential equation modeling are those associated with state space modeling. To examine whether the method described retains the advantages of state space modeling, oscillators with random perturbations to the phase were examined. These oscillators have similar state spaces as the time series previously described, but observed trajectories that differ from a linear oscillator. These time series were generated as described above; however, at each observation a number was drawn from a uniform distribution bounded by 0 and 1. When the number drawn fell below a criterion value, δ was redrawn from a uniform distribution bounded by 0 and 2π. Criterion values were 0.00, 0.02, 0.04, 0.06, 0.08, and 0.10. This provided randomly placed phase shifts in the time series with randomly selected amounts of phase shift. Conditions were crossed with all previously listed conditions and 500 time series were generated per set of conditions. There are 2160 sets of conditions, so a total of 1.08 million time series were examined. Note that when the criterion value is 0.00, a true linear oscillator will be produced; all other criterion values will produce linear oscillators with random phase resets.

Evaluation of bias was based on the recovery of true model parameter ω and the true expected value of ρ. The distributions of ω and ρ estimates were not necessarily expected to be symmetrically distributed around some central tendency. As symmetry cannot be assumed, descriptions of parameter estimates using means and variances may not be ideal. Instead, models were evaluated using median values.* Efficiencies, that is, the mean-squared deviation from the true value, are also reported for the ω estimates.

The results for the τ-corrected estimates were compared to two alternatives based on LLA. It has been shown that the results for LLA depend on the selection of τ, and so estimates based on LLA are given to contrast the τ-corrected results of the method presented in this chapter. In the first alternative, estimates of frequency and R^2 were produced using LLA and a single τ value of 2. In the second alternative, the value of τ that would produce the least bias was selected for each particular time series. This ideal τ is equal to $\sqrt{2}/\omega$, rounded to the nearest integer; for these data, the ideal τ values equalled 1, 2, 4, 8, and 15 for the corresponding values of ω (1.50, 0.75, 0.375, 0.1875, and 0.09375).

8.3.2 Results for ω

The median τ-corrected estimates showed very little bias across conditions, although the estimates tended to be positively skewed. A summary of the difference between all estimated values of ω and the true values of ω, over all conditions, resulted in a median of 0.0039; this is small compared to the true values of ω, which ranged from 1.5 to 0.09375. The mean over

* Additional analyses of the simulation results discussed in this chapter show that the estimates for ω and ρ depart from a normal distribution across a wide range of conditions (Deboeck, 2007). This suggests that the means of these parameters may not clearly reflect the central tendency of the estimates.

TABLE 8.1

Estimates of ω, S:N Ratio of 1:3

Simulation Values		Median				Efficiency x 100			
		τ-Corrected		LLA		τ-Corrected		LLA	
ω	*P*(reset)	3 τ's	10 τ's	τ = 2	τ = Ideal	3 τ's	10 τ's	τ = 2	τ = Ideal
Time Series Length = 50									
1.500	0.000	1.509	1.501	0.791	1.404	15.250	10.912	51.005	1.482
0.750	0.000	0.780	0.751	0.702	0.702	49.683	21.743	0.391	0.391
0.375	0.000	0.392	0.383	0.644	0.352	34.154	32.188	7.375	0.103
0.188	0.000	0.205	0.194	0.621	0.174	32.380	38.886	18.998	0.030
0.094	0.000	0.144	0.094	0.612	0.092	28.445	29.726	26.803	0.006
1.500	0.100	1.518	1.518	0.774	1.409	28.621	32.974	53.313	1.607
0.750	0.100	0.772	0.776	0.709	0.709	48.244	40.360	0.400	0.400
0.375	0.100	0.428	0.415	0.647	0.350	52.808	57.353	7.616	0.128
0.188	0.100	0.334	0.217	0.630	0.176	36.058	66.985	19.865	0.038
0.094	0.100	0.226	0.157	0.616	0.094	43.843	46.947	27.375	0.014
Time Series Length = 200									
1.500	0.000	1.498	1.501	0.791	1.398	0.882	0.033	50.533	1.198
0.750	0.000	0.751	0.748	0.702	0.702	3.743	0.031	0.271	0.271
0.375	0.000	0.374	0.375	0.640	0.351	2.045	0.047	7.042	0.068
0.188	0.000	0.195	0.188	0.619	0.175	2.001	1.417	18.657	0.018
0.094	0.000	0.092	0.094	0.616	0.092	1.743	4.145	27.206	0.001
1.500	0.100	1.506	1.496	0.773	1.404	2.896	1.716	52.995	1.105
0.750	0.100	0.734	0.757	0.702	0.702	6.498	2.515	0.273	0.273
0.375	0.100	0.410	0.369	0.652	0.351	4.927	1.555	7.781	0.071
0.188	0.100	0.286	0.187	0.635	0.175	4.063	2.216	20.090	0.019
0.094	0.100	0.239	0.144	0.630	0.094	5.940	9.968	28.863	0.002

all conditions was 0.0775, indicating that the bias tended to be positively skewed; positive bias is associated with estimation of a frequency that is higher than the true frequency. The first and third quartiles of the estimates minus the true values were −0.0142 and 0.0432, respectively.

Tables 8.1 and 8.2 provide a sample of median estimates of ω. The most biased cases occurred when there was simultaneously a large amount of phase resetting combined with a small true ω value, that is, a low frequency. The use of a small number of τ values exacerbated this situation, although it was less problematic when examining higher frequency signals. Benefits for longer time series and an increased signal-to-noise ratio are apparent for low frequencies, but are less influential for higher frequency signals.

TABLE 8.2

Estimates of ω, S:N Ratio of 3:1

Simulation Values		Median				Efficiency × 100			
		τ-Corrected		LLA		τ-Corrected		LLA	
ω	*P*(reset)	3 τ's	10 τ's	τ = 2	τ = Ideal	3 τ's	10 τ's	τ = 2	τ = Ideal
Time Series Length = 50									
1.500	0.000	1.501	1.500	0.934	1.375	0.036	0.006	32.306	1.646
0.750	0.000	0.750	0.751	0.687	0.687	0.033	0.005	0.409	0.409
0.375	0.000	0.375	0.375	0.475	0.344	0.063	0.008	1.117	0.100
0.188	0.000	0.187	0.188	0.385	0.172	0.311	1.140	4.063	0.026
0.094	0.000	0.098	0.093	0.349	0.088	0.464	1.959	6.739	0.005
1.500	0.100	1.501	1.496	0.894	1.379	0.350	0.848	36.985	1.682
0.750	0.100	0.729	0.757	0.692	0.692	0.510	1.049	0.435	0.435
0.375	0.100	0.405	0.381	0.521	0.347	0.499	1.104	2.523	0.146
0.188	0.100	0.268	0.190	0.454	0.175	1.499	0.655	7.500	0.059
0.094	0.100	0.229	0.144	0.439	0.093	3.057	0.878	12.212	0.028
Time Series Length = 200									
1.500	0.000	1.499	1.500	0.934	1.377	0.006	0.000	32.127	1.538
0.750	0.000	0.750	0.750	0.688	0.688	0.007	0.000	0.391	0.391
0.375	0.000	0.375	0.375	0.474	0.344	0.010	0.096	1.008	0.096
0.188	0.000	0.189	0.187	0.390	0.172	0.057	0.000	4.124	0.024
0.094	0.000	0.097	0.094	0.362	0.088	0.238	0.179	7.278	0.003
1.500	0.100	1.503	1.492	0.896	1.378	0.070	0.116	36.626	1.521
0.750	0.100	0.731	0.756	0.692	0.692	0.147	0.112	0.361	0.361
0.375	0.100	0.409	0.384	0.526	0.348	0.210	0.377	2.394	0.090
0.188	0.100	0.277	0.185	0.464	0.175	0.981	0.051	7.765	0.026
0.094	0.100	0.233	0.141	0.443	0.093	2.140	0.295	12.331	0.005

In comparison, ω estimates were very biased when using a fixed value of τ; this bias is not in a uniform direction. The estimated values were correlated with the true values used to create the time series; however, the variance of the estimates was dramatically less than that of the true frequency values. The estimates of ω using LLA with the ideal value of τ produce nearly unbiased estimates across all conditions. Keep in mind that ideal selection of τ for LLA requires a knowledge of the frequency of oscillation, so it can be difficult to know whether an ideal value of τ has been selected in practice.

Tables 8.1 and 8.2 also provide efficiency estimates for the methods examined. In the τ-corrected method, the use of 10 τ-conditional estimates rather than 3 produced more efficient estimates of ω. As it seems recommendable to use more τ-conditional estimates when applying this method, the following discussion will focus on the results that used 10 τ-conditional estimates. The results for LLA depend on the selection of τ. As the selection of τ approached the ideal, the estimates of ω became very efficient; as the selection of τ departed from the ideal, the estimates became very inefficient. Across most conditions the τ-corrected method was more efficient than LLA, the primary exception being in the case of short time series measured with a large proportion of error and analyzed using the ideal value of τ.

8.3.3 Results for ρ

For the τ-corrected estimates of ρ, across all conditions there was some bias in the estimates. The estimates tended to be negatively skewed and the true signal variance divided by the total variance tended to be underestimated. A summary of all estimates minus the true divided by total variance resulted in a median of -0.0566, which is not insignificant compared to the true values of ρ, which ranged from 0.167 to 0.833. The mean of -0.0951 suggests that the bias tends to be negatively skewed. The first and third quartiles of the estimates minus the true values are -0.1355 and -0.0128, respectively. However, much of the bias depends on a few factors, which gives further insight as to what the ρ parameter is quantifying.

Table 8.3 provides a sample of median estimates of ρ. This table suggests that the largest amounts of bias occur as the probability of phase resetting increases. When the probability of phase resetting is zero, the estimates are approximately unbiased. A summary of all estimated ρ parameters minus the ratio of true variance divided by total variance, when phase resetting is equal to zero, produces a median bias of zero (to six digits of precision) and a mean bias of -0.0094. The mean bias is small compared to the true values of ρ, which range from 0.167 to 0.833. The bias due to increases in the proportion of true score variance and increased number of τ values are contingent on occurrence of phase resetting. Only when there is phase resetting, combined with a high proportion of true score variance and the use of a large number of τ values, do the most biased cases occur. There does seem to be some dependence on ω and time length, although the aforementioned variables seem to dominate.

Table 8.3 also provides estimates of R^2 based on LLA. The LLA estimates are very biased when a non-ideal value of τ is used. The results from the τ-corrected method and LLA with ideal τ are similar when there

TABLE 8.3

Estimates of ρ

Simulation Values		Median, True ω = 1.5				Median, True ω = 0.09375			
		τ-Corrected		LLA		τ-Corrected		LLA	
ω	*P*(reset)	τ = 3	τ = 10	τ = 2	τ = Ideal	τ = 3	τ = 10	τ = 2	τ = Ideal
Time Series Length = 50									
0.833	0.000	0.836	0.833	0.939	0.84	0.849	0.847	0.121	0.844
0.750	0.000	0.747	0.752	0.908	0.766	0.772	0.772	0.175	0.761
0.500	0.000	0.517	0.491	0.825	0.534	0.536	0.532	0.338	0.516
0.250	0.000	0.264	0.248	0.743	0.285	0.306	0.271	0.494	0.284
0.167	0.000	0.217	0.188	0.711	0.226	0.230	0.199	0.553	0.208
0.833	0.100	0.680	0.502	0.900	0.442	0.791	0.698	0.250	0.492
0.750	0.100	0.618	0.468	0.876	0.401	0.728	0.635	0.275	0.444
0.500	0.100	0.406	0.303	0.800	0.298	0.523	0.442	0.401	0.330
0.250	0.100	0.216	0.183	0.727	0.205	0.292	0.250	0.528	0.203
0.167	0.100	0.192	0.166	0.715	0.190	0.228	0.188	0.583	0.189
Time Series Length = 200									
0.833	0.000	0.834	0.833	0.938	0.835	0.833	0.833	0.132	0.836
0.750	0.000	0.752	0.749	0.908	0.755	0.754	0.749	0.185	0.753
0.500	0.000	0.500	0.500	0.820	0.507	0.504	0.500	0.346	0.508
0.250	0.000	0.256	0.248	0.739	0.257	0.266	0.247	0.507	0.255
0.167	0.000	0.168	0.168	0.711	0.175	0.180	0.163	0.560	0.178
0.833	0.100	0.682	0.487	0.900	0.190	0.768	0.659	0.261	0.250
0.750	0.100	0.610	0.435	0.873	0.180	0.693	0.598	0.301	0.233
0.500	0.100	0.403	0.288	0.798	0.129	0.475	0.402	0.416	0.165
0.250	0.100	0.208	0.148	0.730	0.081	0.241	0.204	0.545	0.095
0.167	0.100	0.145	0.099	0.710	0.069	0.168	0.134	0.587	0.073

is no phase resetting occurring—that is, there is no process error. When process error occurs, both methods underestimate the true signal variance. Interestingly, the estimates using the LLA with ideal τ appear to be dependent on the length of the time series, while those for the τ-corrected method do not appear to have this property. The independence of the τ-corrected method's ρ estimate from time series length may prove to be an advantageous property for partitioning error variance in the future.

8.3.4 Discussion

The results suggest that the τ-corrected method has expected ω medians approximately equal to the true values of ω. Furthermore, this conclusion is stable over a wide range of frequencies, signal-to-noise ratios, time series length, and probabilities of phase resets. These results are less biased than across different LLA conditions and, in most cases, more efficient. LLA estimates are more efficient when the ideal value of τ has been selected, which requires prior knowledge regarding the exact frequency of oscillation.

The most problematic cases for the τ-corrected method occur when a small number of τ values is used for analysis; there is a large probability of phase resetting and a high sampling frequency (e.g., 33 or more observations/cycle). Naturally, the number of τ values is researcher controlled, so this element is not problematic. This is not to say that researchers applying these methods need to be concerned about the values of τ selected, as the estimates produced by this method appear to be independent of the τ values selected. Rather, researchers should strive to have time series long enough so that multiple τ-conditional estimates can be made (preferably more than three).

The results suggest that large amounts of phase resetting are more problematic with low frequencies as these resemble faster frequencies when modeled. The presence, however, of either a low frequency or a high probability of phase resetting is not sufficient to seriously bias median estimates. The combination can still be dealt with if the original time series is moderately long, as one could reduce the sampling frequency by analyzing alternating observations thereby reducing the number of observations/cycle and removing one of the conditions that leads to biased results. Researchers applying this method would report the τ-corrected estimate of frequency, but would also be recommended to report the number and range of τ values used to create the τ-conditional estimates as well as the frequency at which the data were sampled. As expected, the variance of the estimates increased as the noise variance increased, as the number of observations decreased, and as the probability of phase resetting (i.e., process error) increased.

The results suggest that the τ-corrected method produces expected ρ medians approximately equal to the ratio of true variance to total variance as long as there is no probability of phase resetting. With no phase resetting this conclusion holds over a wide range of frequencies, signal-to-noise ratios, and time series lengths. However, with phase resetting the ρ parameter is a poor estimate of the true signal variance divided by the total variance. One of the primary advantages of differential equation modeling over trajectory modeling is the ability to model data where events such as phase resetting are expected. Unfortunately, in many cases the ρ parameter may be a poor indicator of the proportion of true signal variance.

However, the results for ρ are still very interesting and useful. It was observed that ρ behaved as expected when the probability of phase resetting was zero, but that estimates of ρ were negatively biased when the probability of phase resetting was nonzero. This suggests that the ρ parameter is capturing not only the measurement error but also errors associated with process error. This would seem to suggest that the ρ parameter is summarizing any deviations in the state space from the prescribed model. Additional work is required to investigate this parameter, as all sources of deviations in the state space seem likely to lead to decreases in the ρ parameter, such as poorly specified models or dynamic parameters or equilibria. Whether these different sources of error can be teased apart remains to be seen. In practice, the ρ parameter is likely to be a useful tool as it provides an overall estimate of how well the state space conforms to the specified model. However, in practice small ρ will lead to some uncertainty, as there are many potential sources of deviations in the state space including measurement error, process error, and poorly specified models. Unless $1 - \rho$ can be partitioned into different sources of error, use of ρ as an indicator of model fit may be limited.

As this simulation involved nonlinear estimation, the topic of convergence should be addressed. In the simulations presented, few problems with convergence were observed. A total of 2.4×10^8 analyses were performed, including some not presented here. For every one of the 2.4×10^8 analyses a solution was identified within the 30 calls to the `optim` function. The maximum number of nonconverging iterations that occurred in any one analysis was 8 out of the 30 calls to `optim`. In 82.2% of analyses, none of the 30 iterations failed to converge. Convergence, therefore, appears to be a relatively minor issue for the method presented.

8.4 NONOSCILLATING TIME SERIES

8.4.1 Methods

To contrast the results of the previous simulation, an additional simulation was run to examine the results produced by the τ-corrected method when the time series of interest does not include a true linear oscillator component. The first set of nonoscillating time series consisted of white noise. Three thousand time series consisting of independent, normally distributed observations with a mean of 0 and a standard deviation of 1 were generated for each of the three time series lengths: 50, 100, and 200 observations. Maximum τ values of 3, 6, 10, and 20 were examined for all time series. The second set of nonoscillating time series consisted of a random walk. A random walk is a process where the value at some given time is dependent on the value at the previous time plus some random perturbation, or $x_{t+1} = x_t + \epsilon$. The values of ϵ were randomly drawn from a normal distribution with a mean of 0 and a standard deviation of 1. Time series consisting of 50, 100, and 200 observations were generated, with the initial observation equal to 0 in all time series. Maximum τ values of 3, 6, 10, and 20 were examined for all times series. Three thousand time series were generated for each time series length. As it is not unusual for random walk time series to result in nonzero means, it should be noted that the mean of each time series was removed as part of the LLA estimation of η_τ. Parameters were estimated using the techniques previously described.

8.4.2 Results

The results for the nonoscillating series are considered in two parts, beginning with the estimates for times series consisting of white noise. Figure 8.4 and Table 8.4 provide summaries of the estimated ω and ρ parameters obtained for white noise time series. The estimated values of ω cover the

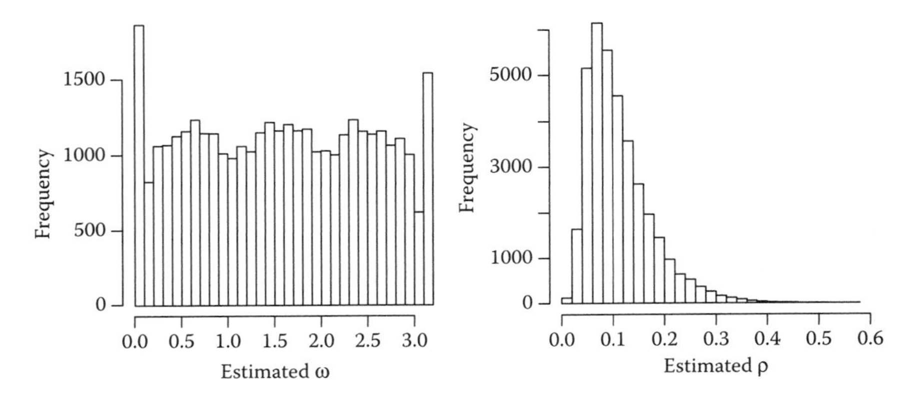

FIGURE 8.4 Histograms for the estimated values of ω and ρ for 9000 time series consisting of white noise.

TABLE 8.4

Estimates for White Noise Time Series

	ω Estimation		ρ Estimation	
Statistic	**τ = 3**	**τ = 10**	**τ = 3**	**τ = 10**
50 Observations				
Median	1.57	1.64	0.16	0.14
Mean	1.57	1.61	0.18	0.15
First, third quartiles	0.69, 2.47	0.82, 2.39	0.11, 0.23	0.11, 0.18
Variance, skew	0.96, −0.02	0.86, −0.06	0.01, 0.77	0.00, 0.91
99% Range	0.00, 3.14	0.00, 3.14	0.02, 0.46	0.05, 0.34
95% Range	0.00, 3.14	0.00, 3.14	0.04, 0.38	0.07, 0.28
90% Range	0.00, 3.14	0.15, 3.01	0.06, 0.34	0.08, 0.26
200 Observations				
Median	1.57	1.57	0.08	0.06
Mean	1.57	1.56	0.09	0.07
First, third quartiles	0.69, 2.46	0.76, 2.35	0.05, 0.11	0.05, 0.08
Variance, skew	0.95, 0.01	0.85, 0.01	0.00, 0.71	0.00, 0.72
99% Range	0.00, 3.14	0.00, 3.14	0.01, 0.22	0.02, 0.14
95% Range	0.00, 3.14	0.00, 3.12	0.02, 0.18	0.03, 0.12
90% Range	0.00, 3.14	0.15, 2.99	0.03, 0.16	0.04, 0.11

Notes: The headings listing the number of observations correspond to the number of observations of the time series generated. The range statistics are intended to give a further impression as to the range over which the majority of the estimated values span.

entire range of possible values, with a central tendency very close to the midpoint of the range. There was some tendency for the ω estimates to occur at the bounds of 0 and π, but other than these extremes the estimated values of ω were almost evenly distributed across the range of possible values. Increasing the number of observations in the time series did not appear to alter the results. As the number of τ values used to estimate ω increased, many values still occur at the bounds, although to a lesser extent than for small values of τ. The distribution of estimated values became more uniform as the number of τ values used for analysis increased.

The estimated values of ρ were distributed in a manner that would seem to reflect a time series with a low signal-to-noise ratio, indicating a very small proportion of signal variance and a large proportion of noise variance. The central tendency generally tended to occur in the range of 0.06 and 0.18; the distributions tended to be positively skewed. Across all conditions, 95% of ρ estimates fell between 0.034 and 0.273. Changes in τ produced very small reductions in the central tendency. The time series length had a large

TABLE 8.5

Estimates for Random Walk Time Series

	ω Estimation		ρ Estimation	
Statistic	$\tau = 3$	$\tau = 10$	$\tau = 3$	$\tau = 10$
50 Observations				
Median	0.21	0.14	0.93	0.84
Mean	0.23	0.15	0.91	0.80
First, third quartiles	0.16, 0.28	0.11, 0.18	0.88, 0.96	0.72, 0.91
Variance, skew	0.01, 0.66	0.01, 3.11	0.01, −1.76	0.02, −1.20
99% Range	0.00, 0.52	0.00, 0.52	0.62, 0.99	0.28, 1.00
95% Range	0.09, 0.44	0.05, 0.33	0.73, 0.99	0.40, 0.98
90% Range	0.10, 0.39	0.07, 0.27	0.77, 0.98	0.48, 0.98
200 Observations				
Median	0.11	0.06	0.98	0.95
Mean	0.11	0.07	0.98	0.94
First, third quartiles	0.08, 0.13	0.05, 0.08	0.97, 0.99	0.92, 0.97
Variance, skew	0.00, 0.71	0.00, 10.43	0.00, −1.86	0.00, −7.40
99% Range	0.03, 0.24	0.02, 0.16	0.90, 1.00	0.72, 1.00
95% Range	0.04, 0.21	0.03, 0.13	0.93, 1.00	0.82, 0.99
90% Range	0.05, 0.18	0.03, 0.11	0.94, 1.00	0.86, 0.99

Notes: The headings listing the number of observations correspond to the number of observations of the time series generated. The range statistics are intended to give a further impression as to the range over which the majority of the estimated values span.

effect on reducing the central tendency of the distribution and dramatically reduced the variability around that central tendency.

The results for the times series consisting of a random walk were very dissimilar from those for time series consisting of white noise. Figure 8.5 and Table 8.5 provide summaries of the estimated ω and ρ parameters obtained for random walk time series. The estimated values of ω tended to be confined to primarily small values, which reflect estimates of low-frequency signals. The central tendency of the results tended to occur between 0.06 and 0.23, depending on both the number of τ values and the length of the time series; the distributions tend to be positively skewed. Across all conditions, 95% of ω estimates fell between 0.03 and 0.33. A relatively small number of estimates occurred at the bound of 0, but this number was small enough to be ignored (134 cases of 36,000, or 0.37%). Increases in the number of τ values examined and the time series length tended to decrease estimates of the central tendency and reduce estimates of the variance. Estimates of skewness increased with an increase in the number

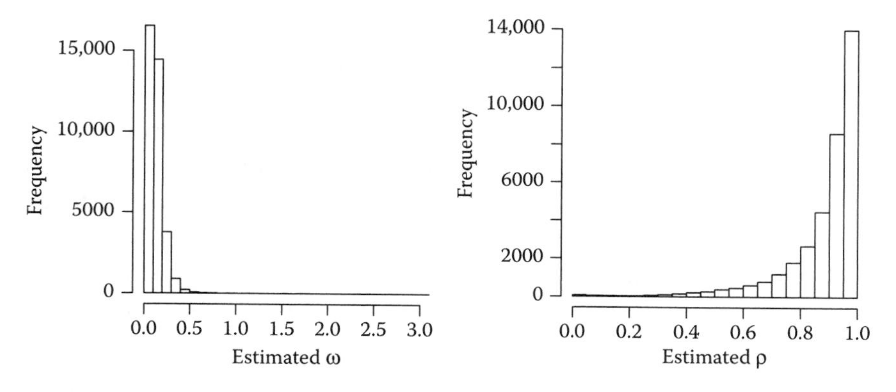

FIGURE 8.5 Histograms for the estimated values of ω and ρ for 9000 time series consisting of a random walk.

of τ values and an increase in the number of observations in the time series.

The estimated values of ρ were distributed in a manner that would seem to reflect a time series with a high signal-to-noise ratio, indicating a very large proportion of signal variance and a small proportion of noise variance. The central tendency generally tended to occur in the range of 0.71 and 0.98; the distributions tended to be negatively skewed. Across all conditions, 95% of ρ estimates fell between 0.478 and 0.994. As the number of τ values increased, the central tendency tended to move away from 1 and estimates of variability tended to increase. As the time series length increased, the central tendency of estimates came closer to 1 and estimates of variability tended to decrease.

8.4.3 Discussion

The results presented for the white noise time series are similar to those that were generally expected. White noise can be defined as the summing of an infinite number of frequencies (Gottman, 1981). It is therefore not surprising that a wide range of frequencies were observed with the estimates of ω. The ρ parameter also behaved as expected, producing estimates consistent with a low signal-to-noise ratio if a signal had been present. While the estimates of ρ tend to be slightly higher than zero, they are generally of small magnitude. This is particularly true as the number of τ values used for analysis increased and the time series length increased. In practice the estimates of ω will not be useful in recognizing time series that are likely to consist of white noise, but the ρ parameter seems likely to be very helpful in this endeavor.

The results presented for the random walk time series are very dissimilar from those of white noise time series. The results for random walk time series are similar to those that would be expected for moderate to low frequencies with a wide range of amounts of measurement error. Over all conditions, 95% of ω estimates fell between 0.03 and 0.33, which correspond to wavelengths of 209.4–19.0 observations/cycle if the time between observations equals 1. This wide range of results does not improve much by increasing the number of τ values used for analysis. The estimated values of ρ span a range of values that seem likely for many applied settings. In other literatures, distinguishing random walks from deterministic systems is not trivial (e.g., Nakamura & Small, 2007; Stephenson, Pavan, & Bojariu, 2000). In practice the estimates of ρ are not likely to be helpful for distinguishing cases that may consist of a random walk. However, the estimates of ω suggest that it may be possible to design studies with sampling frequencies that would make it unlikely that an oscillating system would have estimates similar to a random walk process. It should be noted that only the mean was removed from the random walk time series and that results may differ if a linear trend or another trend were removed.

Unfortunately, these results also suggest that it may be unwise to pursue traditional null hypothesis tests such as $\omega = 0$ or $\rho = 0$. The ω results for the white noise time series suggest that estimates of ω can take the entire range of values, even when there is no signal present in the data. In addition, the ρ results for the random walk time series suggest that it may be very easy for certain time series to produce nonzero estimates of ρ, even when there is no signal present in the data. The results from both nonoscillating time series suggest that there are a wide range of linear oscillator parameters that can occur in systems that do not have the dynamics of a linear oscillator. This suggests that it is unwise to try to conclude whether a set of data behaves in a manner similar to that of the state space being modeled (i.e., that a particular curve "fits" a time series). This is also similar to avoiding trying to conclude whether a particular model is good in some absolute sense. Instead, the focus needs to be placed on the interpretation of the parameters, what they inform one about the system of interest, and exogenous variables that are predictive of those parameters.

8.5 CONCLUSIONS

Differential equation modeling and the concepts related to dynamical systems are promising for psychological research. Unfortunately, the fields in which these techniques and concepts were developed were the ones in which long time series with high sampling rates are frequently easy to collect, and this is frequently not the case in psychology. Efforts are being made to develop techniques for the smaller, noisier data sets common to much of psychological research.

Current methods such as LLA, LDE, and GLLA, when applied to univariate time series can yield very biased estimates of model parameters. For these three methods the results will only be unbiased when a researcher-controlled parameter, τ, is perfectly selected. This parameter is a smoothing parameter that tries to reduce the effects of error variance without obscuring true change of the system of interest. The idea of smoothing time series prior to analysis is one that is common and arose from the same fields in which many dynamical system ideas were first developed, that is fields in which ample data can be collected. Unfortunately, the appropriateness of smoothing time series collected on many psychological constructs is more questionable than many other fields of study, as inappropriate smoothing of a time series can bias model estimates. Alternative methods, such as those developed by Oud and Jansen (2000) and Harvey and Souza (1987), can also produce unbiased estimates of models such as those explored in this chapter. Future research should endeavor to compare the relative merits of these methods and the τ-corrected method, so as to provide clear guidance for applied researchers.

The method presented in this chapter circumvents the problems associated with the selection of smoothing parameters by proposing to study time series by smoothing at multiple time scales simultaneously. Given a model of interest, there are expectations as to how parameter estimates will change depending on the amount of smoothing and the true model parameters. For the linear oscillator model it is shown that biased estimates of the frequency parameter are a function of the amount of smoothing and the true linear oscillator frequency parameter.

The results of the simulations support the functional relationship described for the linear oscillator. The simulations presented demonstrate unbiased estimation of the frequency parameter over a wide range of conditions. The primary exception is low-frequency systems, relative to the sampling frequency, that have frequent phase resetting; these cases tend to produce frequency estimates that are higher than the true frequency. The estimates of the ρ parameter are unbiased estimates of the true signal variance divided by the total signal variance when there is no phase resetting. However, in cases for which there is phase resetting, the ρ parameter captures elements of both measurement error and process error.

For applied research, the method presented offers several distinctive advantages over related methodologies. One advantage is that the method is able to model the state space, even when the state space does not literally conform to the model due to process error such as phase resetting. This means that advantages related to the use of differential equation modeling are retained and a particular trajectory over time does not have to be assumed. Furthermore the method is particularly adept for modeling high-frequency signals, relative to the rate of sampling. While the lowest sampling rate examined corresponded to the collection of 4.19 observations per cycle, additional simulations not presented here suggest that lower sampling rates can be modeled assuming they do not exceed the Nyquist limit. The application of the method presented is also relatively straightforward and requires fewer considerations than methods such as LLA. Finally, the τ-corrected method yields parameters that can be directly interpreted; this was not possible previously because parameter estimates were directly related to the researcher-selected smoothing parameter. This is not to suggest that the parameters should only be interpreted in some absolute sense, for example, in an attempt to demonstrate that time series conform to a particular model. Instead, these parameter estimates will probably be most informative when they can be predicted by exogenous variables.

The primary limitation of the method presented is that the model presented is for a linear oscillator, which relates the position of a variable at some time to its second derivative. This is a very limited example, which raises the question of how easily these methods can be applied to other models of change. Even if these methods can be applied to other models, this still requires a parallel to Equation 8.9 to be developed for each model considered. A second limitation is the ability to interpret the ρ parameter, which takes on different interpretations in the simulations depending on the presence of process error. The ρ parameter appears to capture deviations in the state space from the prescribed model, suggesting that ρ may diverge from 1 due to a host of causes, including measurement error, process error, poorly specified models, a system with dynamic parameters, or a system with a changing equilibrium. Whether different proportions of $1 - \rho$ can be attributed to different sources remains to be seen.

Despite the limitations, the simulations support the concept of modeling time series by relating τ-conditional model parameters to τ-corrected model parameters. This concept is promising for expanding on previous methodology. Furthermore, the considerations required to apply these methods seem to take a step towards increasing accessibility for a wider audience of researchers. The limitations associated with this project are inseparably bound to its future directions, as the limitations only seem to pose additional questions rather than imposing insurmountable obstacles. Therefore, the current presentation and future work are likely to contribute to the questions that can be asked about how individuals change over time, when they do so, and why.

APPENDIX 8.1

It is claimed that the parameter ρ, which is the ratio of $x_{t(\text{true})}$ over $x_{t(\text{total})}$, can be considered an estimate of reliability. In this appendix support for this claim is demonstrated. The relationship $\eta_\tau \tau_\Delta^2 \approx 2\rho \cos(\omega \tau_\Delta) - 2$ can be rewritten such that

$$\rho \approx \frac{\eta_\tau \tau^2 + 2}{2\cos(\omega \tau_\Delta)}. \tag{8.10}$$

Recall that η_τ is estimated using linear regression of x on $\ddot{x}$, where η_τ is the only estimated parameter. In linear regression, $\beta = \sum(X - \overline{X})(Y - \overline{Y}) / \sum(X - \overline{X})^2$ or, in the case being examined,

$$\eta_\tau = \frac{\sum(x_t - \overline{x}_t)(\ddot{x}_t - \overline{\ddot{x}}_t)}{\sum(x_t - \overline{x}_t)^2}. \tag{8.11}$$

The expected values of x_t and $\ddot{x}_t$ are equal to zero, as the models have assumed that the equilibrium is equal to zero. In this case, Equation 8.11

can be simplified to

$$\eta_\tau = \frac{\sum(x_t \ddot{x}_t)}{\sum x_t^2}.$$

Inserting this result into Equation 8.10,

$$\rho \approx \left[\tau^2 \left(\frac{\sum(x_t \ddot{x}_t)}{\sum x_t^2}\right) + 2\right] \Big/ \left[2\cos(\omega\tau_\Delta)\right]. \quad (8.12)$$

Using the LLA approximations of x_t and $\ddot{x}_t$ and defining x_t as $x_t = A_0 \cos(\omega t) + e_t$, Equation 8.12 can be simplified to

$$\rho \approx \left[\sum A_0^2 \cos(\omega t)^2\right] \Big/ \sum x_t^2, \quad (8.13)$$

given the assumption that the errors are uncorrelated with each other and the true values of x_t, and that the errors have an expected mean of zero. Based on the definition of x, Equation 8.13 can be rewritten as

$$\rho \approx \sum x_{\text{true}}^2 \Big/ \sum x_{\text{total}}^2. \quad (8.14)$$

Recall that the expected values of x_t and $\ddot{x}_t$ are equal to zero, so these values can be introduced, such that

$$\rho \approx \sum(x_{\text{true}} - \overline{x}_{\text{true}})^2 \Big/ \sum(x_{\text{total}} - \overline{x}_{\text{total}})^2. \quad (8.15)$$

As the sample sizes for both x_{true} and x_{total} are the same, this equation is approximately equal to the variance of true scores of x divided by the total scores of x. Consequently, ρ can be interpreted as an estimate of reliability.

REFERENCES

Abarbanel, H. D., Brown, R., Sidorowich, J. J., & Tsimring, L. S. (1993). The analysis of observed chaotic data in physical systems. *Reviews of Modern Physics*, *65*(4), 1331–1392.

Arminger, G. (1986). Linear stochastic differential equation models for panel data with unobserved variables. In N. Tuma (Ed.), *Sociological methodology* (pp. 187–212). San Francisco: Jossey-Bass.

Bisconti, T. L., Bergeman, C. S., & Boker, S. M. (2006). Social support as a predictor of variability: An examination of the adjustment trajectories of recent widows. *Psychology and Aging, 21*(3), 590–599.

Boker, S. M. (2002). Consequences of continuity: The hunt for intrinsic properties within parameters of dynamics in psychological processes. *Multivariate Behavioral Research, 37*(3), 405–22.

Boker, S. M., Deboeck, P. D., Edler, C., & Keel, P. K. (2009). Generalized local linear approximation of derivatives from time series. In S.-M. Chow & E. Ferrar (Eds.), *Statistical methods for modeling human dynamics: An interdisciplinary dialogue* (pp. 161–178). Boca Raton, FL: Taylor & Francis.

Boker, S. M., & Graham, J. (1998). A dynamical systems analysis of adolescent substance abuse. *Multivariate Behavioral Research, 33*(4), 479–507.

Boker, S. M., & Laurenceau, J. P. (2005). Dynamical systems modeling: An application to the regulation of intimacy and disclosure in marriage. In T. A. Walls & J. L. Schafer (Eds.), *Models for intensive longitudinal data* (pp. 195–218). Oxford: Oxford University Press.

Boker, S. M., Neale, M. C., & Rausch, J. R. (2004). Latent differential equation modeling with multivariate multi-occasion indicators. In K. V. Montfort, J. Oud, & A. Satorra (Eds.), *Recent developments on structural equation models: Theory and applications* (pp. 151–174). Amsterdam, Kluwer: Kluwer Academic Publishers.

Boker, S. M., & Nesselroade, J. R. (2002). A method for modeling the intrinsic dynamics of intraindividual variability: Recovering the parameters of simulated oscillators in multi-wave panel data. *Multivariate Behavioral Research, 37*(1), 127–160.

Broyden, C. G. (1970). The convergence of a class of double-rank minimization algorithms 2. The new algorithm. *Journal of the Institute for Mathematics and Applications, 6*, 222–231.

Byrd, R. H., Lu, P., Nocedal, J., & Zhu, C. (1995). A limited memory algorithm for bound constrained optimization. *Scientific Computing, 16*, 1190–1208.

Carver, C. S., & Scheier, M. F. (1998). *On the self-regulation of behavior.* New York, NY: Cambridge University Press.

Deboeck, P. R. (2005). *Using surrogate data analysis to estimate τ for local linear approximation of damped linear oscillators.* Unpublished master's thesis, University of Notre Dame.

Deboeck, P. R. (2007). *Smoothing-independent estimation of a linear differential equation model.* PhD in psychology, University of Notre Dame.

Deboeck, P. R., Boker, S. M., & Bergeman, C. S. (2008). Modeling individual damped linear oscillator processes with differential equations: Using surrogate data analysis to estimate the smoothing parameter. *Multivariate Behavioral Research, 43*(4), 497–523.

Duncan, T. E., Duncan, S. C., Strycker, L. A., Li, F., & Alpert, A. (1999). *An introduction to latent variable growth curve modeling.* Mahwah, NJ: Lawrence Erlbaum Associates.

Fletcher, R. (1970). A new approach to variable metric algorithms. *Computer Journal*, 13, 317–322.

Gasquet, C., & Witomski, P. (1999). *Fourier analysis and applications: Filtering, numberical computation*, wavelets. New York: Springer.

Goldfarb, D. (1970). A family of variable-metric methods derived by variational means. *Mathematics of Computation, 24*, 23–26.

Gottman, J. M. (1981). *Time-series analysis: A comprehensive introduction for social scientists.* New York: Cambridge University Press.

Harvey, A. C., & Souza, R. C. (1987). Assessing and modeling the cyclical behavior of rainfall in northeast brazil. *Journal of Climate and Applied Meteorology*, *26*(10), 1339–1344.

Kaplan, D., & Glass, L. (1995). *Understanding nonlinear dynamics*. New York: Springer.

Lorenz, E. N. (1963). Deterministic nonperiodic ow. *Journal of the Atmospheric Sciences*, 20, 130–141.

Maxwell, S. E., & Boker, S. M. (2007). Multilevel models of dynamical systems. In S. M. Boker & M. J. Wenger (Eds.), *Data analytic techniques for dynamical systems in the social and behavioral sciences* (pp. 131–159). Mahwah, NJ: Lawrence Erlbaum Associates.

Molenaar, P. C. M. (2004). A manifesto on psychology as idiographic science: Bringing the person back into scientific psychology, this time forever. *Measurement*, *2*(4), 201–218.

Nakamura, T., & Small, M. (2007). Tests of the random walk hypothesis for financial data. *Physica A*, 377, 599–615.

Nesselroade, J. R. (1991). Interindividual differences in intraindividual change. In L. M. Collins & J. L. Horn (Eds.), *Best methods for the analysis of change* (pp. 92–105). Washington, DC: American Psychological Association.

Nesselroade, J. R., & Ram, N. (2004). Studying intraindividual variability: What we have learned that will help us understand lives in context. *Research in Human Development*, *1*(1 & 2), 9–29.

Oud, J. H., & Jansen, R. A. (2000). Continuous time state space modeling of panel data by means of SEM. *Psychometrica*, *65*(2), 199–215.

R. (2006). Software. http://www.r-project.org/.

Sauer, T., Yorke, J., & Casdagli, M. (1991). Embedology. *Journal of Statistical Physics*, *65*(3,4), 95–116.

Shanno, D. F. (1970). Conditioning of quasi-Newton methods for function minimization. *Mathematics of Computation*, *24*, 647–656.

Stephenson, D., Pavan, V., & Bojariu, R. (2000). Is the north Atlantic oscillation a random walk? *International Journal of Climatology*, *20*, 1–18.

Takens, F. (1985). Detecting strange attractors in turbulence. In A. Dold & B. Eckman (Eds.), *Lectur notes in mathematics 1125: Dynamical systems and bifurcations* (pp. 99–106). Berlin: Springer.

Tipler, P. A. (1998). *Physics for scientists and engineers* (4th ed.). New York, NY: W.H. Freeman & Company.

9

Detrending Response Time Series

Peter F. Craigmile, Mario Peruggia, and Trisha Van Zandt

9.1 INTRODUCTION

In 1850, Hermann von Helmholtz (1821–1894) published his measurements concerning the speed of neural conduction. Franciscus Donders (1818–1889) recognized that if neural conduction took a measurable amount of time, then *thinking* also must take time, and he devised a research program in which tasks were divided into their constituent subtasks and the time required to complete each subtask could then be measured (Donders, 1969). Thus, mental chronometry was born, and now there is not a field in psychology or human performance that does not use response time (RT) measures to evaluate behavior, models of cognition, engineering designs, and even mental and physical health.

Mental chronometry assumes that we can, by mapping out conditions under which RTs speed up or slow down, figure out how the brain is wired together. As Luce (1986) points out, this endeavor is hopelessly optimistic: it is akin to trying to produce a wiring diagram of a computer's motherboard by measuring how long it takes the computer to perform different computations.

However, the use of formal mathematical models, together with the measurement of RTs, has led to several important advances in our understanding of how people process information. We know, for example, that cognitive problems are not solved in a series of discrete steps, as

Donders (1969) originally proposed. Instead, many different processes are undertaken in parallel—in many areas of the brain simultaneously (e.g., Arbib & Arbib, 2003). We also know that in choice tasks, where people are asked to make a selection from a small number of options (usually two) in response to some stimulus, the decision process is well described by a process that resembles an accumulation of information over time. Ratcliff's (Ratcliff, 1978; Ratcliff & Smith, 2004) work, for example, characterizes the decision as a Wiener process with two absorbing boundaries. The state of the system at a point in time t represents the amount of evidence accumulated toward one of two alternatives, and the boundaries represent the amount of evidence required before either of the two responses can be selected. This model simultaneously predicts a person's choice accuracy and RT in a wide range of choice tasks, and has more recently been confirmed in studies examining the neural circuitry of monkey frontal eye fields (e.g., Schall, 2003).

Analyses of RT data have lagged significantly behind state-of-the-art statistical techniques, however. Consider data from an RT experiment in which subjects produce responses to a long sequence of stimuli under different experimental conditions (possibly mixed within blocks of trials). Most treatments of such data assume that an individual i's observations from each condition j are independent and identically distributed (iid; e.g., Ratcliff & Smith, 2004; Van Zandt, Colonius, & Proctor, 2000). Typically, model-fitting and parameter estimation efforts aimed at detecting the effects of experimental conditions focus on analysis of variance or maximum likelihood without regard to serial dependencies across trials.

Time series approaches, however, embrace the notion that sequences of RTs are neither independent nor identically distributed. Work investigating sequential effects, priming, inhibition of return, task switching, and so forth is directed toward understanding how information about previous stimuli and responses influences processing of later stimuli and facilitates or inhibits responses to those stimuli (e.g., Jones, Love, & Maddox, 2006; Meeter & Olivers, 2006; Stewart, Brown, & Chater, 2005). Related work by Gilden and others (Gilden, 1997, 2001; Pressing & Jolley-Rogers, 1997; Thornton & Gilden, 2005; Van Orden, Holden, & Turvey, 2003) has emphasized long-range effects across sequences of trials, or $1/f$ (pink) noise, which has brought more attention to the autocorrelation structure of RT sequences (see also Farrell, Wagenmakers, & Ratcliff, 2006; Wagenmakers, Farrell, & Ratcliff, 2004).

In this article, we consider a series of RTs for a single subject and experimental condition. Following Craigmile, Peruggia, and Van Zandt (2006), we let $\{R_t\}$ be the natural logarithm of the original RT series, where the index t denotes the trial number. Using a popular decomposition (e.g., Priestley, 1981, Section 7.7), we write this process as

$$R_t = \mu_t + \eta_t \tag{9.1}$$

for each t. Here μ_t denotes the trend and η_t denotes a random error component (possibly time-dependent). Although there are many definitions of trend, the one we will use is that of a smoothly varying, deterministic function of t that captures the long-range variations in a time series. This may include, for example, a mean that increases or decreases steadily with time (from fatigue or skill acquisition) or long-range seasonalities. The task structure may introduce a seasonal trend related to scheduled or unscheduled rests between blocks of trials.

The decision about what fraction of the variability in the data should be accounted for by μ_t and what fraction should be accounted for by η_t is as much driven by goodness-of-fit considerations as it is by scientific interest. While cognitive psychologists (RT modelers) see error as a nuisance, psychometricians are frequently most interested in the error component (at least insofar as it reflects interesting individual differences, e.g., Nesselroade, 1991).

Even though sequences of RTs have autocorrelational structure (e.g., Bertelson, 1965; Remington, 1969), most models of cognition ignore the time component completely, focussing instead on predicting main effects, or changes in the marginal mean over experimental conditions. The effect of time is ignored not only because it makes the model-fitting procedure harder, but also because changes in μ_t are not explained by models of the decision process that describe how RT varies over conditions.

For example, Ratcliff and colleagues frequently collect RT data from subjects over days or weeks to ensure large numbers of observations in each experimental condition (e.g., Ratcliff, Van Zandt, & McKoon, 1999). Changes in the estimated parameters of the Wiener decision process model (the drift rate and absorbing boundaries) are explained by changes in stimulus quality and factors that influence a person's willingness to respond. The model (fit to the data under the iid assumption) does not address the trend due to, say, skill acquisition, even though mean RTs may decrease dramatically over the course of the experiment. This kind of analysis seeks to separate trend from random error, but assumes that trend is constant within conditions and that error contains nothing of interest.

Some researchers model explicitly sequential dependencies in the data (Gilden, 1997, 2001; Peruggia, Van Zandt, & Chen, 2002; Thornton & Gilden, 2005; Wagenmakers et al., 2004). This is often accomplished by specifying an autocorrelated error component η_t, which is expected to capture features of RT series that are not necessarily associated with any hypothesized decision process or interesting individual differences. Their analyses, like those of the more traditional model-fitting exercises, either ignore the trend component μ_t (Gilden, 1997; Peruggia et al., 2002) or remove it after assuming that it follows a polynomial functional form estimated via least squares (e.g., Gilden, 2001; Van Orden *et al.*, 2003).

We should bear in mind that any decision concerning the removal of trend has a profound impact on estimates of η_t. In particular, unremoved trend may lead to the appearance of long-range correlation in the error structure. Thus, an important issue is how best to "detrend" RT series. To detrend a time series is to eliminate $\{\mu_t\}$, either by removing it directly, using a technique like differencing, or by estimating its form and subtracting it from the series. However, trends in RT series are not guaranteed to follow a simple functional form and, in the presence of fluctuations and seasonalities induced by experimental structure (rest breaks, intertrial timing, etc.), will be badly approximated by a low-order polynomial.

Also, estimates of μ_t are affected by properties of the marginal distribution of the stochastic component $\{\eta_t\}$ such as symmetry and tail behavior. It is well known and widely appreciated that RT data are skewed (e.g., Luce, 1986). Even after transforming the RT series and subtracting various possible estimates of trend, the marginal distribution of the residual stochastic component remains asymmetric, with heavy tails. In this chapter, we will demonstrate the impact of these issues on the quality of the trend estimates.

Another important issue is how to preprocess the data for analysis. Most researchers begin by removing perceived outliers and closing up the gaps thus created in the series (e.g., Kello, Beltz, Holden, & Van Orden, 2007; Van Orden et al., 2003; Wagenmakers et al., 2004). While in some cases this practice might not noticeably affect the estimates of autocorrelation, it nonetheless changes the dependence structure of the series and, in our opinion, should be avoided.*

Another common preprocessing practice is to subtract away the marginal means for different experimental conditions and transform the series to standard (z) scores. While this practice eliminates the necessity of estimating the variance of the stochastic component, it does nothing to address the problem of asymmetric marginal distributions with heavy tails. One way to reduce the influence of heavy tails on the estimates of trend and correlation is to use a transformation that "squeezes in" the upper tail. The most common approach (not seen in the RT literature) is to analyze the data on a logarithmic scale, an approach that we advocate. Even though this transformation does not produce in general a series with a symmetric marginal distribution (neither for the log RT series nor for the residual η_t series), it has the added benefit of "stretching out" overly fast RTs in the lower tail.

In this chapter, we provide an overview of several methods for removing trend in RT series. (We will not address the role of subtracting condition means from the series.) We introduce a new procedure in which we transform the series to normal quantiles, and then apply smoothing splines to estimate the trend, and contrast this procedure with other methods. We begin by motivating our discussion using actual RT data, and introduce a time series model for $\{\eta_t\}$ that we will use to explore detrending methods. We then describe various detrending methods, demonstrating how each method performs on the actual RT data, as well as on a simulated series. We present the results of Monte Carlo studies to evaluate the effectiveness of each method, and finish with a discussion of our work.

9.2 MOTIVATING SERIES

We now consider a single series of RT data published by Wagenmakers et al. (2004).† The top left panel of Figure 9.1 shows a plot of the log RT series for

* We have performed several simulation studies that demonstrate how the estimates of autocorrelations can be damped by outliers. Removing outliers or Windsorizing the series did not prove sufficient to recover the autocorrelations of the underlying processes (Craigmile, P., "Statistical Methods for Modeling Human Dynamics," University of Notre Dame. May 29, 2007—http://www.stat.osu.edu/~pfc/talks/2007/notre_dame_2007.pdf).

† These data are for Subject 1 in the short condition performing a simple RT task. They can be downloaded from http://users.fmg.uva.nl/ewagenmakers/fnoise/noisedat.html

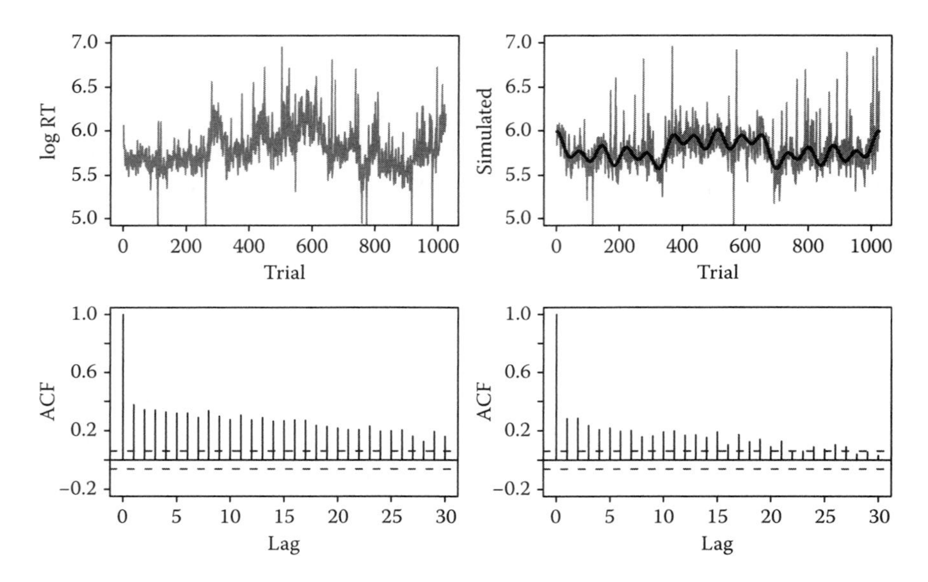

FIGURE 9.1 The top left-hand panel shows a plot of the log RT series for 1024 successive trials from a simple RT task. The bottom left panel shows the ACF of this series. The top right-hand panels shows a realization of the sinusoidal trend model plus noise. Superimposed on the series is the true trend (the line). The bottom right panel shows the ACF of the simulated series.

1024 successive trials of a simple RT task, recorded after 24 practice trials. The subject responded to any numerical stimulus on a screen as quickly as possible by pressing a key. The time between a response and the next stimulus was uniformly distributed between 550 and 950 ms.

The top left panel of Figure 9.1 makes clear a number of features that are common to RT data. From trial 300 to 900, there is evidence of trend (which we consider to be part of $\{\mu_t\}$ in Equation 9.1). Roughly, the log RT level begins low, increases to a maximum at about trial 600, and decreases thereafter. There is also a possibility of an increasing trend from trial 900 until the end of the series. There may also be some seasonality, as evidenced by the slowly changing level, especially after trial 200. The nonstationarity of the RT process, induced by the presence of a deterministic trend, is reflected by the slowly decaying character of the autocorrelation function (ACF, shown in the bottom left panel of Figure 9.1).

There are two other features in the log RT series that should not be ignored. First, there are "bursts" in the series that suggest the presence of substantial dependence between nearby trials. This may be caused by carry-over effects, from either the stimuli or the errors from the subject. Second, there are many long and short RTs that contribute to the long upper and lower tails of the marginal distribution on the logarithmic scale. These features suggest that it may be reasonable to specify a long-tailed distribution with an adequate dependence structure for the errors $\{\eta_t\}$. Before we can examine the error process, however, we must model the trend $\{\mu_t\}$ and eliminate it. Our intention in this article is to investigate methods for the estimation or elimination of trend that can handle these features present in RT data.

9.2.1 A Model of RT Series

We now define a time series model that shares with real RT data the characteristics that we identified above (trend, dependence, and long tails). We will use this model as a basis for investigating different methods of trend estimation.

Building on decomposition (9.1), we let $\{\mu_t\}$ denote the deterministic trend for the log RT series $\{R_t\}$. Following Craigmile et al. (2006), we specify for the error process the mixture model (e.g., Titterington, Smith, & Makov, 1985)

$$\eta_t = X_t + \delta_{Y,t} Y_t - \delta_{Z,t} Z_t, \quad t = 1, \ldots, N. \tag{9.2}$$

The time series $\{X_t\}$ is a Gaussian autoregressive process of order one, AR(1), that captures trial by trial dependencies. To define this process, let $\{U_t\}$ be an iid $\mathrm{N}(0, \sigma^2)$ process. For $t > 2$, let

$$X_t = \phi X_{t-1} + U_t. \tag{9.3}$$

(This process is stationary for $|\phi| < 1$ when we assume $X_1 = U_1/\sqrt{1-\phi^2}$.)

The $\delta_{Y,t} Y_t$ and $-\delta_{Z,t} Z_t$ terms in (9.2) capture the long upper and lower tail behavior seen in RT series. Both $\{Y_t\}$ and $\{Z_t\}$ are iid shifted (mean zero) exponential processes with rates λ_Y and λ_Z, respectively. (These distributions for $\{Y_t\}$ and $\{Z_t\}$ differ slightly from those used in Craigmile et al., 2006.) The process $\{\boldsymbol{\delta}_t\}$ controls which elements (if any) of the tail process are active for any trial. Specifically, for each t, $\boldsymbol{\delta}_t = (\delta_{N,t}, \delta_{Y,t}, \delta_{Z,t})^{\mathrm{T}}$ is an iid multinomial$(1, \boldsymbol{p})$ random vector, where $\boldsymbol{p} = (p_N, p_Y, p_Z)^{\mathrm{T}}$ is a vector of probabilities that sum to one. Then, with probability p_N, $\boldsymbol{\delta}_t = (1,0,0)^{\mathrm{T}}$ and $\eta_t = X_t$ (AR only), with probability p_Y, $\boldsymbol{\delta}_t = (0,1,0)^{\mathrm{T}}$ and $\eta_t = X_t + Y_t$ (AR plus upper tail), and with probability p_Z, $\boldsymbol{\delta}_t = (0,0,1)^{\mathrm{T}}$ and $\eta_t = X_t - Z_t$ (AR minus lower tail).

To generate prototype series of length $N = 1024$, we set $\sigma^2 = 0.01$ and $\phi = 0.35$ in the model for $\{X_t\}$. In the component for the tail behavior, we let $\lambda_Y = 5$, $\lambda_Z = 0.7$, and $\boldsymbol{p} = (0.68, 0.32, 0.02)^{\mathrm{T}}$. (These values are compatible with the parameter estimates for the log RT series from Wagenmakers et al., 2004.)

The right-hand panels of Figure 9.1 summarize one realization of this model with a sinusoidal trend $\{\mu_t\}$ shown as a dark gray line. The form of this trend is

$$\mu_t = \alpha_0 + \sum_{j=1}^{5} \beta_j \cos(2\pi f_j t), \quad t = 1, \ldots, N, \tag{9.4}$$

with $\alpha_0 = 5.78$, $\beta = (-0.06, 0.08, 0.05, 0.06, 0.08)^{\mathrm{T}}$, and $f = (1, 2, 5, 8, 14)^{\mathrm{T}}$. (A constant plus five sinusoids visually captures the trend in the log RT series for the data from Wagenmakers et al., 2004.) The simulated data present features of trend, autocorrelation, and tail behavior typical of RT data.

In the next section, we present several methods for detrending time series, using the actual and simulated data in Figure 9.1. Our Monte Carlo experiments that follow later use the parameters for the sinusoidal trend simulations presented here.

9.3 DETRENDING METHODS

We begin by discussing regression-based detrending techniques, which are probably the methods most widely used in the RT literature. We then contrast those techniques with smoothing techniques, and this leads naturally to our new procedure. We evaluate the performance of the various estimators of trend by their mean squared error (MSE). At each time point t, the MSE of the estimated trend, $\widehat{\mu}_t$, is defined by

$$\mathrm{MSE}(\widehat{\mu}_t) = E\left([\widehat{\mu}_t - \mu_t]^2\right) = \mathrm{var}\,(\widehat{\mu}_t) + [E\,(\widehat{\mu}_t - \mu_t)]^2. \tag{9.5}$$

That is, the MSE is equal to the variance of the estimator plus its squared bias. Our primary interest is to find an estimator of the trend with small MSE.

9.3.1 Regression Methods

Most published RT analyses remove trend in the form of linear or quadratic regression. We can estimate polynomial (or sinusoidal) trends using standard least-squares methods. We can also use local regression methods (which are an offshoot of linear regression methods).

9.3.1.1 Least-Squares Regression

A polynomial trend model of degree K for $\{R_t\}$ is given by

$$\mu_t = \sum_{k=0}^{K} \alpha_k t^k, \quad t = 1, \ldots, N.$$

(A linear regression has $K = 1$, and a quadratic regression has $K = 2$.) In the least-squares method, we choose the values of $\{\alpha_k\}$ to minimize the residual sum of squares $\sum_{t=1}^{N} (R_t - \mu_t)^2$. We assume that this procedure will be performed on the RT series only after appropriate transformation. Failing to transform the raw data will result in estimates that are affected by the tails of the marginal RT distribution.

Figure 9.2 shows the least-squares estimates of trend modeled by a fifth degree polynomial for Wagenmaker's data (top panel) and the simulated data (bottom panel). The true trend component is plotted as a dark gray curve with the estimated polynomial trend for the simulated data. While the low-frequency components of the trend are well captured by the polynomial estimate, the high-frequency components are not. This remaining trend will influence any later analysis of correlational structure in the series.

The major weakness of polynomial regression is that it ignores seasonal and high frequency variation. Such variations can be introduced in an RT series by way of scheduled or unscheduled rests, fluctuations of attention, changes in cognitive strategy, and so forth. Thus, focussing only on polynomial trend may result in inaccurate conclusions about the correlation structure of the error sequence. Such trends are common in RT data, and so focussing only on polynomial trend will result in inaccurate conclusions about correlation structure.

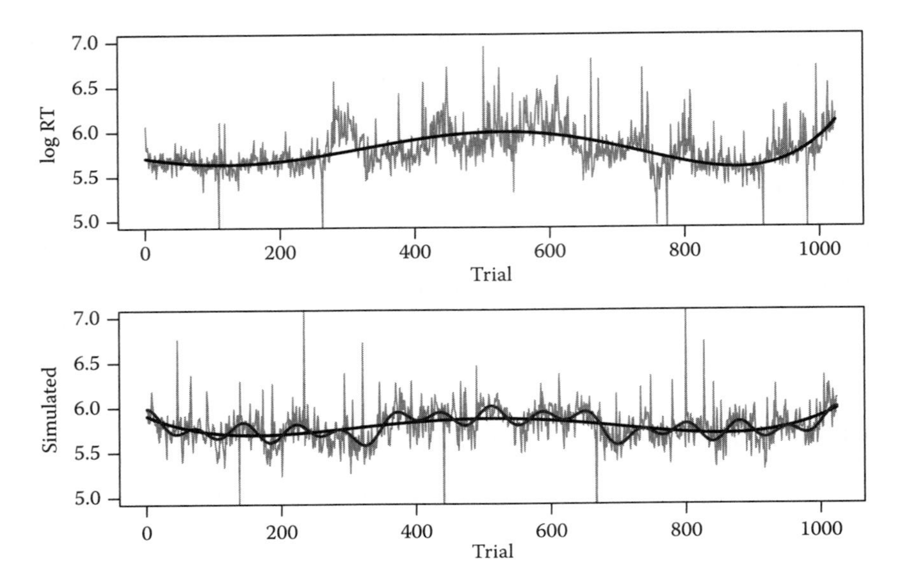

FIGURE 9.2 The top panel shows the polynomial ($K = 5$) estimate of the trend (black line) superimposed on Wagenmaker's log RT data. The bottom panel shows the same for the simulated data. The dark gray line in the bottom panel is the true trend.

An alternative strategy is to fit a *harmonic regression* model that uses sine and cosine functions evaluated at different frequencies as the regressors (e.g., Percival & Walden, 1993, Chapter 10). Selection of the appropriate frequencies of these sinusoids is a hard problem in practice (e.g., Percival & Walden, 1993; Quinn & Hannan, 2001) and we do not address it here.

9.3.1.2 Local Regression Methods

One alternative to polynomial regression is local regression, where we assume that the contribution of $R_s, s \neq t$, to the estimate $\widehat{\mu}_t$ will be weighted according to how close s is to t, with R_s values observed closer in time contributing the most. Local polynomial regression (loess) uses weighted least squares to fit a polynomial of degree k to observations within a neighborhood of t. The weights can be computed in several ways, but are usually derived from a Gaussian kernel, the standard deviation of which determines the size of the effective neighborhood around t.

Because we model trend in local neighborhoods, there is rarely any need to consider polynomials of degree greater than two. Furthermore, there are a number of plug-in methods to choose the standard deviation of the kernel (or other bandwidth, e.g., Ruppert, Sheather, & Wand 1995). The interested reader can consult Cleveland (1979) and Loader (1999) for more details.

Local polynomial regression is implemented in the R package's loess and locpoly routines. Using default control parameters and the bandwidth selector suggested by Ruppert et al. (1995), the loess estimates for Wagenmaker's data (top panel) and the simulated data (bottom panel) are shown in Figure 9.3. The true trend is shown as a dark gray line. While the local regression method does a better job of picking up high-frequency fluctuations than polynomial regression, it is still missing the highest-frequency trend components.

9.3.2 Smoothing Methods

Smoothing is accomplished by applying a filter to the series. It is a nonparametric approach to estimating trend. After the application of the filter, the resulting smoothed series is the estimated trend.

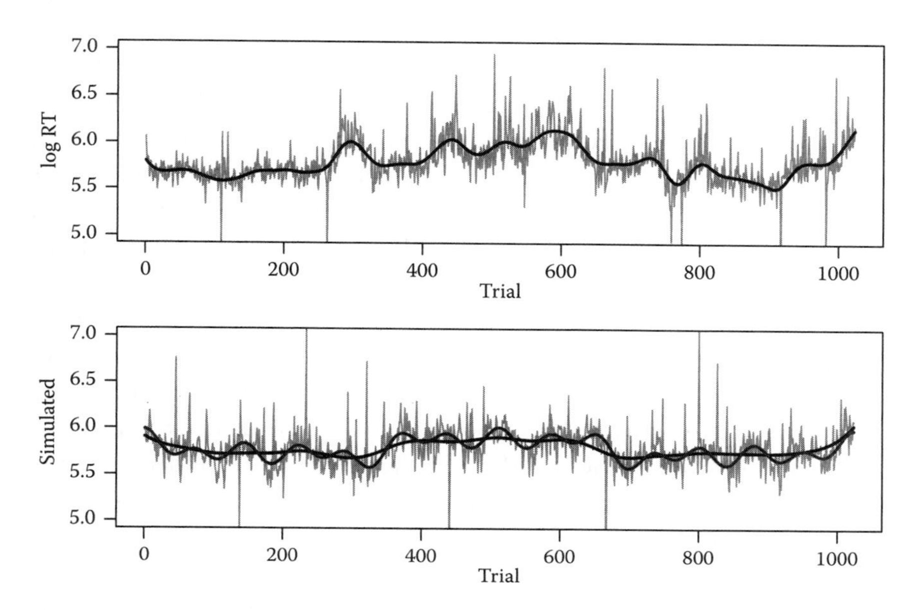

FIGURE 9.3 The top panel shows the *loess* estimate of the trend (black line) for Wagenmaker's log RT data. The bottom panel shows the same for the simulated data. The dark gray line in the bottom panel is the true trend.

9.3.2.1 Filtering

There are several ways to smooth the series $\{R_t\}$. The most straightforward is the moving average (MA) filter of order q defined by

$$\widehat{\mu}_t = (2q+1)^{-1} \sum_{k=-q}^{q} R_{t-k}, \quad q+1 \leq t \leq n-q.$$

Here, $2q+1$ is the width of the filter. Such a filter removes the high-frequency components of the series, but retains the low-frequency components. In particular, it preserves linear and locally linear trends (e.g., Brockwell & Davis, 2002, Chapter 1). Writing the filter more generally as

$$\widehat{\mu}_t = \sum_{i=-q}^{q} a_i R_{t-i},$$

we may choose the coefficients $\{a_i\}$ such that polynomial trends (of a given degree) or sinusoids (of a given period) are retained.

There are many such filters to choose from, each of which varies in terms of the weights applied to $\{R_t\}$, as well as more complicated filters, such as the Wiener filter, Kalman filters, kernel methods, stochastic filters, and so on. Yet another method uses Fourier transforms. The series $\{R_t\}$ is transformed (via fast Fourier transform or some other algorithm) from the time to the frequency domain, and all high-frequency components are given an amplitude of 0. The truncated Fourier series is then transformed back to the time domain, giving a time series in which all rapid fluctuations have been removed.

Misapplying a filter may result in an estimated trend that bears no resemblance to the actual trend, and subsequent modeling efforts will produce inaccurate parameter estimates in the model for η_t. The choice of a filter width is crucial in this respect. Too wide a width and the series will be oversmoothed; too narrow a width and the series will be undersmoothed (or overfit). Cross-validation (e.g., Efron & Tibshirani, 1993, Chapter 17) is one way in which we might select the filter width. In cross-validation, the data are partitioned (either systematically or at random) into two sets. Filtering based on a given width is applied to the first set (the training set) and the MSE resulting from predicting the data points in the second set (the validation set) by means of the estimated trend is calculated. The procedure is repeated for several partitions and an overall measure of predictive accuracy corresponding to the given filter width is derived. The width yielding the best overall performance is eventually selected. For the case of time series data, however, the application of the filtering to the training set raises nontrivial issues connected to the disruption in the serial dependencies that results from omitting the data points reserved for validation.

Figure 9.4 shows the smoothed series estimated by an MA filter of order $q = 32$ for Wagenmaker's data (top panel) and the simulated data (bottom panel). The MA technique does a much better job of recovering the true trend than any of the regression techniques considered above, although it, like the regression techniques, underestimates the high-frequency trend components.

9.3.2.2 Smoothing Splines

The methods we now discuss make use of splines. Splines are piecewise polynomials of a given degree k joined at a finite number m of fixed points called *knots*. The splines are constrained so that at each knot their

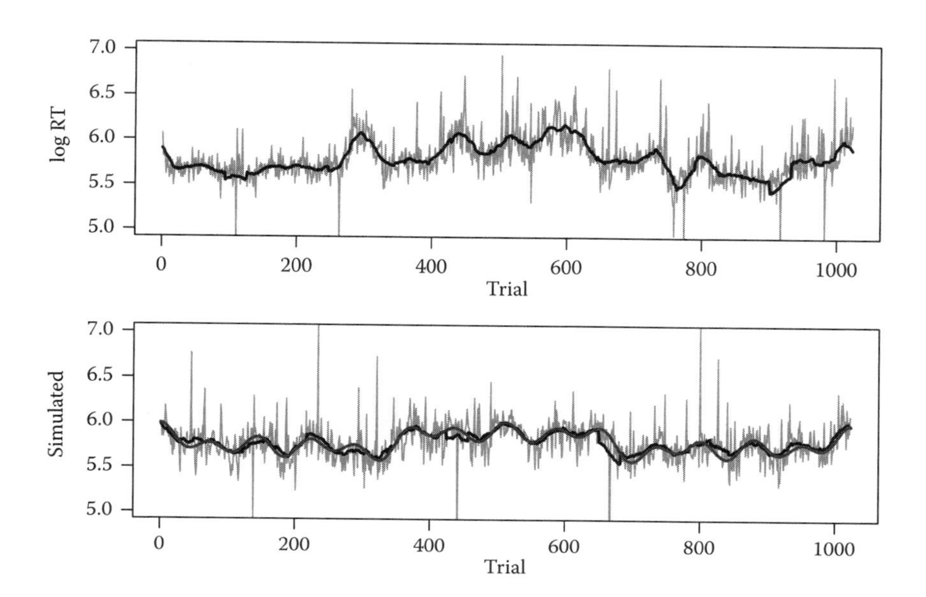

FIGURE 9.4 The top panel shows the MA filter of order $q = 32$ estimate of the trend (black line) superimposed on Wagenmaker's log RT data. The bottom panel shows the same for the simulated data. The dark gray line (bottom panel) is the true trend.

derivatives up to order k are equal. Letting $\alpha_1, \ldots, \alpha_m$ be these m knots, polynomials of degree k,

$$\psi_j(t) = \begin{cases} (t - \alpha_j)^k, & (t - \alpha_j) > 0, \\ 0, & (t - \alpha_j) \leq 0, \end{cases}$$

are called *basis functions*, and the smoothed estimate can be written as

$$\widehat{\mu}_t = \sum_{j=1}^{m} c_j \psi_j(t)$$

for appropriately chosen c_j.

The degree of smoothness of the resulting estimates (obtained by a criterion that balances goodness of fit and roughness) can be controlled by the value of tuning parameters (like the MA filter width) that are typically chosen by cross-validation techniques. These techniques are optimal when the errors $\{\eta_t\}$ are independent. If the errors are dependent, the estimates can be badly distorted (Wang, 1998). We fit cubic smoothing splines, using a generalized cross-validation measure to select the optimal smoothing parameter (Wahba, 1990). The top panel of Figure 9.5 shows Wagenmaker's data and its estimated trend, and the bottom panel shows the simulated data together with the true and estimated trend. As with the MA and regression methods, the trend is oversmoothed and the high-frequency components of the trend are not well captured.

9.3.2.3 Normalization with Smoothing Splines

One problem common to all the methods we have presented is that, even after the log transformation, the data are neither independent nor symmetrically distributed. Independence and symmetry facilitate the estimation of trend. To improve on these methods, we normalized the observations in the series by converting them to Gaussian quantiles by inversion of their empirical cumulative distribution function.

Let $q(\alpha)$ denote the αth quantile of the standard normal distribution. For example, if $\alpha = 0.975$, then $q(0.975) = 1.96$. For the log RT sequence $\{R_t\}$, let $\{S_t\}$ denote the associated ranks of each observation in the sequence. For example, if $\{R_t\} = \{5.3, 4.9, 5.6, 5.2\}$, then $\{S_t\} = \{3, 1, 4, 2\}$.

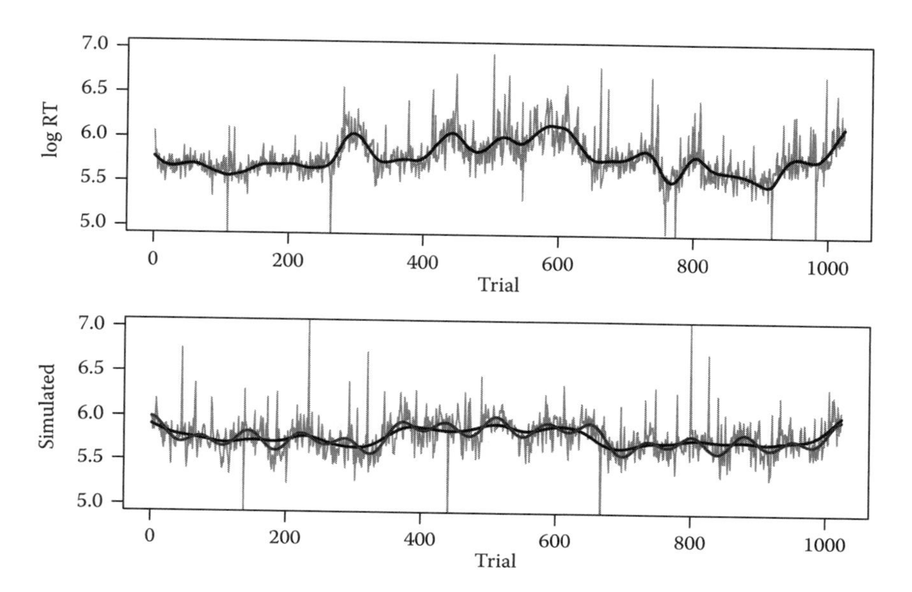

FIGURE 9.5 The top panel shows the smoothing spline estimate of the trend (black line) superimposed on Wagenmaker's log RT data. The bottom panel shows the same for the simulated data. The dark gray line (bottom panel) is the true trend.

The normalized data are then given by $\{G_t = q((S_t - 1/2)/N): t = 1, 2, \ldots, N\}$. For the simple example above, $N = 4$ and so

$$\begin{aligned}\{G_t\} &= \left\{q\left(\frac{1}{4}\left(S_t - \frac{1}{2}\right)\right)\right\},\\ &= q\left(\{0.625, 0.125, 0.875, 0.375\}\right),\\ &= \{0.319, -1.150, 1.150, -0.319\},\end{aligned}$$

which is a set of symmetric normal quantiles with ranks equal to the ranks of the original data.

Figure 9.6 shows the estimates of $\{\mu_t\}$ obtained by applying a smoothing spline to the normalized data $\{G_t\}$ and transforming the estimates back to the log RT scale using the empirical cumulative distribution function and linear interpolation. The top panel shows Wagenmaker's data and the bottom panel shows the simulated data, together with the estimated and true trend. While slight oversmoothing can still be detected, the estimates seem better than any we have previously encountered.

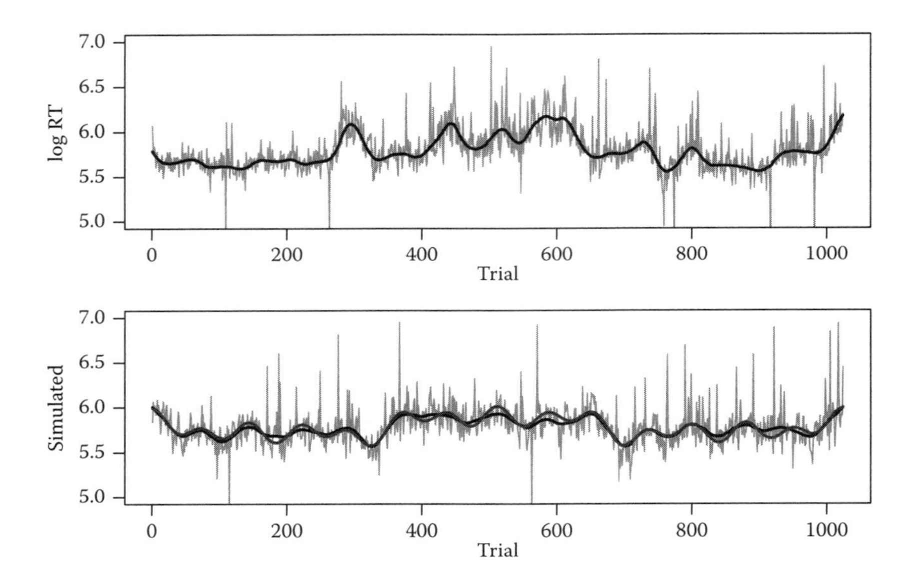

FIGURE 9.6 The top panel shows the normalized smoothing spline estimate of the trend (black line) superimposed on Wagenmaker's log RT data. This method assumes that the errors on the transformed scale are uncorrelated. The bottom panel shows the same for the simulated data. The dark gray line (bottom panel) is the true trend.

A procedure that smooths dependent data was presented by Wang (1998). In this procedure, cubic smoothing splines are fit to Gaussian data and the dependence structure is modeled with an AR(1) process. Wang adjusts the standard (uncorrelated) smoothing spline method to allow for correlation and demonstrates, using reproducing kernel methods, how to rewrite the problem into one that can be solved using linear mixed-effects models. This is implemented in the R package **assist** using the `ssr` function. Rather than using cross-validation, the smoothing parameter is estimated via Gaussian maximum likelihood. This is a valid modeling approach, since our method uses Gaussian quantiles to obtain the normalized data $\{G_t\}$. Figure 9.7 shows the trend estimates obtained by applying this function to the normalized data $\{G_t\}$, assuming a Gaussian AR(1) process, and then transforming back to the original log RT scale as before. The top panel of the figure shows Wagenmaker's data with the estimated trend, and the bottom panel shows the simulated data with both the estimated and the true trend. This estimate looks very similar to the estimate obtained without consideration of the correlated error.

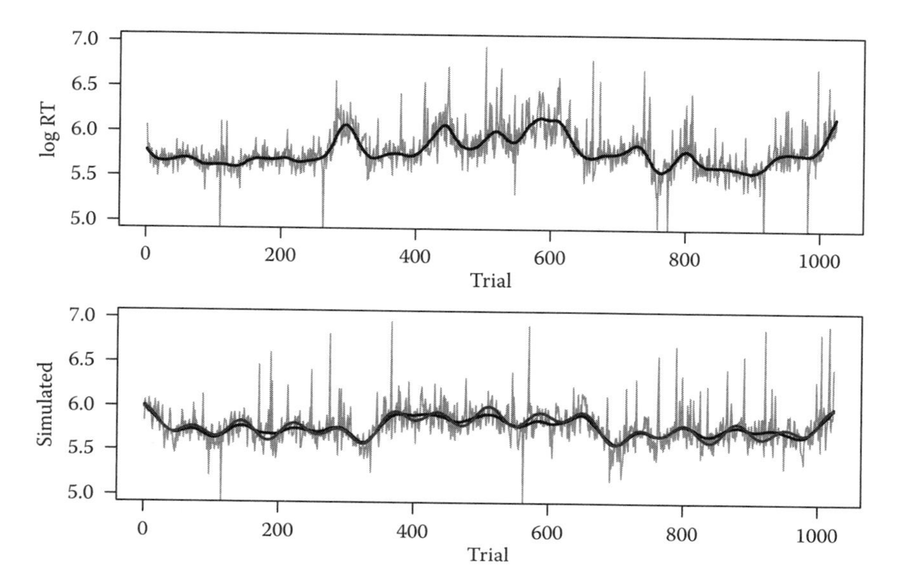

FIGURE 9.7 The top panel shows the normalized smoothing spline estimate of the trend (black line) superimposed on Wagenmaker's log RT data. This method assumes that the errors on the transformed scale come from an AR(1) process. The bottom panel shows the same for the simulated data. The dark gray line (bottom panel) is the true trend.

9.3.3 Summary

We have presented several examples of regression and smoothing methods for estimating (and eliminating) trend in time series. Of these techniques, only our normalization procedure produced good estimates of trend.

It is clear from the examples we have shown that some procedures are more accurate than others, and that it will be difficult to determine each procedure's strengths and weaknesses on the basis of an analysis of a single time series. For this reason, we next present the results of a simulation study we conducted to evaluate the different detrending procedures.

9.4 A SIMULATION STUDY

In this section, we evaluate the performance of the various trend estimators in terms of their MSEs defined by Equation 9.5. Our study is based on 200 replicates of the log RT series generated by four models that follow the decomposition given in Equation 9.1. They are as follows:

i. A linear trend $\mu_t = 5.5 + 0.5t$ plus a parametric error $\{\eta_t\}$ that follows the model specified by Equation 9.2. The parameters for the error model are specified in the paragraphs following the model description.
ii. A quadratic trend $\mu_t = 5.5 + (t - 0.5)^2$ plus the same error model as for the linear trend.
iii. A sinusoidal trend, defined by Equation 9.4, plus the same error model as for the linear trend.
iv. An empirical estimate of trend for the Wagenmaker data presented earlier. This estimate was computed by fitting a time series model to the data (Craigmile et al., 2006).* For each series replicate, the error component was generated by bootstrapping a series from the residuals (the log RT values minus the trend). (Because the residuals are correlated, we used a moving block bootstrap with block size $B = 4$.†)

Figure 9.8 shows each of these trends. The linear and quadratic trend models represent the assumptions made by those researchers who use least-squares regression methods for detrending. The sinusoidal and empirical trend models represent the more realistic and complex trends seen in RT data.

For each of the 200 realizations simulated from each model, we estimated the trend using the following methods:

1. Least-squares regression fitting polynomial trends of degrees 1, 2, and 5 (`deg1, deg2, deg5`).
2. Loess fits using locally weighted quadratic regression and neighborhoods that span 25%, 50%, and 75% of the series (`loess25, loess50, loess75`).

* The time series model used is a regression model in which a wavelet basis is used to estimate the trend, and the errors are explained by a model similar in form to Equation 9.2.

† In the moving block bootstrap, we break a stationary time series into K overlapping blocks of length B. We then randomly sample blocks, arranging them sequentially to generate a new time series. Sampling blocks preserve the dependence inherent in the stationary series. See Lahiri (2003) for further details on the moving block bootstrap procedure.

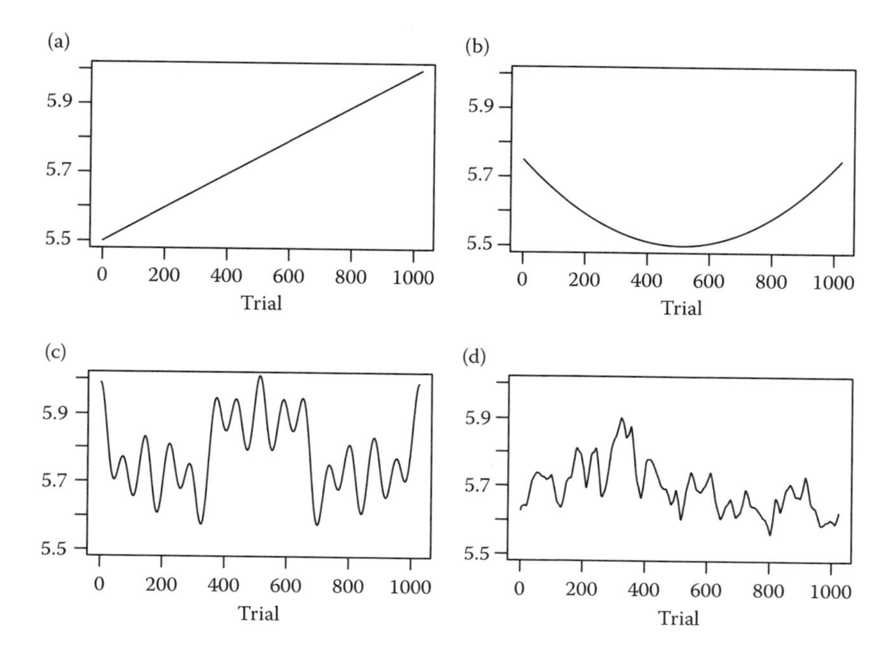

FIGURE 9.8 The four trends that are used in the simulations: (a) linear; (b) quadratic; (c) sinusoidal; and (d) empirical.

3. MA filters of order $q = 16$ (`MA16`), $q = 32$ (`MA32`), and $q = 64$ (`MA64`).
4. Cubic smoothing splines fit to the original data assuming iid errors (`SS`) and AR(1) errors (`SSAR1`).
5. Cubic smoothing splines fit to the normalized data assuming iid errors (`normSS`) and AR(1) errors (`normSSAR1`).

For a given simulation and estimation method, let $\widehat{\mu}_t$ be the estimator of the trend μ_t at time t and let $\widehat{\mu}_{k,t}$ be its realized value for replicate k. Define $\overline{\mu}_t = \sum_{k=1}^{200} \widehat{\mu}_{k,t}/200$. Then, we estimated the bias of $\widehat{\mu}_t$ as

$$\widehat{\text{bias}}(\widehat{\mu}_t) = \overline{\mu}_t - \mu_t,$$

and its variance as

$$\widehat{\text{var}}(\widehat{\mu}_t) = \frac{1}{199} \sum_{k=1}^{200} (\widehat{\mu}_{k,t} - \overline{\mu}_t)^2.$$

Finally, we estimated the MSE as $\widehat{\text{MSE}}(\widehat{\mu}_t) = \widehat{\text{var}}(\widehat{\mu}_t) + (\widehat{\text{bias}}(\widehat{\mu}_t))^2$.

TABLE 9.1

The Estimated Bias, Variance, and MSE Averaged Over Time of Different Methods of Estimating a Linear and Quadratic Trend

	(i) Linear Trend			(ii) Quadratic Trend		
Method	Bias^2	Variance	MSE	Bias^2	Variance	MSE
deg1	<0.0001	0.1	0.1	5.6	0.1	5.7
deg2	<0.0001	0.2	0.2	<0.0001	0.2	0.2
deg5	<0.0001	0.5	0.5	<0.0001	0.4	0.4
loess25	<0.0001	0.9	0.9	<0.0001	0.8	0.8
loess50	<0.0001	0.5	0.5	<0.0001	0.4	0.4
loess75	<0.0001	0.3	0.3	<0.0001	0.3	0.3
MA16	0.4	4.5	4.8	<0.0001	4.6	4.6
MA32	0.7	2.3	2.9	<0.0001	2.3	2.3
MA64	1.3	1.2	2.5	<0.0001	1.1	1.2
SS	<0.0001	0.2	0.2	<0.0001	0.3	0.3
SSAR1	<0.0001	0.2	0.2	<0.0001	0.3	0.3
normSS	<0.0001	0.1	0.1	0.1	0.2	0.3
normSSAR1	<0.0001	0.1	0.1	0.1	0.1	0.3

Note: The values in the table have been multiplied by 1000 to aid comparison. Each set of estimates are based on 200 simulated series.

Tables 9.1 and 9.2 show estimated squared bias, variance, and MSE (multiplied by 1000 to aid comparison) averaged over time ($t = 1, \ldots, 1024$) for each model and method. From Table 9.1, for both the linear trend model (i) and the quadratic trend model (ii), the MSE is determined almost entirely by the variance of the estimator, except for the MA filters. The linear regression method has the smallest squared bias ($<5 \times 10^{-7}$) when applied to the linear trend model, but when this method is applied to the quadratic trend model, the squared bias is very large. This is because the linear regression method is consistent with the true trend for the linear trend model, but a very poor approximation to the quadratic trend model. Our normalized smoothing splines method, applied to either the linear or quadratic trend models, does almost as well as the regression methods with appropriately selected polynomials.

The sinusoidal (iii) and empirical (iv) trend models provide a real challenge for the trend estimation methods. Table 9.2 shows that all the methods have large (relative to Table 9.1) squared biases for these more difficult problems, especially the three regression (`deg`) methods, the three local regression (`loess`) methods, and the smoothing spline methods. The

TABLE 9.2

The Estimated Bias, Variance, and MSE Averaged Over Time, of Different Methods of Estimating a Sinusoidal and Empirical Trend

	(iii) Sinusoidal Trend			(iv) Empirical Trend		
Method	Bias^2	Variance	MSE	Bias^2	Variance	MSE
`deg1`	11.3	0.2	11.4	3.7	0.1	3.8
`deg2`	10.6	0.2	10.9	3.3	0.2	3.5
`deg5`	6.3	0.4	6.7	2.2	0.3	2.6
`loess25`	4.3	0.8	5.1	1.4	0.6	2.0
`loess50`	5.8	0.4	6.2	2.0	0.3	2.4
`loess75`	7.0	0.3	7.3	2.4	0.2	2.6
`MA16`	0.1	4.4	4.5	0.2	3.2	3.4
`MA32`	0.3	2.2	2.5	0.4	1.6	2.0
`MA64`	2.7	1.1	3.8	1.0	0.8	1.8
`SS`	1.8	1.8	3.5	1.6	0.6	2.2
`SSAR1`	2.9	1.5	4.4	1.8	0.5	2.3
`normSS`	0.3	1.0	1.3	0.9	0.4	1.2
`normSSAR1`	0.6	0.9	1.5	1.2	0.3	1.5

Note: The values in the table have been multiplied by 1000 to aid comparison. Each set of estimates are based on 200 simulated series.

smallest squared bias, which comes at the expense of a much larger variance, belongs to the MA smoothing filters of small order. The important finding is that our normalized smoothing spline method has the smallest MSE of any of the other methods.

Thus, while the true trend influences how well each method performs, our smoothing spline method applied to normalized data leads consistently to optimal or nearly optimal performance. We further quantify this claim by reporting summaries of the percentage "improvement" that our smoothing spline method achieved over the other methods at each time point t. Letting $\widehat{\text{MSE}}_t(\texttt{method})$ denote the estimated MSE for a given `method` at time t, we calculated several quantiles of the set of percentage improvements over time:

$$\left\{ \frac{\widehat{\text{MSE}}_t(\texttt{method}) - \widehat{\text{MSE}}_t(\texttt{normSSAR1})}{\widehat{\text{MSE}}_t(\texttt{method})} \times 100\%\colon\ t = 1, \ldots, 1024 \right\}.$$

Positive percentages indicate that the `normSSAR1` method is preferable in terms of MSE.

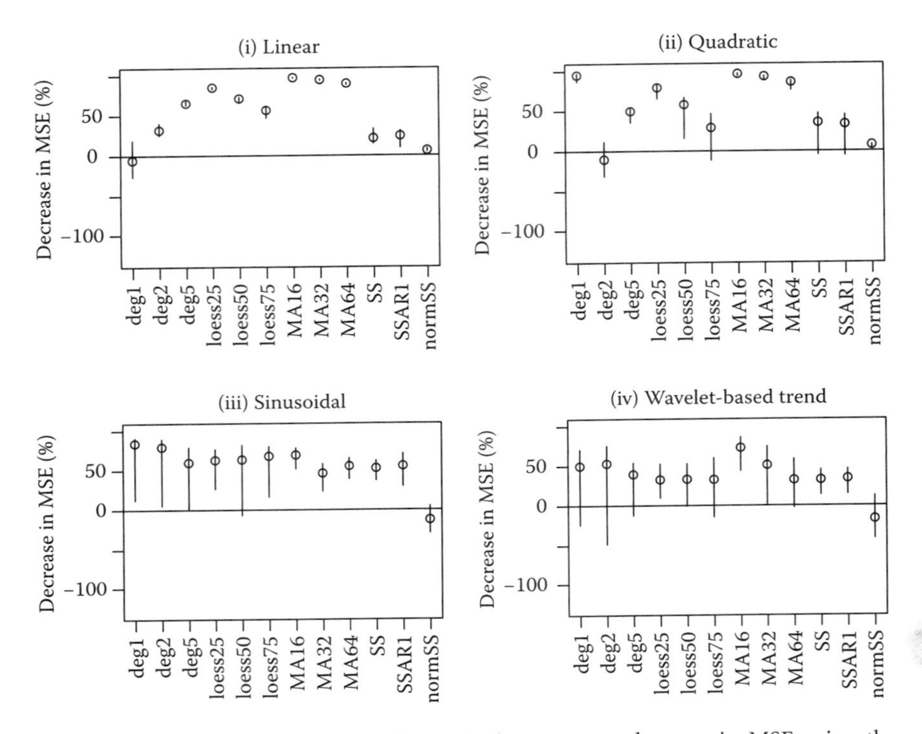

FIGURE 9.9 Plots of the median (over time) percentage decrease in MSE using the `normSSAR1` method relative to every other trend estimation method. The vertical line around each point connects lower and upper quantiles of the decrease. Each panel shows the results for a different model for the true underlying trend.

The results are summarized in Figure 9.9. For each trend model and trend estimation methods, the figure displays the lower and upper quartile (the endpoints of the line segment) and the median (the circle) of the percentage improvements attained by our normalized smoothing splines method with AR(1) errors (the `normSSAR1` method). For the linear trend model (i), only the linear regression method exhibits a negative percentage improvement at more than 50% of the time points. In all other cases, the `normSSAR1` method beats its competitors at more than 75% of the time points. For the quadratic trend model (ii), only the quadratic regression method exhibits a negative percentage improvement at more than 50% of the time points. In all other cases, the `normSSAR1` method beats its competitors at more than 50% of the time points. This further illustrates the fact that the efficiency of any particular detrending method will depend on the true underlying trend.

For the sinusoidal (iii) and empirical (iv) trend models, both the `normSS` and `normSSAR1` outperform the other methods at a majority of time points. The `normSS` method tends to beat the `normSSAR1` method.

We conclude that normalizing the log RT series before applying smoothing splines helps to reduce the MSE of the trend estimators. The evidence is mixed for the claim that using a trend estimation procedure that models the autocorrelation of the errors with an AR(1) process will reduce the MSE even more.

To investigate further the need for modeling the autocorrelation in the error, we restricted our comparisons to the `normSS` and `normSSAR1` methods. We calculated several quantiles of the set of percentage improvements in the squared bias relative to the MSE as a function of the autocorrelation parameter ϕ:

$$\left\{ \frac{\widehat{\text{bias}}_t^2(\texttt{normSS}) - \widehat{\text{bias}}_t^2(\texttt{normSSAR1})}{\widehat{\text{MSE}}_t(\texttt{normSSAR1})} \times 100\%: \ t = 1, \ldots, 1024 \right\}.$$

This is shown in the left panel of Figure 9.10. These calculations are based on 200 realizations of sinusoidal trend plus noise, for values of $\phi = 0$ (corresponding to iid noise), 0.2, 0.4, and 0.6. We did the same for the percentage improvements in the variance and MSE (middle and right panels of Figure 9.10, respectively). In each panel, the circles denote the median values, and the endpoints of the line segments denote the lower and upper quartiles.

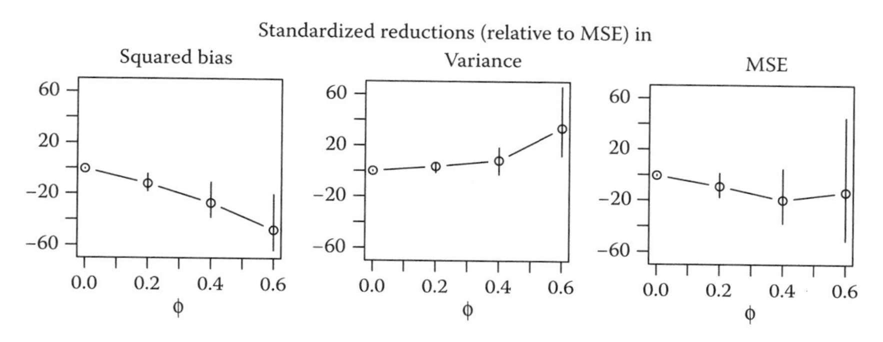

FIGURE 9.10 From left to right, plots of the median percentage improvements in squared bias, variance, and MSE, respectively, when using the `normSSAR1` method relative to the `normSS` method, as the amount of autocorrelation ϕ in the AR(1) error process increases. The vertical lines connect the lower and upper quantiles of the improvements. These simulations are based on 200 realizations of sinusoidal trend plus noise.

As the autocorrelation in the errors increases, there is an improvement in squared bias using the `normSS` method (i.e., assuming the errors of the normalized data are uncorrelated) compared with the `normSSAR1` method (i.e., assuming the errors of the normalized data follow an AR(1) model). This squared bias reduction is not offset by a large increase in the variance; so the `normSS` method gives smaller MSEs than the `normSSAR1` method.

The lack of any significant improvement in the estimated MSE using the `normssAR1` method, even as the degree of autocorrelation increases, might be explained in several ways. First, converting to normalized scores can change the correlation structure of the errors, especially in the presence of long tails like those in RT data. If the errors are AR(1) on the original scale, they need not be AR(1) after transforming to the normalized scale.

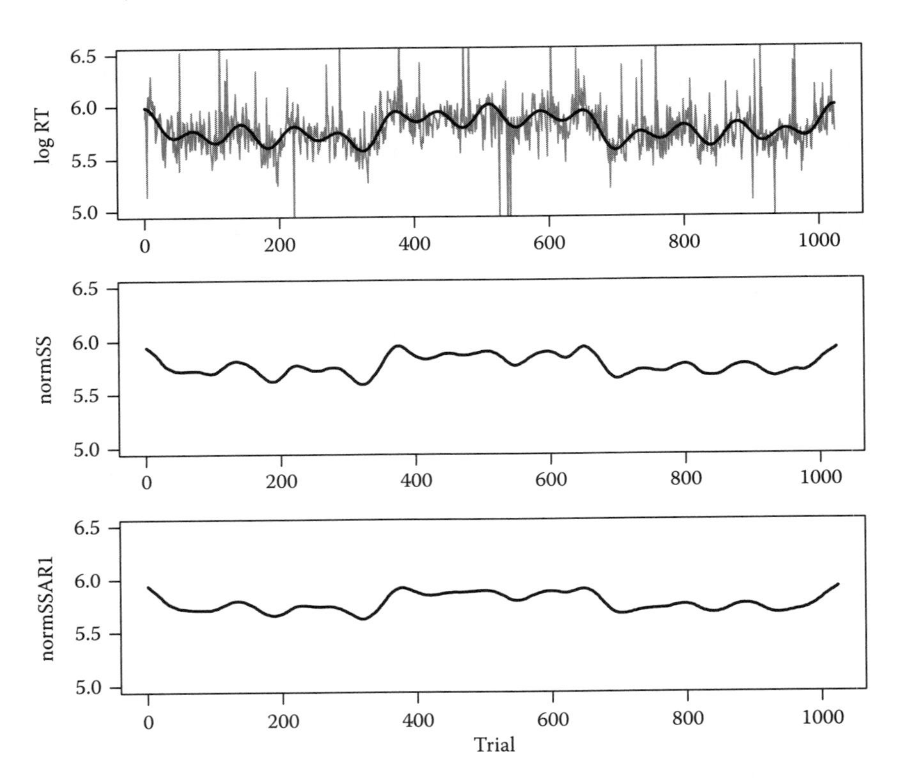

FIGURE 9.11 The top panel of the figure shows a realization of sinusoidal trend plus error with an autocorrelation parameter of $\phi = 0.4$. The solid line shows the true trend. The middle panel shows the estimated trend using the `normSS` method and the bottom panel shows the estimated `normSSAR1` trend.

Second, and more importantly, it is very hard to model correlated data with splines, because there is a trade-off between local trends and correlation in the errors. Figure 9.11 demonstrates this trade-off. The top panel shows a realization of the sinusoidal trend model with an autocorrelation parameter of $\phi = 0.4$ with the true trend superimposed as a black line. The middle and bottom panels show the estimated trend using the `normSS` and `normSSAR1` methods, respectively. The `normSSAR1` method removes more of the local dependence, leaving a smoother (more biased, but less variable) estimate of the trend, while the `normSS` method removes less. The middle panel of the figure shows that, for this example, `normSS` leads to oversmoothing of the trend component. Including an AR(1) error term in the procedure (bottom panel) apportions an additional part of the total variability to the error, leading to even more oversmoothing of the trend.

It appears that, at least for the models we have explored in this chapter, smoothing spline methods designed for correlated error structures do not contribute much additional benefit for estimating trend.

9.5 DISCUSSION AND CONCLUSIONS

In this chapter, we presented and evaluated several methods for detrending RT series. These included least-squares polynomial regression methods, local polynomial regression methods, MA filtering, and smoothing splines. In particular, we presented a new method using smoothing splines, the important component of which involves transforming the log RT series to Gaussian quantiles.

Most published studies of RT series suffer from several deficiencies. First, analyses are performed on the raw RTs: no attempt is made to transform the data to reduce the effect of heavy tails and skewness on the estimates of trend and autocorrelation. Second, outliers are removed and the resulting gaps in the series are closed, corrupting the autocorrelation structure in the data. Third, attempts to model and remove trend are focussed only on overly simplistic assumptions, usually linear or low-degree polynomial trend. These deficiencies result in inaccurate estimates of trend, meaning that when the estimated trend is removed from the series, it has not been removed completely. Therefore, conclusions about autocorrelation structure are inaccurate.

We showed that least-squares polynomial regression methods are effective only when the true trend is polynomial. While these methods may be effective for more complex trend, the resulting estimates are highly variable and therefore must be viewed with suspicion. In contrast, the normalized smoothing spline method performs well consistently.

One issue we discovered involves the attempt to model autocorrelation in the errors when using normalized smoothing splines for trend estimation. The R implementation of the procedure in Wang (1998) assumes a Gaussian AR(1) error structure. Our simulated data did not conform to this assumption and this additional step in the estimation procedure was rarely beneficial in the calculation of our estimates of trend.

In summary, we conclude that normalizing the log-transformed RT data provides considerable benefits in recovering accurate estimates of trend. Estimates based on smoothing splines were as good as, or better (in an MSE sense) than, any other procedure we considered. Thus, until other detrending methods demonstrate better accuracy than our normalized smoothing spline method, we advocate the following procedure for detrending RT series:

1. Transform the raw RT data to the log scale
2. Do not remove or trim outliers
3. Transform the log RT data to Gaussian quantiles
4. Estimate trend for the Gaussian quantiles using smoothing splines
5. Transform the trend back to the log RT scale using the inverse empirical cumulative distribution function and linear interpolation.

ACKNOWLEDGMENTS

This work is supported by the National Science Foundation under award numbers DMS-0604963, DMS-0605052, SES-0214574, and SES-0437251. The authors are grateful to E.J. Wagenmakers for making his data available for inclusion in this chapter. This work was supported in part by an allocation of computing time from the Ohio Supercomputer Center. R functions for the detrending of RT sequences can be downloaded from http://www.stat.osu.edu/~pfc/software.

REFERENCES

Arbib, M. A., & Arbib, P. H. (Eds.). (2003). *The handbook of brain theory and neural networks* (2nd ed.). Cambridge, MA: The MIT Press.

Bertelson, P. (1965). Serial choice reaction-time as a function of response versus signal-and-response repetition. *Nature, 206*, 217–218.

Brockwell, P. J., & Davis, R. A. (2002). *Introduction to time series and forecasting*. New York: Springer.

Cleveland, W. (1979). Robust locally weighted regression and smoothing scatterplots. *Journal of the American Statistical Association, 74*, 829–836.

Craigmile, P. F., Peruggia, M., & Van Zandt, T. (2006). *An autocorrelated mixture model for sequences of response time data*. Department of Statistics Technical Report Number 778, The Ohio State University.

Donders, F. C. (1969). On the speed of mental processes. *Acta Psychologica, 30*, 412–431. (Original work published in 1868. Translated by W. G. Koster)

Efron, B., & Tibshirani, R. (1993). *An introduction to the bootstrap*. Boca Raton: Chapman & Hall.

Farrell, S., Wagenmakers, E.-J., & Ratcliff, R. (2006). 1/f noise in human cognition: Is it ubiquitous, and what does it mean? *Psychonomic Bulletin & Review, 13*, 737–741.

Gilden, D. L. (1997). Fluctuations in the time required for elementary decisions. *Psychological Science, 8*, 296–301.

Gilden, D. L. (2001). Cognitive emissions of $1/f$ noise. *Psychological Review, 108*, 33–56.

Jones, M., Love, B. C., & Maddox, W. T. (2006). Recency effects as a window to generalization: Separating decisional and perceptual sequential effects in category learning. *Journal of Experimental Psychology: Learning, Memory, and Cognition, 32*, 316–332.

Kello, C. T., Beltz, B. C., Holden, J. G., & Van Orden, G. C. (2007). The emergent coordination of cognitive function. *Journal of Experimental Psychology: General, 136*(4), 551–568.

Lahiri, S. (2003). *Resampling methods for dependent data*. New York: Springer.

Loader, C. (1999). *Local regression and likelihood*. New York: Springer.

Luce, R. D. (1986). *Response times: Their role in inferring elementary mental organization*. New York: Oxford University Press.

Meeter, M., & Olivers, C. N. L. (2006). Intertrial priming stemming from ambiguity: A new account of priming in visual search. *Visual Cognition, 13*, 202–222.

Nesselroade, J. R. (1991). Interindividual differences in intraindividual change. In L. Collins & J. Horn (Eds.), *Best methods for the analysis of change* (pp. 92–106). Washington, DC: American Psychological Association.

Percival, D., & Walden, A. (1993). *Spectral analysis for physical applications*. Cambridge: Cambridge University Press.

Peruggia, M., Van Zandt, T., & Chen, M. (2002). Was it a car or a cat i saw? An analysis of response times for word recognition. *Case Studies in Bayesian Statistics*, 6 , 319–334.

Pressing, J., & Jolley-Rogers, G. (1997). Spectral properties of human cognition and skill. *Biological Cybernetics, 76*, 339–347.

Priestley, M. B. (1981). *Spectral analysis and time series* (Vol. 1). *Univariate series*. London: Academic Press.

Quinn, B. G., & Hannan, E. J. (2001). *The estimation and tracking of frequency*. Cambridge: Cambridge University Press.

Ratcliff, R. (1978). A theory of memory retrieval. *Psychological Review, 85,* 59–108.

Ratcliff, R., & Smith, P. L. (2004). A comparison of sequential sampling models for two-choice reaction time. *Psychological Review, 111,* 333–367.

Ratcliff, R., Van Zandt, T., & McKoon, G. (1999). Comparing connectionist and diffusion models of reaction time. *Psychological Review, 106,* 261–300.

Remington, R. J. (1969). Analysis of sequential effects on choice reaction times. *Journal of Experimental Psychology, 82,* 250–257.

Ruppert, D., Sheather, S. J., & Wand, M. P. (1995). An effective bandwidth selector for local least squares regression. *Journal of the American Statistical Association, 90,* 1257–1270.

Schall, J. D. (2003). Neural correlates of decision processes: neural and mental chronometry. *Current Opinion in Neurobiology, 12,* 182–186.

Stewart, N., Brown, G. D. A., & Chater, N. (2005). Absolute identification by relative judgment. *Psychological Review, 112,* 881–911.

Thornton, T. L., & Gilden, D. L. (2005). Provenance of correlations in psychological data. *Psychonomic Bulletin and Review, 12,* 409–441.

Titterington, D. M., Smith, A. F. M., & Makov, U. E. (1985). *Statistical analysis of finite mixture distributions.* Chichester: Wiley.

Van Orden, G. C., Holden, J. G., & Turvey, M. T. (2003). Self-organization of cognitive performance. *Journal of Experimental Psychology: General, 132,* 331–350.

Van Zandt, T., Colonius, H., & Proctor, R. W. (2000). A comparison of two response time models applied to perceptual matching. *Psychonomic Bulletin and Review, 7,* 208–256.

Wagenmakers, E.-J., Farrell, S., & Ratcliff, R. (2004). Estimation and interpretation of $1/f$ noise in human cognition. *Psychonomic Bulletin and Review, 11,* 569–612.

Wahba, G. (1990). *Spline models for observational data.* Philadelphia: SIAM (Society for Industrial and Applied Mathematics).

Wang, Y. (1998). Smoothing spline models with correlated random errors. *Journal of the American Statistical Association, 93,* 341–348.

10

Dynamic Factor Analysis with Ordinal Manifest Variables

Guangjian Zhang and Michael W. Browne

10.1 INTRODUCTION

Change is an important question in psychology (Boker & Wegner, 2007; Collins & Sayer, 2001; Walls & Schafer, 2005). Studying change requires measuring the same individual at multiple times. These measurements often form a time series. Because perfect measures of many psychological constructs such as moods and personality states do not exist, time series of psychological variables are usually contaminated by measurement error. Dynamic factor analysis (DFA) (Browne & Nesselroade, 2005; Browne & Zhang, 2007; Engle & Watson, 1981; Geweke & Singleton, 1981; Molenaar, 1985; Nesselroade, McArdle, Aggen, & Meyers, 2002) is a combination of factor analysis and time-series analysis and is an ideal tool for modeling multivariate time series with measurement error.

DFA is routinely applied to questionnaire data in practice (Ferrer & Nesselroade, 2003). Questionnaire data are ordinal, but most estimation methods of DFA were derived for continuous manifest variables; see Browne and Zhang (2007) and Molenaar (1985) for the lagged correlation approach,[†] Engle and Watson (1981) for the Kalman filter approach, and Geweke and Singleton (1981) for the frequency-domain approach.

[†] The DFA model can also be fitted to lagged covariances, but fitting the model to lagged correlations often leads to simpler interpretation.

Thus, modifications of the estimation methods are needed to accommodate ordinal manifest variables.

There have been a number of efforts to factor-analyze ordinal variables in the usual between-subject situation;[†] see Wirth and Edwards (2007) for a review. One popular approach is to assume that a continuous variable underlies each ordinal manifest variable. The factor analysis model is fitted to the correlation matrix of the underlying continuous variables rather than to that of the ordinal manifest variables. The correlation between two underlying continuous variables, often referred to as the polychoric correlation, is estimated from a contingency table formed from observations on the two ordinal manifest variables (Jöreskog, 1994; Olsson, 1979).

The purpose of the present chapter is to extend the polychoric correlation approach to the situation where the data are multivariate time series of ordinal variables. In the between-subject factor analysis, polychoric correlations are estimated from measurements made on many individuals at one time point. In DFA, polychoric correlations are estimated from measurements made on a single individual at multiple time points. In particular, estimation of the lagged polychoric correlation, a correlation between two underlying continuous variables where one variable lags behind another, is crucial in DFA, but is a nonissue in the usual between-subject factor analysis.

When DFA is applied to multivariate time series of ordinal variables in psychological research, the fact that ordinal variables are discrete is often ignored: Pearson's product moment correlations and lagged correlations are computed from ordinal variables directly as if they were continuous variables. In contrast, the polychoric approach takes into account the fact that ordinal variables are discrete: it estimates polychoric correlations and lagged correlations of underlying continuous variables. The two approaches proceed in the same way after lagged correlation matrices are obtained. For example, a Fortran program DyFA 2.03 (Browne & Zhang, 2005) can be used to estimate the DFA model by minimizing the distance between sample lagged correlation (Pearson's product moment or polychoric) matrices and the model implied lagged correlation matrices. The polychoric approach is more plausible than Pearson's product moment approach, because a linear function of continuous factors cannot result in

[†] Data are collected from multiple individuals in the between-subject situation. It seems reasonable to assume that data from different individuals are independent.

a discrete manifest variable. The polychoric approach has been shown to be superior to the Pearson's product moment approach in the usual between-subject factor analysis (Dolan, 1994). A simulation study will be carried out to compare these two approaches for DFA with multivariate time series of ordinal variables.

The chapter focusses on point estimation of the DFA model with ordinal manifest variables. Standard error and model testing in DFA are more difficult than those in the usual between-subject factor analysis, because the distribution of polychoric lagged correlations is intractable. Zhang (2006) used the parametric bootstrap to estimate the standard error and the test statistic of the DFA model with ordinal manifest variables but coverage of this work is beyond the scope of the chapter.

Independent work carried out by Rijn (2008) showed how LISREL may be employed to fit a process factor analysis model to lagged polychoric correlation coefficients. Virtually, the only resemblance between this method and our work is that both fit some type of process factor analysis correlation structure to polychoric correlation coefficients. There are substantial differences between the two approaches in the parameterization of the correlation structure, the polychoric correlations that are computed, the discrepancy function used, and the manner in which standard errors are obtained.

The rest of the chapter is organized as follows. We first describe the DFA model and its estimation for continuous manifest variables. We then consider the DFA model for ordinal manifest variables. In particular, we provide details about estimating lagged polychoric correlation matrices from ordinal variables where some variables lag behind others. We next illustrate the proposed procedure using both a simulation study and an empirical data set. The chapter ends with a few concluding comments.

10.2 DFA MODELS AND THEIR ESTIMATION

Two kinds of DFA models have been proposed for analyzing multivariate time series: the process factor analysis model (Browne & Nesselroade, 2005; Browne & Zhang, 2007; Engle & Watson, 1981; Immink, 1986; Nesselroade et al., 2002) and the shock factor analysis model (Browne & Nesselroade, 2005; Geweke & Singleton, 1981; Molenaar, 1985; Nesselroade et al., 2002).

The process DFA model consists of two parts. The factor analysis part relates the multivariate time series of manifest variables $\boldsymbol{y}_t$ to the multivariate latent factors $\boldsymbol{f}_t$,

$$\boldsymbol{y}_t = \boldsymbol{\mu} + \boldsymbol{\Lambda}\boldsymbol{f}_t + \boldsymbol{e}_t. \tag{10.1}$$

Here $\boldsymbol{\mu}$ is the mean vector of the manifest variables $\boldsymbol{y}_t$, $\boldsymbol{\Lambda}$ is an $m \times k$ factor loading matrix, and $\boldsymbol{e}_t$ is a vector of measurement errors. Integers m and k indicate the dimensions of $\boldsymbol{y}_t$ and $\boldsymbol{f}_t$, respectively. The subscript t denotes the tth measurement occasion. Note that $\boldsymbol{\mu}$ and $\boldsymbol{\Lambda}$ do not have the subscript t because they remain invariant across time. The second part of the model is the time-series part. The factors $\boldsymbol{f}_t$ follow a vector ARMA(p, q) process,

$$\boldsymbol{f}_t = \sum_{i=1}^{p} \boldsymbol{A}_i \boldsymbol{f}_{t-i} + \boldsymbol{z}_t + \sum_{j=1}^{q} \boldsymbol{B}_j \boldsymbol{z}_{t-j}. \tag{10.2}$$

Here $\boldsymbol{A}_i$ is the ith order autoregressive weight matrix representing the influence of $\boldsymbol{f}_{t-i}$ on $\boldsymbol{f}_t$, $\boldsymbol{B}_j$ is the jth order moving average weight matrix representing the influence of $\boldsymbol{z}_{t-j}$ on $\boldsymbol{f}_t$, and $\boldsymbol{z}_t$ is a vector of shock variables. The integers p and q represent the AR order and the MA order, respectively. Different components of $\boldsymbol{z}_t$ can correlate with each other within the same time point but not across different time points. A key characteristic of this model is that the latent factors $\boldsymbol{f}_t$ directly affect only the concurrent manifest variables, $\boldsymbol{y}_t$. The influence of factors $\boldsymbol{f}_t$ on later manifest variables $\boldsymbol{y}_{t+s} (s > 0)$ is through their influence on later factors $\boldsymbol{f}_{t+s}$.

Another extension of the common factor model specifies that manifest variables $\boldsymbol{y}_t$ are dependent directly upon the concurrent common factors, $\boldsymbol{u}_t$, and previous common factors, $\boldsymbol{u}_{t-1}, \boldsymbol{u}_{t-2}, \ldots, \boldsymbol{u}_{t-l}$,

$$\boldsymbol{y}_t = \sum_{i=0}^{l} \boldsymbol{\Lambda}_i \boldsymbol{u}_{t-i} + \boldsymbol{e}_t. \tag{10.3}$$

The common factors $\boldsymbol{u}_t$ are like the shock variables $\boldsymbol{z}_t$ in Equation 10.2: different components of $\boldsymbol{u}_t$ can correlate with each other within the same time point but not across different time points. Thus, the model has been referred to as the shock factor analysis model (Browne & Nesselroade, 2005) and the white noise factor score model (Nesselroade et al., 2002). The shock variables $\boldsymbol{z}_t$ in Equation 10.2 affect concurrent and all future manifest variables, but the influences are indirect. In contrast, the shock variables $\boldsymbol{u}_t$ affect the concurrent and future manifest variables at the next l time points, and the influences are direct. For example, the factor matrix $\boldsymbol{\Lambda}_0$ indicates the influence of $\boldsymbol{u}_t$ on $\boldsymbol{y}_t$, $\boldsymbol{\Lambda}_1$ the influence of $\boldsymbol{u}_t$ on $\boldsymbol{y}_{t+1}$, and $\boldsymbol{\Lambda}_l$ the influence of $\boldsymbol{u}_t$ on $\boldsymbol{y}_{t+l}$. The shock variables $\boldsymbol{u}_t$ have no influence on manifest variables at time points later than $t + l$.

Comparisons of these two models may be found in Browne and Nesselroade (2005), Nesselroade et al. (2002), and Molenaar and Nesselroade (2001). Conceptually, Molenaar (1985, p. 185, lines 17–18) made use of a representation of DFA that is similar to the shock factor analysis model in Equation 10.3 but replaces the finite number of lags, l, by ∞. Browne and Nesselroade (2005, pp. 447–448, Equations 26 and 27) show how the infinite lag representation of a DFA model is a consequence of the classic Wold decomposition (Hamilton, 1994, pp. 108–109), which represents any stationary time series by an infinite lag moving average time series. It is conceptually interesting that the infinite lag representation will not only include all finite lag ARMA-based process factor analysis models defined by Equations 10.1 and 10.2 but also all possible process factor analysis models defined by Equation 10.1 with Equation 10.2 replaced by any stationary time series. Although the infinite lag representation is of theoretical interest, it is not a usable statistical model because it involves infinitely many parameters and estimation is impossible.

For practical use, Molenaar (1985, Equation 3) truncated the infinite lag representation of a latent time series at a finite number of lags to yield the finite lag shock factor model given here in Equation 10.3. Unlike the infinite lag representation, Molenaar's finite lag shock factor analysis model will no longer contain the finite lag process factor analysis model as a special case if $p > 0$ (Browne & Nesselroade, 2005, p. 448). A finite shock factor analysis model may only be regarded as an approximation to a process factor analysis model. Because the approximating shock model requires more parameters than the process model that is approximated, the shock factor analysis approximation will not satisfy the parsimony principle, also known as Occam's razor (Everitt, 2006).

Molenaar (1985) fitted the shock DFA model to a Block Toeplitz matrix consisting of lagged correlation matrices using standard SEM software. The same approach can be used with the process DFA model (Nesselroade et al., 2002). In this approach, the maximum Wishart likelihood estimation option of SEM computer programs has been employed. Because the Wishart likelihood function is inappropriate for lagged correlation matrices, the estimates and test statistic do not have the desirable asymptotic properties of maximum likelihood. Consequently, this estimation process has been referred to as pseudo-maximum likelihood (Molenaar & Nesselroade, 1998).†

Du Toit and Browne (2007, Equation 11, p. 78) derived the covariance structure of a multivariate ARMA time series. Their derivation involves an initial state vector that encapsulates the influences of the preceding time series. The covariance matrix of this initial state vector is a nonlinear function of autoregressive weight matrices, moving average weight matrices, and the shock variable covariance matrix (Du Toit & Browne, 2007, Equation 21, p. 81). The covariance structure of a VARMA process can be employed both for manifest variables and for latent variables. In Browne and Zhang (2007, Equations 13.19 and 13.20 on p. 276), this covariance structure was simplified into a recurrence relation for the lagged correlation function of a stationary latent VARMA time series and employed in DFA. Methods for obtaining estimates were also described (Browne & Zhang, 2007, Equation 13.14, p. 273). These were implemented in the computer program DyFA 2.03 (Browne & Zhang, 2005).

The aforementioned model specification and estimation are suitable for continuous manifest variables. In psychological research, manifest variables are often ordinal variables like questionnaire items. It is natural to assume that a continuous variable underlies an ordinal manifest variable and that the underlying continuous variables satisfy a DFA model. Next, we describe how to estimate lagged correlation matrices of underlying continuous variables from ordinal manifest variables.

10.3 POLYCHORIC LAGGED CORRELATIONS

Many applications of DFA, or its precursor, the P technique, involve questionnaire data (Borkenau & Ostendorf, 1998; Ferrer & Nesselroade, 2003; Lebo & Nesselroade, 1978). In these studies, participants select one response from a few alternatives, for example, "strongly disagree," "disagree," "neutral," "agree," and "strongly agree." In practice, questionnaire data are often treated as if they were continuous and Pearson's product

† In statistics, a product of independent conditional likelihoods is often referred to as a pseudo-likelihood (Upton & Cook, 2006).

moment correlations are computed in the usual manner. Because the data are discrete, it is natural to assume that the DFA model is satisfied by underlying continuous variables y^* that underlie ordinal manifest variables y (Jöreskog, 1994; Olsson, 1979),

$$y_t^* = \mathbf{\Lambda} f_t + e_t. \tag{10.4}$$

Note that ordinal manifest variables y_t in general do not satisfy the model.

If the ordinal manifest variable involves c categories, its relation with the underlying continuous variable y^* can be expressed[†] as

$$\begin{aligned} y &= 1 \quad \text{if } y^* < \tau_1, \\ &\vdots \\ y &= i \quad \text{if } \tau_{i-1} \leq y^* < \tau_i, \\ &\vdots \\ y &= c \quad \text{if } \tau_{c-1} \leq y^*. \end{aligned}$$

The correspondence involves $c - 1$ thresholds $\tau_1, \ldots, \tau_i, \ldots, \tau_{c-1}$. Although the underlying continuous variables are not measured directly, their correlations can be estimated from the corresponding ordinal variables. These correlations are referred to as polychoric correlations (Bollen, 1989, pp. 441–442). Procedures for estimating polychoric correlations also produce threshold estimates as a by-product.

Because DFA involves modeling lagged correlations among variables at different time points, more notation are needed to accommodate the lagged relations. Let $y_{t,i}$ be the ith ordinal manifest variable at time t and $y_{t,i}^*$ be its underlying continuous variable. The most general case is the polychoric cross-correlation $\rho_{l,i,j}$ between $y_{t+l,i}^*$ and $y_{t,j}^*$, which is the correlation between two variables separated by l time points. The ith variable lags the jth variable l time points. On the other hand, if the jth variable lags the ith variable l time points, the polychoric cross-correlation becomes $\rho_{l,j,i}$. These two correlations are in general different.

When l is zero, there is no time lag between these two variables. Thus, the polychoric cross-correlation becomes a polychoric correlation $\rho_{0,i,j}$. When

[†] We omit the subscript t, because the correspondence between observed discrete variables and underlying continuous variables remains invariant at different time points.

i and j are equal, the polychoric cross-correlation becomes a polychoric autocorrelation, which is the correlation of a variable with itself at l time points later.

For multivariate time series of ordinal variables $\boldsymbol{y}_t$, their polychoric lagged correlations form polychoric lagged correlation matrices, $\boldsymbol{R}_l = \text{corr}(\boldsymbol{y}_{t+l}, \boldsymbol{y}'_t)$. Note that the $m \times m$ polychoric lagged correlation matrix at lag l contains both polychoric autocorrelations $\rho_{l,i,i}$ (diagonal elements) and polychoric cross-correlations $\rho_{l,i,j}$ (off-diagonal elements). The lag 0 polychoric correlation matrix is symmetric, but polychoric lagged correlation matrices at $l > 0$ are nonsymmetric.

The lagged correlation coefficients are estimated using the contingency tables formed from observations on pairs of ordinal variables. To construct a contingency table, we first rearrange the two observed ordinal variables in the following way:

$$\begin{bmatrix} y_{1,i} & y_{1+l,j} \\ y_{2,i} & y_{2+l,j} \\ y_{3,i} & y_{3+l,j} \\ \vdots & \vdots \\ y_{T-l-1,i} & y_{T-1,j} \\ y_{T-l,i} & y_{T,j} \end{bmatrix}.$$

These two columns of discrete scores are then treated as if they were scores from $T - l$ different individuals. A contingency table as shown in Table 10.1 is constructed. The entry at the ath row and the bth column represents the number of cases where $y_{t,i} = a$ and $y_{t+l,j} = b$. An estimate of the probability $P(y_{t,i} = a, y_{t+l,j} = b)$ is then given by the proportion

$$\widehat{P}(y_{t,i} = a, y_{t+l,j} = b) = \frac{n_{ab}}{n_{11} + n_{12} + \cdots + n_{cc}}.$$

Olsson (1979) described two methods for estimating the polychoric correlation from a contingency table: a single-stage method and a two-stage method. The single-stage method estimates the polychoric correlation and thresholds simultaneously. On the other hand, the two-stage method first estimates thresholds from univariate normal distributions,

$$p(y \leq a) = \Phi(y^* < \tau_a). \tag{10.5}$$

It then estimates the polychoric correlation with thresholds fixed at the values obtained at the first stage.

TABLE 10.1

Contingency Table for Estimating $\rho_{h,j,i}$

		$y_{t+h,j}$					
		1	2	$\cdots$	b	$\cdots$	c
$y_{t,i}$	1	n_{11}	n_{12}	$\cdots$	n_{1b}	$\cdots$	n_{1c}
	2	n_{21}	n_{22}	$\cdots$	n_{2b}	$\cdots$	n_{2c}
	$\vdots$	$\vdots$	$\vdots$	$\ddots$	$\vdots$	$\ddots$	$\vdots$
	a	n_{a1}	n_{a2}	$\cdots$	n_{ab}	$\cdots$	n_{ac}
	$\vdots$	$\vdots$	$\vdots$	$\ddots$	$\vdots$	$\ddots$	$\vdots$
	c	n_{c1}	n_{c2}	$\cdots$	n_{cb}	$\cdots$	n_{cc}

Note: Each variable has c categories. The sum of all entries is $T - h$.

The two-stage method is usually preferred for three reasons (Jöreskog, 1994, p. 384). First, a major disadvantage of the single-stage method is that the same ordinal variable has different threshold estimates when it is paired with different other variables. Second, the two-stage method is computationally simpler than the one-stage method. Third, the two methods produce similar polychoric correlation estimates. We consequently use the two-stage method to estimate polychoric lagged correlation matrices for multivariate time series of ordinal variables.

We now summarize the polychoric approach for estimating the DFA model with ordinal manifest variables.

1. Construct contingency tables for every pair of the ordinal variables at every lag.
2. Use the two-stage method to estimate the polychoric lagged correlations from the contingency tables.
3. Arrange the polychoric lagged correlations properly to form the polychoric lagged correlation matrices.
4. Estimate the DFA model by minimizing the ordinary least squares discrepancy function (Browne & Zhang, 2007, pp. 277–283).

10.4 A SIMULATION STUDY

10.4.1 Design and Population Parameter Values

A simulation study was carried out to illustrate the polychoric correlation approach for estimating DFA models with ordinal variables and to compare the polychoric approach and Pearson's product moment approach. The process factor analysis model (Equations 10.1 and 10.2) was employed in the simulation study. It involved three time-series lengths ($T = 100$, 200, and 1000), three category numbers ($c = 2$, 3, and 5), and two ways of estimating lagged manifest variable correlations (polychoric correlations and Pearson product moment correlations). In each condition, $N = 1000$ multivariate time series of ordinal variables were generated.

The model involves 10 variables and 2 factors. The factor loading matrix used is

$$\mathbf{\Lambda} = \begin{bmatrix} 0.5 & 0.6 & 0.7 & 0.8 & 0.9 & 0 & 0 & 0 & 0 & 0 \\ 0 & 0 & 0 & 0 & 0 & 0.5 & 0.6 & 0.7 & 0.8 & 0.9 \end{bmatrix}'$$

and the variances of the independently and normally distributed error variables $\boldsymbol{e}_t$ are

$$\boldsymbol{\sigma}_\epsilon^2 = \begin{bmatrix} 0.75 & 0.64 & 0.51 & 0.36 & 0.19 & 0.75 & 0.64 & 0.51 & 0.36 & 0.19 \end{bmatrix}.$$

The two factors follow an AR(1) process with AR weight matrix $\boldsymbol{A}^\dagger$ given by

$$\boldsymbol{A} = \begin{bmatrix} 0.40 & 0.32 \\ 0 & 0.60 \end{bmatrix}.$$

Shock variables $\boldsymbol{Z}_i$ are distributed as $N_2(\mathbf{0}, \mathbf{\Psi})$,‡ where

$$\mathbf{\Psi} = \begin{bmatrix} 0.73 & -0.17 \\ -0.17 & 0.64 \end{bmatrix}.$$

It follows from Browne and Zhang (2007, p. 270, Equation 13.8) that the initial state vector implied by the stationary time series is distributed as $N_2(\mathbf{0}, \mathbf{\Theta})$, where

$$\mathbf{\Theta} = \begin{bmatrix} 0.27 & 0.20 \\ 0.20 & 0.36 \end{bmatrix}.$$

Note that elements of $\mathbf{\Theta}$ are not parameters but functions of the AR weight matrix and shock variable covariance matrix.

† The complete notation for the AR weight matrix should be $\boldsymbol{A}_1$. For simple presentation, we omit the subscript.

‡ The symbol $N_p(\boldsymbol{\mu}, \mathbf{\Sigma})$ denotes the p variate normal distribution with the mean vector $\boldsymbol{\mu}$ and covariance matrix $\mathbf{\Sigma}$.

These distributional assumptions imply that the marginal distributions of the continuous variables underlying the ordinal manifest variables are the standard normal distribution. Converting continuous variables to ordinal variables involves comparing the continuous variables with thresholds. Figure 10.1 displays the thresholds for two-category, three-category, and five-category ordinal variables.

10.4.2 Data Generation

Multivariate time series of ordinal manifest variables were generated by a three-step method: generation of continuous factors, generation of continuous manifest variables, and conversion of continuous manifest variables to ordinal manifest variables.

At the first step, multivariate time series of continuous factors were generated according to Equation 10.2. Generation of the factors at the first

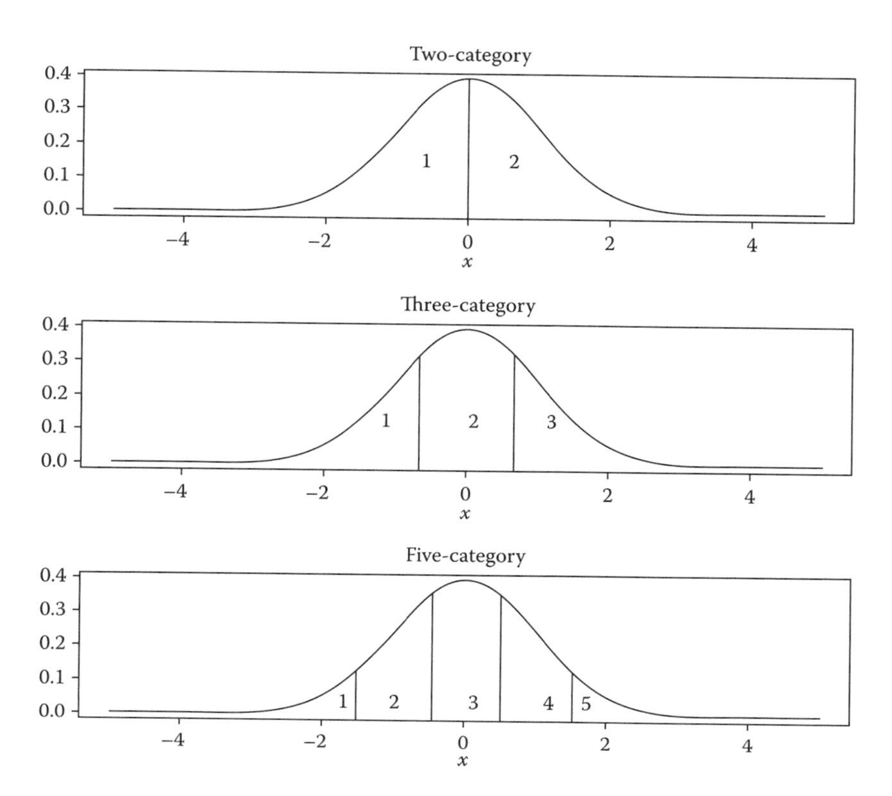

FIGURE 10.1 Correspondence of continuous variables and ordinal variables.

time point, f_1, required the initial state vector, x (Browne & Zhang, 2007, Equation 13.5),

$$f_1 = x + z_1. \tag{10.6}$$

The initial state vector x was generated from $N_2(\mathbf{0}, \mathbf{\Theta})$. Shock variables z_1 were generated from $N_2(\mathbf{0}, \mathbf{\Psi})$. Factors at other time points, $f_2, f_3, \ldots, f_T$, were generated by applying Equation 10.2 where the corresponding z_i was generated from $N_2(\mathbf{0}, \mathbf{\Psi})$.

At the second step, multivariate time series of continuous manifest variables $y_1^*, y_2^*, \ldots, y_T^*$ were generated according to Equation 10.1. The factor scores $f_1, f_2, \ldots, f_T$ were generated at the first step. Measurement error variables e_i were generated from independent univariate normal distributions $N_1(0, \sigma_{\epsilon,i}^2)$.

At the third step, multivariate time series of continuous manifest variables $y_1^*, y_2^*, \ldots, y_T^*$ were converted to multivariate time series of ordinal manifest variables $y_1, y_2, \ldots, y_T$ by the scheme displayed in Figure 10.1. For example, three-category ordinal variables involve two thresholds: -0.67 and 0.67. If the continuous variable $y_{t,i}^*$ is less than -0.67, the ordinal variable $y_{t,i}$ is 1; if the continuous variables $y_{t,i}^*$ lies between -0.67 and 0.67, the ordinal variable $y_{t,i}$ is 2; if the continuous variable $y_{t,i}^*$ is larger than 0.67, the ordinal variable $y_{t,i}$ is 3.

10.4.3 Model Estimation

The polychoric approach and Pearson's product moment approach differ in the way manifest variable lagged correlation matrices are computed. Polychoric lagged correlations are estimated from contingency tables formed from ordinal manifest variables. Pearson's product moment lagged correlations are computed from ordinal manifest variables directly as if they were continuous variables. After manifest variable lagged correlation matrices are obtained, the two procedures proceed in the same way. Both polychoric lagged correlation matrices and Pearson's product moment lagged correlation matrices were estimated using the Fortran program DyFA 2.03 (Browne & Zhang, 2005). Estimation of the DFA model with lagged correlation matrices was carried out using the same program.

The fitted model is a two-factor exploratory factor analysis model with dynamic factors following an AR(1) process. A two-stage estimation method was used (Browne & Zhang, 2005, p. 10): factor loadings were estimated from the lag 0 correlation matrix, and the AR weight matrix and shock variable covariance matrix were estimated from lagged factor correlation matrices at lags 1 and 2. Oblique target rotation (Browne, 2001) was used. The target matrix was constructed from the aforementioned factor loading matrix: factor loadings of zero were specified as zero in the target matrix and other loadings were unspecified. Note that target rotation in exploratory factor analysis differs from confirmatory factor analysis: in target rotation, elements of the factor loading matrix that correspond to zero target elements are made close to zero in a least squares sense, whereas they are forced to be equal to zero in confirmatory factor analysis.

10.4.4 Results

One thousand multivariate time series of ordinal manifest variables were generated for each combination of time-series lengths and category numbers. The polychoric approach and Pearson's product moment approach each produced $N = 1000$ replications of the rotated factor loading matrix, factor AR matrix, and shock variable covariance matrix. Means and standard deviations of parameter estimates in each condition were computed from the $N = 1000$ replications.

Table 10.2 shows the estimate means and standard deviations of three factor loadings, λ_{11}, λ_{31}, and λ_{51}. Other factor loadings have a similar pattern. Also shown in Table 10.2 are an autoregressive weight, $\boldsymbol{A}_{11}$, and a shock variable variance, $\boldsymbol{\Psi}_{11}$. Other time-series parameters have a similar pattern.

We highlight four aspects of the means and standard deviations of the factor loading estimates. First, the polychoric factor loading estimates are essentially unbiased, but Pearson's product moment factor loading estimates are biased. For example, the population value of λ_{51} is 0.9 and the mean of the polychoric estimates is 0.89 but the mean of Pearson's product moment estimates is 0.75 in the condition where the time-series length T is 100 and ordinal manifest variables have two categories. Second, the polychoric factor loading estimates have smaller mean-squared errors than the corresponding Pearson's product moment factor loading estimates. Mean-squared error is a measure of estimator accuracy, and it consists of two parts: the estimator bias and variance. Mean-squared errors of polychoric factor loading estimates are mainly due to estimator variances; mean-squared errors of Pearson's product moment factor loading

TABLE 10.2

Means and Standard Deviations of Parameter Estimates: A Simulation Study

	True	Poly2	PM2	Poly3	PM3	Poly5	PM5
				$T = 100$			
λ_{11}	0.50	0.50 (0.13)	0.40 (0.11)	0.50 (0.11)	0.45 (0.10)	0.50 (0.10)	0.48 (0.09)
λ_{31}	0.70	0.70 (0.11)	0.57 (0.10)	0.70 (0.08)	0.63 (0.08)	0.70 (0.07)	0.67 (0.07)
λ_{51}	0.90	0.89 (0.08)	0.75 (0.08)	0.89 (0.06)	0.81 (0.06)	0.89 (0.05)	0.85 (0.05)
$\boldsymbol{A}_{11}$	0.73	0.73 (0.12)	0.76 (0.11)	0.73 (0.11)	0.74 (0.10)	0.73 (0.10)	0.74 (0.10)
$\boldsymbol{\Psi}_{11}$	0.40	0.36 (0.13)	0.34 (0.13)	0.36 (0.12)	0.35 (0.11)	0.37 (0.11)	0.36 (0.11)
				$T = 200$			
λ_{11}	0.50	0.50 (0.09)	0.39 (0.08)	0.50 (0.07)	0.45 (0.07)	0.50 (0.07)	0.48 (0.06)
λ_{31}	0.70	0.70 (0.08)	0.57 (0.07)	0.70 (0.06)	0.63 (0.05)	0.70 (0.05)	0.67 (0.05)
λ_{51}	0.90	0.90 (0.06)	0.76 (0.06)	0.90 (0.04)	0.82 (0.04)	0.90 (0.04)	0.86 (0.03)
$\boldsymbol{A}_{11}$	0.73	0.73 (0.08)	0.75 (0.08)	0.73 (0.08)	0.74 (0.08)	0.73 (0.08)	0.73 (0.08)
$\boldsymbol{\Psi}_{11}$	0.40	0.38 (0.09)	0.36 (0.09)	0.39 (0.08)	0.38 (0.08)	0.39 (0.08)	0.38 (0.08)
				$T = 1000$			
λ_{11}	0.50	0.50 (0.04)	0.39 (0.03)	0.50 (0.03)	0.45 (0.03)	0.50 (0.03)	0.48 (0.03)
λ_{31}	0.70	0.70 (0.03)	0.57 (0.03)	0.70 (0.03)	0.63 (0.02)	0.70 (0.02)	0.67 (0.02)
λ_{51}	0.90	0.90 (0.03)	0.76 (0.03)	0.90 (0.02)	0.82 (0.02)	0.90 (0.02)	0.86 (0.02)
$\boldsymbol{A}_{11}$	0.73	0.73 (0.04)	0.75 (0.04)	0.73 (0.04)	0.74 (0.04)	0.73 (0.04)	0.73 (0.04)
$\boldsymbol{\Psi}_{11}$	0.40	0.40 (0.04)	0.38 (0.04)	0.40 (0.04)	0.39 (0.04)	0.40 (0.03)	0.40 (0.03)

Note: Poly2, Poly3, and Poly5 represent the polychoric approach with two-category, three-category, and five-category manifest variables, respectively; PM2, PM3, and PM5 represent the product moment approach with two-category, three-category, and five-category manifest variables, respectively. Standard deviations are shown in parentheses. T represents time-series lengths.

estimates are due to both estimator biases and variances. Third, as the time-series length increases, the factor loading standard deviations decrease. The reduction in factor loading estimate standard deviations is proportional to the square root of the increase in time-series lengths. For example, the polychoric estimate standard deviations for $\widehat{\lambda}_{11}$ are 0.13, 0.09, and 0.04 at time-series lengths $T = 100$, 200, and 1000, respectively. Increasing the time-series length has little effect on parameter estimate means. For example, Pearson's product moment estimate means for $\widehat{\lambda}_{11}$ are 0.40, 0.39, and 0.39 at time-series lengths $T = 100$, 200, and 1000, respectively. Fourth, increasing categories brings about two benefits. The first benefit is the decrease in biases of Pearson's product moment factor loading estimates. The second benefit is the decrease in standard deviations for both polychoric factor loading estimates and Pearson's product moment factor loading estimates.

Also shown in Table 10.2 are two time-series parameters: the AR weight A_{11} and the shock variable variance Ψ_{11}. Like the estimates of factor loadings, the polychoric estimates of time-series parameters are essentially unbiased. As the sample size increases, estimate standard deviations decrease. The rate of standard deviation decrease is proportional to the square root of sample size increase. The beneficial effect of increasing manifest variable categories are also observed with time-series parameters. For example, Pearson's product moment estimate means for $\widehat{A}_{11}$ at $T = 200$ are 0.75, 0.74, and 0.73 for two-category, three-category, and five-category ordinal manifest variables. Increasing the number of categories also leads to a reduction in estimate standard deviations. For example, the polychoric estimate standard deviations of $\widehat{A}_{11}$ at $T = 100$ are 0.12, 0.11, and 0.10 for two-category, three-category, and five-category ordinal manifest variables. The beneficial effects of increasing ordinal manifest variable categories seem more substantial for factor loadings than for time-series parameters.

The biases of Pearson's product moment time-series parameter estimates are less substantial than those of Pearson's product moment factor loading estimates. Furthermore, the biases of Pearson's product moment time-series parameter estimates diminish as the time-series length increases. For example, Pearson's product moment estimate means for Ψ_{11} of the two-category case are 0.34, 0.36, and 0.38 at time-series lengths of $T = 100, 200,$ and 1000.

Because the simulation study involves only one set of parameters, the results should be viewed with caution. Nevertheless, it suggests that the polychoric approach provides consistent estimates for DFA. At short time-series lengths like $T = 100$, mean-squared errors of polychoric estimates are reasonable. We next illustrate the polychoric approach using an empirical example.

10.5 AN EMPIRICAL EXAMPLE

The multivariate time series of the empirical example is a part of a study† (Borkenau & Ostendorf, 1998, Individual # 9) on the big five personality states. The time series consists of daily ratings of 30 adjectives on 90 days.

† We are indebted to the authors for making their data available to us.

These adjectives are listed in Table 10.3. The ratings range from 0 to 6. Figure 10.2 displays the time series of four adjectives, "irritable," "reserved," "selfish," and "industrious." The four time series show substantial day-to-day variation. Time series of other adjectives are similar.

An exploratory DFA model specifying a VAR(1) time series for the five factors was fitted to these data. The computer program DyFA 2.03 (Browne & Zhang, 2005) was used to estimate the model using both the

TABLE 10.3

The Factor Loading Matrix: The Polychoric Approach

	N	E	A	C	I
Irritable	**0.83**	−0.10	−0.07	0.13	0.12
Bad tempered	**0.03**	−0.18	−0.53	0.18	−0.25
Vulnerable	**0.90**	−0.16	0.09	0.04	−0.02
Emotionally stable	**−0.80**	−0.10	−0.22	0.08	−0.05
Calm	**−0.61**	−0.23	−0.05	0.14	0.24
Resistent	**−0.77**	0.20	0.01	−0.17	−0.07
Dynamic	−0.05	**0.83**	−0.01	0.22	0.00
Sociable	−0.17	**0.71**	0.04	0.11	0.11
Lively	−0.04	**0.87**	−0.18	0.07	0.08
Shy	0.05	**−0.73**	−0.03	0.08	−0.08
Silent	−0.10	**−0.62**	−0.21	−0.07	−0.15
Reserved	0.00	**−0.91**	0.05	−0.03	−0.01
Good natured	0.15	0.03	**0.35**	−0.02	0.60
Helpful	0.15	0.20	**0.22**	0.18	0.33
Considerate	0.05	−0.03	**0.59**	0.16	0.19
Selfish	0.01	0.08	**−0.70**	−0.16	0.10
Domineering	−0.07	0.03	**−0.93**	0.01	0.22
Obstinate	−0.05	0.00	**−0.71**	0.28	0.30
Industrious	0.20	0.27	−0.18	**0.70**	−0.10
Persistent	−0.04	0.35	−0.12	**0.35**	0.31
Responsible	−0.15	−0.30	0.32	**0.66**	0.09
Lazy	−0.19	−0.32	0.16	**−0.72**	0.27
Reckless	0.04	0.53	−0.34	**−0.45**	−0.19
Changeable	0.22	0.05	−0.28	**0.13**	0.02
Witty	0.00	−0.03	0.33	0.27	**0.27**
Knowledgeable	0.07	0.18	−0.35	0.12	**0.59**
Prudent	−0.21	0.40	0.13	0.41	**0.01**
Unresourceful	0.00	−0.58	−0.43	0.14	**−0.13**
Uninformed	−0.02	−0.12	0.11	0.03	**−0.49**
Unimaginative	−0.04	−0.56	−0.42	−0.02	**0.04**

Note: N, E, A, C, and I represent neuroticism, extraversion, agreeableness, conscientiousness, and intellect, respectively. Factor loadings in bold face were expected to be substantial and other factor loadings were expected to be small.

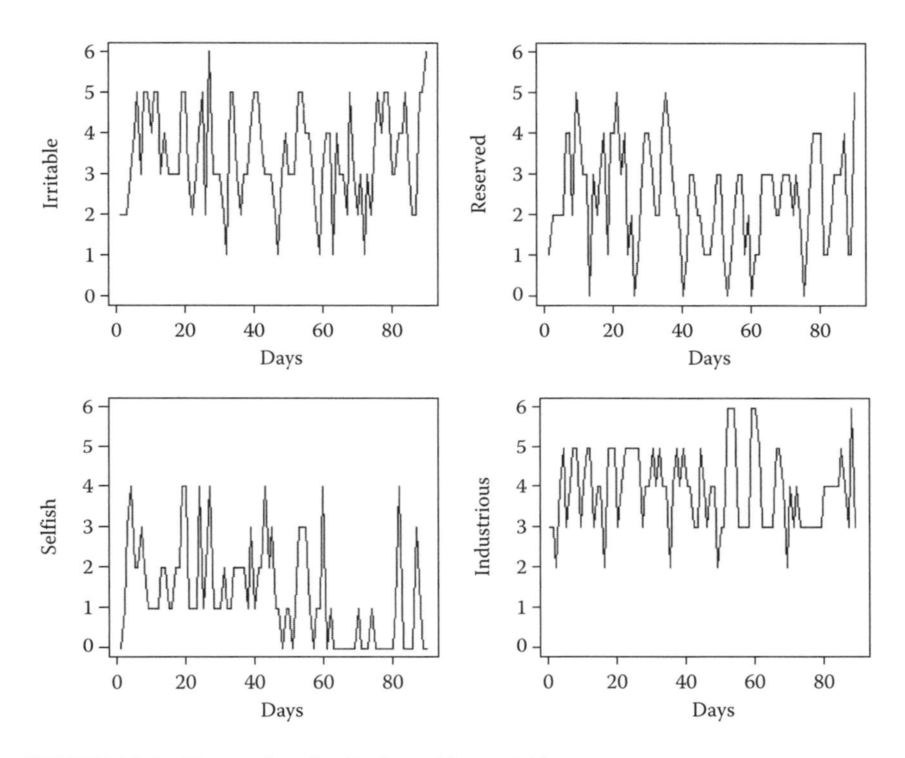

FIGURE 10.2 Time series of ordinal manifest variables.

polychoric approach and Pearson's product moment approach. A two-stage method was employed. First, factor loadings were estimated from lag 0 manifest variable correlation matrices. Secondly, the AR weight matrix, shock variable covariance matrix, and predicted variable covariance matrix were estimated from lag 1 and lag 2 manifest variable correlation matrices. A target rotation was carried out to aid interpretation and identification. The target matrix was specified to reflect the fact that the 30 adjectives are marker variables of the big five factors: these loadings were expected to be substantial and are shown in bold face in Table 10.3.

Factor loading estimates of the polychoric approach are shown in Table 10.3. Four factors, "neuroticism," "extraversion," "agreeableness," and "conscientiousness," are well represented by their corresponding marker variables. For example, all six markers load substantially on the factor extraversion and the smallest one is −0.62. Some loadings of marker variables on their factors are small: the loadings of "witty," "prudent,"

TABLE 10.4

The AR Matrix and the Predicted Factor Covariance Matrix: The Polychoric Approach

	N	E	A	C	I
			$\widehat{A}$		
Neuroticism	0.44	0.22	−0.08	−0.06	−0.16
Extraversion	−0.42	0.28	0.29	0.15	0.08
Agreeableness	0.05	0.12	0.81	−0.07	−0.09
Conscientiousness	−0.24	−0.10	−0.09	0.30	0.32
Intellect	−0.09	0.05	0.03	−0.02	0.41
			$\widehat{\Theta}_{11}$		
Neuroticism	0.25	−0.16	−0.01	−0.15	−0.09
Extraversion	−0.16	0.39	0.24	0.14	0.13
Agreeableness	−0.01	0.24	0.68	−0.13	0.03
Conscientiousness	−0.15	0.14	−0.13	0.27	0.16
Intellect	−0.09	0.13	0.03	0.16	0.18

Note: N, E, A, C, and I represent neuroticism, extraversion, agreeableness, conscientiousness, and intellect, respectively.

"unresourceful," and "unimaginative" on the factor "intellect" are 0.27, 0.01, −0.13, and 0.04, respectively. Several large factor loadings were unexpected. For example, the loading of "bad tempered" on "agreeableness" is −0.53; the loading of "good natured" on "intellect" is 0.60; the loading of unresourceful on extraversion is −0.58; the loading of unimaginative on extraversion is −0.56. This factor loading matrix represents the specific pattern for this particular individual. Other individuals may have different patterns.[†]

Estimates of the factor AR weight matrix and predicted factor covariance matrix of the polychoric approach are shown in Table 10.4. Elements of the AR weight matrix indicate the influence of yesterday's factors on today's factors. For example, the AR weight of agreeableness on itself is 0.81: the more agreeable the participant was on a certain day, the more agreeable the participant tended to be on the next day. The predicted factors capture the influence of preceding factors on the current factors (Browne & Zhang, 2007, Equations 21 and 22). In particular, each diagonal element of the predicted factor covariance matrix indicates the amount of variances of the

† An example of a somewhat different factor loading pattern for Borkenau and Ostendorf's (1988) subject # 1 is given by Browne and Zhang (2007, Table 1).

factor at the current point accounted for by factors at preceding time points (Browne & Zhang, 2007, Equation 23). Thus, preceding factors account for 68% of variance in agreeableness and preceding factors account for less than 50% of variances of the other four factors.

Estimates of factor loadings of Pearson's product moment approach are shown in Table 10.5. Most Pearson's product moment factor loading estimates are smaller than their corresponding polychoric factor loading estimates shown in Table 10.3. For example, the loading of "domineering" on agreeableness is −0.78 under Pearson's product moment approach but is −0.93 under the polychoric approach; the loading of industriousness on conscientiousness is 0.60 under Pearson's product moment approach but is 0.70 under the polychoric approach. They are consistent with a result of the simulation studies: Pearson's product moment approach with ordinal variables gives biased factor loading estimates. A few Pearson's product moment factor loading estimates are larger than the corresponding polychoric factor loading estimates, however. For example, the factor loading of "uninformed" on intellect is −0.64 under Pearson's product moment approach but is −0.49 under the polychoric approach. Because the number of such exceptions is small, they might be due to random error.

Estimates of the factor AR weight matrix and predicted factor covariance matrix of Pearson's product moment approach are shown in Table 10.6. A comparison with the upper panel of Table 10.4 shows that the AR weight estimates under these two approaches are similar. For example, the regression weight of agreeableness at t on itself at $t + 1$ is 0.75 under Pearson's product moment approach and the weight is 0.81 under the polychoric approach; the regression weight of conscientiousness at t on itself at $t + 1$ is 0.37 under Pearson's product moment approach and it is 0.30 under the polychoric approach. A comparison of the lower panels of Tables 10.4 and 10.6 shows that the estimates of the predicted factor covariance matrix are similar under these two approaches. For example, the proportion of variance in agreeableness accounted for by preceding factors is 60% under Pearson's product moment approach and it is 68% under the polychoric approach.

To summarize, most polychoric factor loading estimates were larger than their corresponding Pearson's product moment factor loading estimates, but the two approaches yielded similar estimates for the AR weight matrix and predicted factor covariance matrix.

TABLE 10.5

The Factor Loading Matrix: Pearson's Product Moment Approach

	N	E	A	C	I
Irritable	**0.79**	−0.08	−0.05	0.11	0.09
Bad tempered	**0.06**	−0.14	−0.51	0.16	−0.24
Vulnerable	**0.88**	−0.17	0.09	0.01	−0.03
Emotionally stable	**−0.78**	−0.06	−0.20	0.10	−0.08
Calm	**−0.60**	−0.20	−0.03	0.14	0.19
Resistent	**−0.76**	0.17	0.00	−0.15	−0.02
Dynamic	−0.05	**0.82**	−0.01	0.20	−0.02
Sociable	−0.17	**0.69**	0.02	0.07	0.14
Lively	−0.05	**0.85**	−0.17	0.06	0.09
Shy	0.06	**−0.68**	−0.05	0.07	−0.06
Silent	−0.12	**−0.59**	−0.23	−0.08	−0.07
Reserved	−0.02	**−0.89**	0.06	0.01	−0.06
Good natured	0.12	0.00	**0.37**	0.02	0.47
Helpful	0.13	0.19	**0.24**	0.23	0.24
Considerate	0.05	−0.03	**0.59**	0.19	0.10
Selfish	0.02	0.03	**−0.64**	−0.16	0.13
Domineering	−0.09	0.04	**−0.78**	0.01	0.14
Obstinate	−0.02	0.01	**−0.61**	0.33	0.25
Industrious	0.21	0.32	−0.20	**0.60**	−0.06
Persistent	−0.04	0.33	−0.07	**0.33**	0.26
Responsible	−0.15	−0.21	0.34	**0.69**	0.00
Lazy	−0.15	−0.40	0.21	**−0.58**	0.21
Reckless	0.04	0.50	−0.32	**−0.47**	−0.12
Changeable	0.24	0.04	−0.28	**0.07**	0.08
Witty	0.01	0.01	0.34	0.25	**0.14**
Knowledgeable	0.03	0.07	−0.27	0.10	**0.63**
Prudent	−0.14	0.29	0.10	0.20	**0.07**
Unresourceful	0.00	−0.52	−0.39	0.18	**−0.19**
Uninformed	0.00	0.00	0.10	0.09	**−0.64**
Unimaginative	−0.04	−0.55	−0.39	0.03	**0.03**

Note: N, E, A, C, and I represent neuroticism, extraversion, agreeableness, conscientiousness, and intellect, respectively. Factor loadings in bold face were expected to be substantial, other factor loadings were expected to be small.

10.6 CONCLUDING COMMENTS

Two approaches for estimating DFA models with ordinal data have been described: the polychoric approach and Pearson's product moment

TABLE 10.6

The AR Matrix and the Predicted Factor Covariance Matrix: Pearson's Product Moment Approach

	N	E	A	C	I
			$\widehat{A}$		
Neuroticism	0.41	0.22	−0.09	−0.06	−0.13
Extraversion	−0.40	0.31	0.29	0.17	0.00
Agreeableness	0.06	0.09	0.75	−0.12	−0.05
Conscientiousness	−0.26	−0.14	−0.09	0.37	0.22
Intellect	−0.06	0.09	0.03	−0.05	0.42
			$\widehat{\Theta}_{11}$		
Neuroticism	0.22	−0.13	−0.03	−0.14	−0.05
Extraversion	−0.13	0.36	0.22	0.09	0.10
Agreeableness	−0.03	0.22	0.60	−0.14	0.05
Conscientiousness	−0.14	0.09	−0.14	0.26	0.10
Intellect	−0.05	0.10	0.05	0.10	0.20

Note: N, E, A, C, and I represent neuroticism, extraversion, agreeableness, conscientiousness, and intellect, respectively.

approach. They differ in how the lagged correlation matrices are estimated.† The use of polychoric correlations implies that the DFA model applies to underlying continuous variables rather than to the ordinal manifest variables. Consequently, the polychoric approach is theoretically more justifiable than Pearson's product moment approach. Our simulation study demonstrated that factor loading estimates of the polychoric approach are unbiased, but factor loading estimates of Pearson's product moment approach are biased.

A key step in the polychoric approach is to estimate the polychoric lagged correlation matrices. The Fortran program DyFA 2.03 (Browne & Zhang, 2005) provides facilities of estimating polychoric lagged correlation matrices and fitting the DFA model to them. The program is available free of charge on the Internet and the distribution package includes a user guide and many illustrations.

The polychoric approach is computationally more expensive than Pearson's product moment approach, because each element in the polychoric

† A reviewer points out that missing data arise frequently in collecting time series with ordinal variables and suggests hot deck imputation to deal with them.

lagged correlation matrices has to be estimated separately using an iterative algorithm. Nevertheless, the polychoric approach is feasible with a typical PC even for a large model. For example, Pearson's product moment approach with the empirical example took 0.89 s; the polychoric approach took 6.03 s.[†] The empirical example was nontrivial: it involved 30 manifest ordinal variables and 5 factors, and more than 2000 polychoric correlations were estimated.

ACKNOWLEDGMENTS

The chapter is based in part on the first author's dissertation (Zhang, 2006) supervised by the second author. We thank the editors and reviewers for helpful comments. We also thank Ying Cheng for reading and commenting on an earlier draft.

REFERENCES

Boker, S., & Wegner, M. (2007). *Data analytic techniques for dynamical systems in the social and behavioral sciences*. Mahwah, NJ: Lawrence Erlbaum Associates.

Bollen, K. A. (1989). *Structural equations with latent variables*. New York: Wiley.

Borkenau, P., & Ostendorf, F. (1998). The big five as states: How useful is the five factor model to describe intraindividual variations over time? *Journal of Research in Personality, 32*, 202–221.

Browne, M. W. (2001). An overview of analytic rotation in exploratory factor analysis. *Multivariate Behavioral Research, 36*, 111–150.

Browne, M. W., & Nesselroade, J. R. (2005). Representing psychological processes with dynamic factor models: Some promising uses and extensions of arma time series models. In A. Maydeu-Olivares & J. J. McArdle (Eds.), *Advances in psychometrics: A festschrift for Roderick P. McDonald* (pp. 415–452). Mahwah, NJ: Erlbaum.

Browne, M. W., & Zhang, G. (2005). *DyFA 2.03 user guide*. Retrieved from http://quantrm2.psy.ohiostate.edu/browne/software.htm

Browne, M. W., & Zhang, G. (2007). Developments in the factor analysis of individual time series. In R. Cudeck & R. C. MacCallum (Eds.), *Factor analysis at 100: Historical developments and future directions* (pp. 265–291). Mahwah, NJ: Lawrence Erlbaum Associates.

Collins, L. M., & Sayer, A. G. (2001). *New methods for the analysis of change*. Washington, DC: American Psychological Association.

[†] The analyses were carried out using a Lenovo X60 laptop.

Dolan, C. V. (1994). Factor analysis of variables with 2, 3, 5, and 7 response categories: A comparison of categorical variable estimators using simulated data. *British Journal of Mathematical and Statistical Psychology, 47*, 309–326.

Du Toit, S., & Browne, M. W. (2007). Structural equation modeling of multivariate time series. *Multivariate Behavioral Research, 42*, 67–101.

Engle, R., & Watson, M. (1981). A one-factor multivariate time series model of metropolitan wage rates. *Journal of the American Statistical Association, 76*, 774–781.

Everitt, B. S. (2006). *The Cambridge dictionary of statistics* (3rd ed.). Cambridge, UK: Cambridge University Press.

Ferrer, E., & Nesselroade, J. R. (2003). Modeling affective process in dyadic relations via dynamic factor analysis. *Emotion, 3*, 344–360.

Geweke, J. F., & Singleton, K. J. (1981). Maximum likelihood "confirmatory" factor analysis of economic time series. *International Economic Review, 22*, 37–54.

Hamilton, J. D. (1994). *Time series analysis.* Princeton, NJ: Princeton University Press.

Immink, W. (1986). *Parameter estimation in Markov models and dynamic factor analysis.* Doctoral dissertation, University of Utrecht, Utrecht.

Jöreskog, K. G. (1994). On the estimation of polychoric correlations and their asymptotic covariance matrix. *Psychometrika, 59*, 381–389.

Lebo, M. A., & Nesselroade, J. R. (1978). Intraindividual difference dimensions of mood change during pregancy identified in five P-technique factor analyses. *Journal of Research in Personality, 12*, 205–224.

van Rijn, P. W. (2008). *Categorical time series in psychological measurement.* Doctoral dissertation, University of Amsterdam, Amsterdam, Netherlands.

Molenaar, P. C. M. (1985). A dynamic factor analysis model for the analysis of multivariate time series. *Psychometrika, 50*, 181–202.

Molenaar, P. C. M., & Nesselroade, J. R. (1998). A comparison of pseudo-maximum likelihood and asumptotically distribution-free dynamic factor analysis parameter estimation in fitting covariance-structure models to block-toeplitz matrices representing single subject multivariate time series. *Multivariate Behavioral Research, 33*, 313–342.

Molenaar, P. C. M., & Nesselroade, J. R. (2001). Rotation in the dynamic factor modeling of multivariate stationary time series. *Psychometrika, 66*, 99–107.

Nesselroade, J. R., McArdle, J. J., Aggen, S. H., & Meyers, J. M. (2002). Dynamic factor analysis models for representing process in multivariate time-series. In D. Moskowitz & S. L. Hershberger (Eds.), *Modeling intraindividual variability with repeated measures data: methods and applications* (pp. 235–265). Mahwah, NJ: Erlbaum.

Olsson, U. (1979). Maximum likelihood estimation of the polychoric correlation coefficient. *Psychometrika, 44*, 443–460.

Upton, G., & Cook, I. (2006). *Oxford dictionary of statistics* (2nd ed.). Oxford, UK: Oxford University Press.

Walls, T. A., & Schafer, J. L. (2005). *Models for intensive longitudinal data.* New York: Oxford University Press.

Wirth, R. J., & Edwards, M. C. (2007). Item factor analysis: Current approaches and future directions. *Psychological Methods, 12*, 58–79.

Zhang, G. (2006). *Bootstrap procedures for dynamic factor analysis.* Doctoral dissertation, Ohio State University, Columbus, OH.

11

Measuring Intraindividual Variability with Intratask Change Item Response Models

Ryan P. Bowles

11.1 INTRODUCTION

Dynamics in human behavior can often be described not just by a trajectory, but also by variability around that trajectory. Individuals may differ in both the predictable trajectory and the magnitude of variability, and both may be reliable traits of the individual (Fiske & Rice, 1955). Put another way, an individual's observed scores over time on some repeated measure may reflect a general time-related trend, as well as time-unstructured intraindividual variability, or IIV, which is a manifestation of a time-independent random process with an individual-specific magnitude of variation. Thus, IIV can be considered a reliable trait that reflects an individual's tendency to be inconsistent across measurement occasions.

Fiske and Rice (1955) provide the following conditions for IIV:

1. The individual "is exposed to the same stimulus or to objectively indistinguishable stimuli" at each measurement occasion (p. 217).
2. The environment in which observations are made is the same on all occasions.
3. The order of responses is irrelevant. That is, there is no serial dependence or systematic trend in the data.

Nesselroade (1991) highlighted that changes due to IIV are transient and are therefore "reversible." He also noted that IIV is asynchronous across individuals, in part to differentiate it from short-term shocks shared by multiple individuals (i.e., period effects). Other forms of partially structured individual variability are possible, such as those involving serially dependent random processes, such as moving averages, or reversible systematic change, such as oscillators. In this chapter, I focus only on unstructured, time-independent IIV.

The simplest and most common index of IIV is the individual standard deviation (ISD). The ISD is defined as the standard deviation of an individual's scores around that individual's mean across time. Alternatively, if there is a structured time-dependent trend, each individual's data can be detrended before the standard deviation is calculated. Other indices of IIV are possible, such as coefficients of variation (e.g., Sosnoff & Newell, 2006; Vega-Lopez, Ausman, Griffith, & Lichtenstein, 2007) or approximate entropy (Pincus, 1991; Pincus & Goldberger, 1994) that address shortcomings of the ISD. The ISD, however, has advantages both in interpretability and in ease of calculation because of general familiarity of the standard deviation as a measure of variability (Estabrook, Grimm, & Bowles, 2008). In this chapter, I focus on the ISD, although the methods described could incorporate alternative indices of IIV.

IIV has many psychological interpretations, depending on the particular research questions being addressed. Ram, Rabbitt, Stollery, and Nesselroade (2005) identified a number of terms used in the extant literature, including instability, error, wobble, lability, inconsistency, noise, or the particularly elegant "steady-state hum" (Nesselroade & Ford, 1985). IIV can predict human behavioral outcomes as well as, or in addition to, the mean or structured trajectory (Butler, Hokanson, & Flynn, 1994; Jensen, 1992). To name just a few examples: IIV in infants' heart rate is predictive of later temperament (Kagan, 1994); IIV in simple reaction time is predictive of neurological disorders (Hultsch & MacDonald, 2004; Fuentes, Hunter, Strauss, & Hultsch, 2001; Schretlen, Munro, Anthony, & Pearlson, 2003); IIV in self-esteem is predictive of susceptibility to depression (Butler, Hokanson, & Flynn, 1994); IIV in affect is predictive of neuroticism (Eid & Diener, 1999); and IIV in perceived control is predictive of impending mortality (Eizenman, Nesselroade, Featherman, & Rowe, 1997).

A key issue in the interpretation of IIV is the time frame across which it is measured (Hultsch & MacDonald, 2004; Newell, Liu, & Mayer-Kress, 2001; Slifkin & Newell, 1998). IIV over short time frames can reflect different mechanisms than IIV over long time frames. For example, Huxhold, Li, Schmiedek, and Lindenberger (2007) found that older adults had higher moment-to-moment, trial-to-trial, and day-to-day variability at all time frames on a measure of postural control. They theorized that moment-to-moment variability reflects losses in signal-to-noise processes, while day-to-day variability reflected both cascading effects of shorter-term IIV and environmental effects.

One time frame of particular interest is instantaneous variability or variability that occurs across infinitesimal time intervals (Nesselroade & Ford, 1985). Measuring instantaneous variability is of course impossible, but it can be approximated with trial-by-trial variability when the trials are (a) identical or "objectively indistinguishable" and (b) closely spaced. These conditions are typically able to be met in physiological or physical measurements, such as physical force (Slifkin & Newell, 1999) or heart rate (Fox & Porges, 1985), which can be measured repeatedly within very short time intervals. In psychological research, these conditions are often met with reaction time, the most common outcome of IIV research.

Much psychological research, however, is based on constructs most readily or validly measured with categorical outcomes, such as correct/incorrect or rating scales, which are combined, usually by summing, into a single score. These measurement instruments are not conducive to the measurement of IIV at short intervals because it is not possible to have closely spaced indistinguishable trials. First, a single item cannot be repeatedly administered because it cannot span a construct; that is, it cannot provide a sufficiently complete picture of an individual's trait or ability level. For example, a single vocabulary item is not sufficient to measure an individual's vocabulary knowledge. Second, the meaning of an item response may change as it is administered repeatedly. For example, the initial administration of a list of words to be remembered measures a aspect of memory different from the third administration of the same list (Karpicke & Roediger, 2007; Tulving, 1967).

The workaround to this dilemma has been to expand the distance between observations (such as day-to-day), yet maintain an interpretation in terms of variability at very short time frames (e.g., Butler et al., 1994;

Eid & Diener, 1999). However, as different time frames can yield differing estimates and interpretations of IIV for the same individual (Huxhold et al., 2007; Newell et al., 2001), this workaround is decidedly unsatisfying. In this chapter, I propose a solution that rests on the partial relaxation of the assumption of identical repeated trials. This allows for the measurement of IIV within a single measurement occasion by using nonrepeated items that together span a construct and avoid complications associated with repeated measurement of the same item.

11.1.1 Item Response Theory models

The key concept underlying this proposed method is the statistical modeling of characteristics of the nonrepeated items, such that, after adjusting for these characteristics, each response to an item can be considered identical conditional on the item characteristics. Such methods are widely available in nondynamic systems through the family of item response theory (IRT) models (Baker, 2001; Embretson & Reise, 2000). Differences among items are accounted for by introducing parameters that describe or define the functioning of an item, such as item difficulty. Including these parameters "controls" for variability among the items, such that remaining variability across individuals reflects only variability in the underlying construct. The simplest common IRT model is the Rasch (1960/1980) model, also called the one (item)-parameter logistic model:

$$P(X_{ni} = 1) = \frac{\exp(\theta_n - \beta_i)}{1 + \exp(\theta_n - \beta_i)}, \tag{11.1}$$

where $P(X_{ni} = 1)$ is the probability of a correct response to item i by person n, θ_n is the stable trait level for person n and β_i is the difficulty of item i. This logistic model is virtually indistinguishable, up to a scaling parameter, from the less common normal ogive version:

$$P(X_{ni} = 1) = \Phi[\theta_n - \beta_i], \tag{11.2}$$

where Φ is the normal cumulative distribution function. Many generalizations of these models have been proposed, usually by adding parameters associated with each item (discrimination and/or basal rate of correct response; Birnbaum, 1968), parameters to account for rating scales (category thresholds; Andrich, 1978; Masters, 1982), or both.

IRT models require the construct to be stable across the entire measurement occasion (i.e., task administration) and are therefore not appropriate for the assessment of IIV. I have proposed a new family of intratask change item response models (ICIRMs; Bowles, 2008; see also Klauer & Sydow, 2001; Verhelst & Glas, 1993, 1995), which incorporate dynamic models into item response models. Because these models relax the standard requirement that the underlying trait is stable across the entire measurement occasion, they may be capable of assessing IIV within a single occasion. To date, the models have been used only to assess the structured trajectory of change occurring during the task administration. In this chapter, I explore the use of these models to assess IIV. I first describe ICIRMs and how they could be used to measure IIV. I then present a brief example of the use of ICIRMs to measure IIV on a working memory task and a set of simulations to examine the accuracy and precision of IIV estimates within ICIRMs. I conclude with a discussion of the potential benefits and challenges of using ICIRMs to measure IIV.

11.2 INTRATASK CHANGE ITEM RESPONSE MODELS

ICIRMs incorporate dynamic models of behavior into standard item response models. The general form of the model is

$$P(X_{nit} = 1) = \Phi[f(t, \Theta_n, Z_{t-1}) - \beta_i], \tag{11.3}$$

where $P(X_{nit} = 1)$ is the probability of a correct response by person n to item i at time t, β_i is the difficulty of item i, Φ is the normal cumulative distribution function, and $f_{nt} = f(t, \Theta_n, Z_{t-1})$ is a dynamic function dependent on a vector of person-specific parameters Θ_n, and a vector of feedback from previous responses Z_{t-1}. Alternative formulations of the item response model aspect of ICIRMs can be readily incorporated, such as adding rating scale parameters. I call f_{nt} the *effective trait level* of person n at time t, in that it is the trait level determining the probability of a correct response at time t, analogous to the single stable trait level in most item response models. Typically, time is indexed by the order of item presentation, such that the first item presented is $t = 1$, the second $t = 2$, and so on. In this chapter, I do not consider serial dependence, which is incorporated through the feedback vector Z_{t-1}. Therefore, I drop Z_{t-1} from the arguments of f_{nt}.

Many dynamic models can be used for the effective trait level function (Bowles, 2008). To assess IIV, define f_{nt} as

$$f_{nt} = f(t, \Theta_n) = \theta_n + \varepsilon_{nt}, \tag{11.4}$$

where θ_n is the mean level of the underlying construct that is stable across item administrations and ε_{nt} is the unpredictable aspect of behavior that occurs at each time t. ε_{nt} is assumed to be IID and normally distributed with mean 0 and person-specific variance σ_n^2. That is, $\varepsilon_{nt} \sim N(0, \sigma_n^2)$. Taking the square root of σ_n^2, $\sqrt{\sigma_n^2} = \sigma_n$, yields the intratask ISD for person n. Alternatively, the mean level, θ_n, can be replaced with a deterministic function of a vector of person parameters and time. For example, linear change with IIV can be defined as

$$f_{nt} = \theta_{1n} + t\theta_{2n} + \varepsilon_{nt}. \tag{11.5}$$

Figure 11.1 demonstrates how an ICIRM with IIV functions for two individuals, one with a relatively low mean level ($\theta_n = -0.5$) and the other with a relatively high mean level ($\theta_n = 0.5$), both taking a task consisting of 10 items. The columns display the effect of IIV: the left column involves no IIV ($\sigma_n = 0$), whereas the right column involves IIV, with the low mean level individual having a high variability ($\sigma_n = 0.4$) and the high mean level individual having a low variability ($\sigma_n = 0.2$). The first row of Figure 11.1 displays this system of trait levels. In the second row, the trait levels are converted to a probability metric for a task with constant difficulty ($\beta_i = 0$ for all i). Note that the right column in this row displays the effect of IIV on probability: there is a consistent average probability of correct response ($\sim$0.31 and 0.69), with variation around that level. In the third row, I add variability in the items, with item difficulty selected from a uniform distribution $[-0.5, 0.5]$ ($\beta_i = [0.19, -0.26, 0.10, -0.32, 0.41, -0.15, -0.28, -0.45, -0.49, 0.37]$). Variation in probability thus reflects random variation associated with IIV and variation due to changes in the item behavior as reflected in the item difficulty. Finally, in the fourth row, item responses are simulated based on the probabilities from the third row. For each item administration, a random number was selected from a uniform [0,1] distribution. If this number was

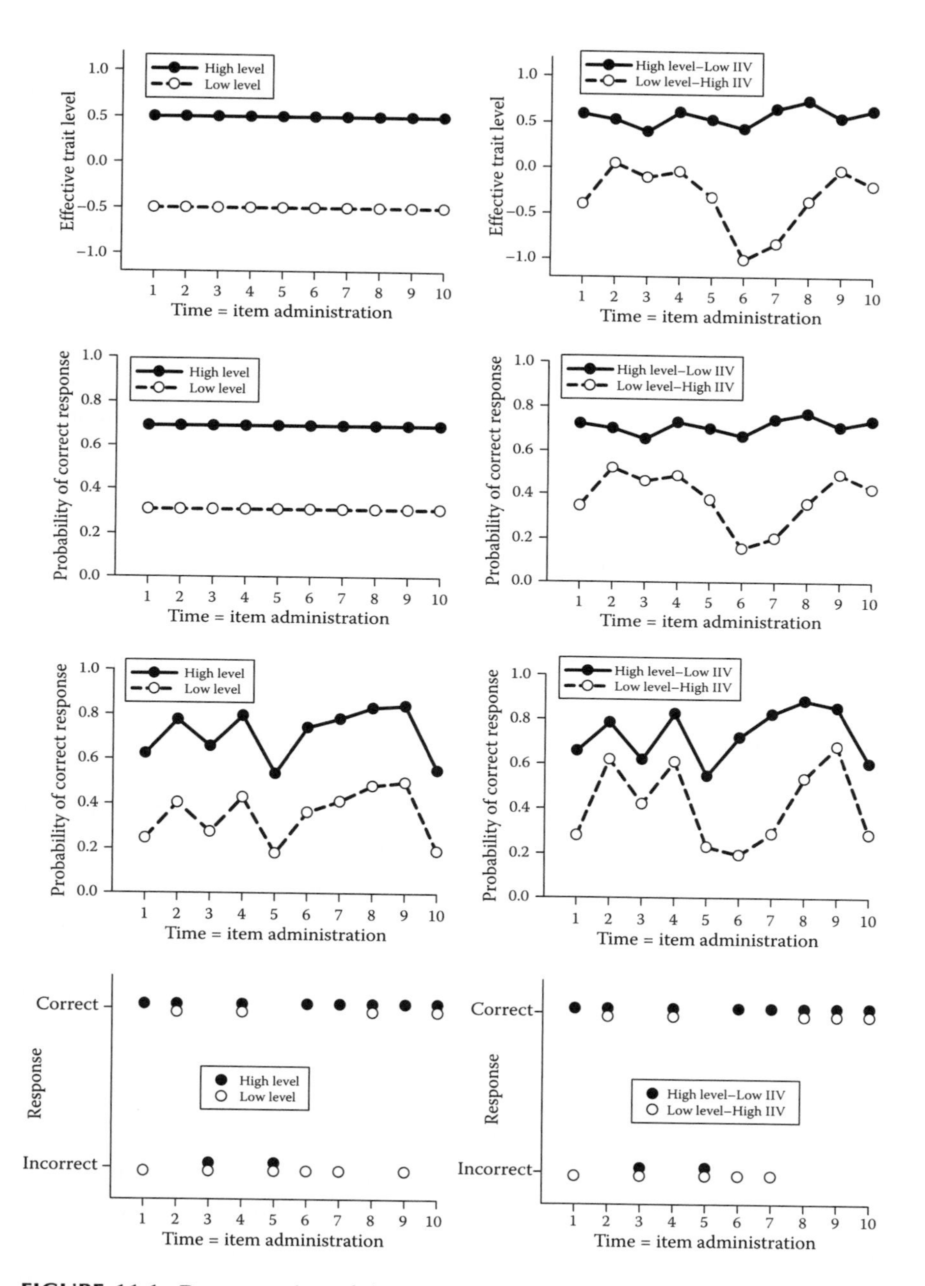

FIGURE 11.1 Demonstration of the impact of IIV on observed item responses using an ICIRM.

less than the probability, then the item response was correct; otherwise, it was incorrect. To maintain consistency, the same random number was used for both individuals, whether IIV was included or not. Thus, variation in the item responses in this row reflects differences in level across individuals, variability due to IIV, and variability in item difficulty, but not variation due to the outcome of the probabilistic system. The goal of ICIRMs that incorporate IIV is to derive estimates of the level and intratask ISD (row 1) from the observed item responses (row 4). Note that in row 4, only one item response changed as a result of the addition of IIV (item administration 9 for the low level–high IIV individual), suggesting that accurate measurement of intratask IIV may be especially challenging although not impossible (see simulations below; *cf.* Estabrook et al., 2008).

The illustration highlights that assessing intratask IIV is quite an analytical challenge. Among the most important challenges:

1. Only one dichotomous observation is available for each individual at any effective trait level. Thus, there is very limited information available.
2. There are two change processes occurring simultaneously: item difficulty changes at the same time the individual's trait level is changing. Separately identifying simultaneously occurring change is difficult (Ferrer, Salthouse, Stewart, & Schwartz, 2004).
3. ICIRMs include two forms of nonlinearity: the normal ogive link function and the effective trait level function. Typical estimation programs associated with, for example, IRT, structural equation modeling, or hierarchical linear modeling, are not capable of estimating such a complex system.

Dealing with these challenges requires consideration of methods of estimation and identification using experimental design.

In this chapter, I employ a general Bayesian estimation program, WinBUGS (Spiegelhalter, Thomas, Best, & Lunn, 2004; available free at http://www.mrc-bsu.cam.ac.uk/bugs/), called from within SAS using a script developed by Zhang, McArdle, Wang, and Hamagami (2006) and macros by Sparapani and Hayat (2007). Bayesian estimation is somewhat different from typical maximum likelihood or least squares estimation, in that each parameter must have a prior distribution that describes prior knowledge about the value for the parameter. A common practice is to use a very uninformative prior, reflecting very little knowledge about the value of the parameter, in which case the Bayesian solution is similar in value and interpretation to a maximum likelihood estimate.

Estimation in WinBUGS uses Monte Carlo Markov chain estimation with a version of Gibbs sampling (Geman & Geman, 1984). Estimation occurs in two stages. The goal of the first stage, called the burn-in, is to reach a type of convergence upon the conditional posterior distribution of each parameter, which is a combination of the likelihood and prior distribution conditional on the values of all other parameters. In this chapter, convergence was assessed with the modified Gelman–Rubin convergence statistic (Brooks & Gelman, 1998), which is available in WinBUGS. Convergence is achieved when the statistic approaches 1 and its components achieve stability. Once convergence is reached, each additional iteration yields a sample value from the posterior distribution for every parameter. Combining the values from a large number of estimation iterations yields an estimated empirical posterior distribution. The mean (or median) of this distribution can be considered a point estimate of the parameter, and the center 95% of values is analogous to a standard 95% confidence interval. Throughout all analyses in this chapter, I used 10,000 estimation iterations. I used all default values in WinBUGS (including no thinning) with one exception: I changed the method UpdaterDFreeARS for log concave to Updater-Slice in the WinBUGS configuration file Updater/Rsrc/Methods.odc. This change has been shown to eliminate convergence issues in some cases. For more details about the estimation technique, please see the WinBUGS user manual (Spiegelhalter, Thomas, Best, & Lunn, 2004).

An example script for estimating an ICIRM with IIV in WinBUGS is in Figure 11.2. The associated SAS script is included on the CD included with this book. I highlight some aspects of the WinBUGS script. Lines 2 and 3 reflect iterating through each person n (in this case, for 403 individuals) and time t (for 15 item administrations). In line 4, *betaa, betab, . . . , and betag* are the item difficulties for item a, item b, . . . , and item g, respectively. Each is a coefficient on a dummy indicator variable (e.g., *item* $b[n, t]$) equal to 1 if person n was administered the item at time t. Expressing item difficulty as a weighted sum of dummy indicators is necessary to eliminate cross-nesting of item responses within both individuals and items. For larger numbers of items, it is possible to express this as a summation. Note also that there is no *betae*. In this script, item e serves both as the reference

```
1.    model{
2.        for (n in 1:403) {
3.            for (t in 1:15) {
4.                p[n,t]<-phi(theta[n,t]-betaa*itema[n,t]-betab*itemb[n,t]-
                      betac*itemc[n,t]-betad*itemd[n,t]-betaf*itemf[n,t]-
                      betag*itemg[n,t])
5.                itemscorec[n,t] ~ dbern(p[n,t])
6.                theta[n,t] ~ dnorm(mu_theta[n],tau_theta[n])
7.            }
8.            mu_theta[n] ~ dnorm(mu_mu_theta,tau_mu_theta)
9.            tau_theta[n] ~ dgamma(A,B)
10.           sig_theta[n]<-1/tau_theta[n]
11.       }
12.
13.       #priors
14.       betaa ~ dnorm(0,1.0E-6)
15.       betab ~ dnorm(0,1.0E-6)
16.       betac ~ dnorm(0,1.0E-6)
17.       betad ~ dnorm(0,1.0E-6)
18.       betaf ~ dnorm(0,1.0E-6)
19.       betag ~ dnorm(0,1.0E-6)
20.
21.       mu_mu_theta ~ dnorm(0,1.0E-6)
22.       tau_mu_theta ~ dgamma(.01,.01)
23.       A ~ dexp(1)
24.       B ~ dgamma(.01, .01)
25.   }
```

FIGURE 11.2 WinBUGS script for the estimation of an ICIRM with IIV. Numbers along the left side are line numbers for illustration and are not included in the script.

category for the item indicators and as the identification constraint necessary in item response models to fix the origin of the theta parameters.* Finally, I highlight that the relevant measure of IIV is *sig_theta[n]*.

Model identification is also a key challenge in using ICIRMs in the study of IIV. The effective trait level is changing at the same time the items are and separately identifying simultaneous change processes is problematic (Ferrer et al., 2004). I have identified three ways to break the concurrent dependence of both effective trait level and item identity on time indexed by item administration (see Bowles, 2008, for a complete discussion). First,

* Another form of identification is evident in the additive nature of the effective trait level and the item parameters, which allows the ISDs to be estimated without any further identification constraint. This model is equivalent to a form of multigroup factor model with categorical outcomes, where each individual is a group. The additive form is equivalent to constraining all factor loadings to 1, so the variances of each individual (i.e., the ISD) can be identified. To continue this mapping, constraining the difficulty of one item to 0 is equivalent to constraining one threshold parameter to 0, which identifies the mean (i.e., level) for each individual.

a constrained change function for item difficulty can be introduced into the model, such that the effective trait level and item difficulty follow different and separable dynamic trends. This potential solution may not be a good option, because it is crucially dependent on selecting the correct model for the changes in item difficulty, and even subject matter experts tend to be poor judges of item difficulty (Bejar, 1983). Second, the items can be administered in random order so that, across individuals, there is no pattern to item difficulty. This option may be computationally intensive and yield imprecise parameter estimates if there are a large number of items with few observations for each item. Third, a static model for item difficulty can be introduced, where item difficulty is a known function of item characteristics (Fischer, 1973), with the item characteristics varying across presentation order even if the items themselves do not. In the simulations and empirical example that follow, I employ both the second and third methods by including both random presentation order and constraining item difficulty to be a function of a single item characteristic (e.g., number of pieces of information to be remembered). This allows for randomization while minimizing the number of item difficulty parameters.

11.3 SIMULATIONS

I ran a series of simulations to assess the accuracy and precision of estimates of the ISD generated from the ICIRM with IIV. I varied two parameters in a 3 by 2 simulation design based on the most important aspects identified by Estabrook et al. (2008): the ratio of the mean ISD (σ_n) to the standard deviation of the level (θ_n), that is, the within-to-between ratio, and the number of item administrations (occasions). The generating parameters for the simulations were based on typical values for item difficulty and typical empirical ISD values (Estabrook et al., 2008). Nine item difficulties were simulated at equal intervals from -2 to 2. Sample size was set to 400 for all simulations; Estabrook et al. found that sample size had almost no effect on estimation of IIV. Level was sampled from a normal distribution with mean = 0 and SD = 1. The ratio of mean ISD to SD of level was set to three values, 0.5, 1.0, or 1.5. Consistent with Estabrook et al., the SD of the ISD was set to 0.3 times the mean ISD.

11.3.1 Results

Correlations between the true level and ISD and estimated values are reported in Table 11.1. Correlations increased with additional numbers of items, as well as with the true within-to-between ratio. In the least favorable condition, 15 items with a 0.5 within-to-between ratio, the correlation was not distinguishable from 0. In the most favorable condition, 50 items and a 1.5 within-to-between ratio, the correlation was substantially higher, 0.53. The low correlation is consistent with previous research on across-occasion IIV (Estabrook et al., 2008), although somewhat lower for the same number of occasions, reflecting the limited information available in dichotomous items. On the other hand, the level was estimated well in all conditions, with a minimum correlation of 0.83. In all but one condition, the mean ISD was overestimated dramatically, but the overestimation generally decreased as the conditions for estimating the ISD improved. The variability of the level was also generally overestimated, but to a lesser degree. A key aspect of the nature of the IIV, the within-to-between ratio, is therefore overestimated by an average factor of approximately 1.5. These simulations highlight the challenge and promise of estimating IIV using ICIRMs. The accuracy and precision of the estimates are below generally acceptable levels. However, the estimates tended to correlate moderately with the true underlying values, suggesting that important relations with IIV may be identifiable under certain conditions (e.g., large effect sizes) or with an alternative estimation technique.

TABLE 11.1

Simulation Results

Simulated W–B Ratio	Items	Correlation with True ISD	Correlation with True Level	Mean ISD	SD of Level	W–B Ratio	Overestimation Factor
	15	0.11	0.90	11.64	9.86	1.18	2.36
0.5	50	0.09	0.97	0.30	0.90	0.33	0.67
	TRUE			0.50	1.00	0.50	
	15	0.25	0.88	14.71	9.03	1.63	1.63
1.0	50	0.40	0.96	3.93	2.78	1.41	1.41
	TRUE			1.00	1.00	1.00	
	15	0.32	0.83	14.33	6.20	2.31	1.54
1.5	50	0.53	0.94	9.29	4.59	2.02	1.35
	TRUE			1.50	1.00	1.50	

Notes: W–B ratio is the ratio of average intraindividual variance to interindividual variance in the level. Underestimation factor is the ratio of the true W–B ratio to the estimated W–B ratio. TRUE refers to the true values used in the simulations.

11.4 EXAMPLE: IIV AND WORKING MEMORY

The example comes from a study of working memory and aging (Bowles, 2008). These data have been used with ICIRMs to examine structured intratask change, yielding a conclusion that performance increases during the task at a decelerating rate and that there is no apparent relation between age and intratask change. In this chapter, I re-examine these data in the context of IIV to assess whether, consistent with previous research examining age effects on variability in response times (e.g., Hale, Myerson, & Smith, 1988; Anstey, 1999; Deary & Der, 2005), there is an age-related increase in IIV in working memory.

The data consist of 403 individuals who took an online version of a standard working memory span task, operation span (Turner & Engle, 1989; Unsworth, Heitz, Schrock, & Engle, 2005). Items consisted of a series of simple arithmetic problems followed by a to-be-remembered letter. After two to eight arithmetic problem–letter combinations, participants recalled the letters in the order in which they were presented. A correct response consisted of correct recall of the letter sequence, regardless of the responses to the arithmetic problems. Some previous studies using this task have eliminated participants with less than 85% correct responses to the arithmetic problems (Unsworth et al., 2005), but this had no effect on these analyses and so all data are used. In order to distinguish changes in the individuals separately from changes in the items, the order of presentation varied randomly across participants. Item difficulty (β_i) was assumed to be dependent only on the number of letters to be remembered, not on the particular letters. The total number of item administrations was 15. The difficulty of a series of length 6 was set to 0 as an identification constraint (i.e., implicitly, *betae* is constrained to 0 in the script in Figure 11.2).

11.4.1 Results

Parameter estimates are presented in Table 11.2. As expected, item difficulty increases as the number of letters to be remembered increases. Based on the estimates of θ_n and σ_n for each individual, the mean average level was 6.60 with a standard deviation of 10.12, while the ISD had a mean of 15.30 with a standard deviation of 4.06. The ratio $15.30^2/10.12^2 = 2.29$ indicates that average within-person variance is about twice as large as across-person variance in mean level. This is on the high end of the range

TABLE 11.2

Estimates from Empirical WM Span Example

Parameter	Estimate	95% confidence interval
Difficulty of item length 2	−27.57	[−47.53, −10.25]
Difficulty of item length 3	−20.48	[−30.50, −7.61]
Difficulty of item length 4	−16.34	[−27.42, −6.18]
Difficulty of item length 5	−8.68	[−15.17, −3.17]
Difficulty of item length 6	=0	
Difficulty of item length 7	8.59	[3.11, 15.35]
Difficulty of item length 8	18.82	[6.92, 31.89]
Mean level	6.60	[2.32, 12.04]
SD level	8.89	[4.53, 20.13]
Mean ISD	15.28	
SD ISD	4.06	

Notes: The difficulty of item length 6 was set to 0 as an identification constraint. The mean and SD of ISD are derived from individual estimates, so no empirical confidence intervals are available.

of typical empirical within-to-between ratios for across-occasion studies of IIV (Estabrook et al., 2008).

Figure 11.3 graphs the relation between age and level (left side) and age and ISD (right side). A regression of the individual level on age yielded a significant age-related linear decline in average intratask working memory span (standardized $b = -0.16, t_1 = 3.29, p < 0.01$). This is an effect of age lower than that typically found in empirical studies; for example, a meta-analysis indicated that the standardized effect of age is −0.27 (Verhaeghen & Salthouse, 1997). The smaller effect is probably due to the nature of Internet sampling, which tends to yield oversamples of high functioning older

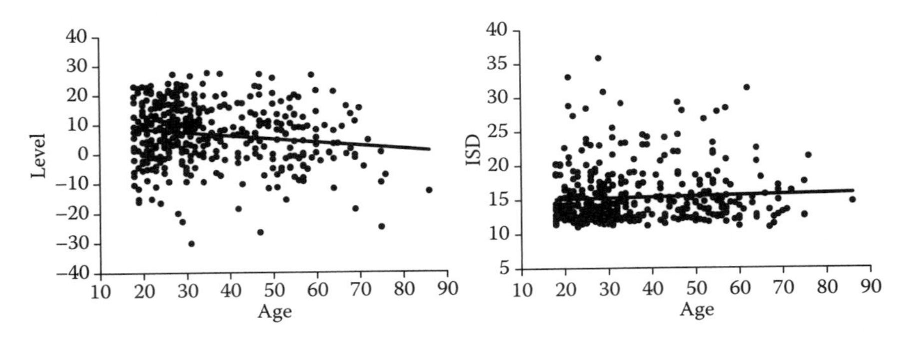

FIGURE 11.3 Relation between age and level (left side) and ISD (right side) for the empirical WM span example.

adults (Lenhart et al., 2003). A regression of ISD on age was not significant (standardized $b = 0.04, t_1 = 0.91, p = 0.36$), which is not consistent with previous research. As indicated in Figure 11.3, the intratask ISD was highly skewed with a floor around 10. Transforming the ISD by taking the square root or the inverse did not change the outcome. Thus, based on these results, the conclusion is that there is no relation between age and short-term IIV in working memory. However, these results should in no way be considered definitive: (1) the Internet sample was not representative; (2) previous results indicate that there is a systematic intratask change trend, which was ignored in this analysis; and (3) 15 items are likely insufficient to yield reliable estimates of the ISD (see simulations). Nonetheless, this analysis provides an example of the use of ICIRMs to assess IIV using a single measurement occasion.

11.5 DISCUSSION

In this chapter, I described a new method for measuring unstructured IIV at short time scales with nonrepeated categorical item responses. This method uses ICIRMs incorporating a change model with random item-by-item variability. The intratask variability has a person-specific magnitude and is measured by the ISD around the typical or average trait level during the task. The ISD can then be used as a predictor or outcome in further analyses; for example, I examined the effect of age on IIV in the empirical example.

11.5.1 Challenges

Three major challenges make the application of this method difficult. First, these models are complex and require less well-known estimation software. In this chapter, I used the general purpose Bayesian estimation program WinBUGS using macros developed within SAS. I included the WinBUGS script in Figure 11.2, and the SAS script is available on the CD associated with this book. Nonetheless users must be able to adapt the WinBUGS script to their own needs, and must be proficient in using a general statistical package that can call WinBUGS, such as SAS or R. This form of estimation takes a very long time because of the need to iterate tens of thousands of times through several hundred parameters, primarily reflecting each individual's level and ISD. The simulations took more than 2 days on a moderately fast computer.

There is no evidence that WinBUGS provides the most efficient or accurate estimation method (whether Bayesian or not) available for this type of model. The simulations suggest that the resulting estimates can be quite different from the true underlying values. It may be possible to develop a specialized estimation program that provides better estimates of the parameters of the ICIRM with IIV. This remains a topic for future research.

The second challenge in estimating IIV is that a large number of item responses may be necessary to yield even modestly precise estimates of IIV. Exactly how many items are necessary to yield acceptable estimates of the ISD remains an open question. Previous research indicates that the number of occasions and the ratio of average IIV to across-individual variability in the average level (the within-to-between ratio) can have strong effects on the reliability of the across-occasion ISD estimates (Estabrook et al., 2008). Regardless of the condition, the correlation between the true parameter values and their estimates is not above a generally acceptable value. However, the correlations for the ISD are not out of line with those based on repeated observations of continuous variables (Estabrook et al., 2008). It appears that the challenge in estimating IIV lies only in part with the use of ICIRMs; the measurement of IIV is a difficult endeavor in general.

The need for large numbers of item responses should come as no surprise when considering Cattell's (1988) databox, which highlights the interactive nature of variables, persons, and occasions. Sample size requirements when considering across-person statistics are analogous to number of occasions requirements when considering across-occasion statistics. Researchers would not typically make conclusions about interindividual differences based on an analysis with only 15 individuals and likewise should not expect reasonable conclusions about IIV with only 15 occasions or item administrations. In fact, even for the simplest IRT models, sample sizes of 300 are often considered a lower bound for robust estimates, which may be analogous to 300 item administrations for IIV with ICIRMs. The fact that a number of empirical studies have found statistically significant effects involving IIV with few occasions suggests that the importance of IIV is quite large and likely underestimated given the low reliability of measures of IIV.

A concern with administering a large number of items within a single occasion, however, is that the meaning of an item response may change over the course of the session. Participants can get fatigued or bored when confronted with a long test, which can reduce the validity of the test as well as the model used to analyze the responses (Yen, 1993). Responses to later presented items may reflect fatigue in addition to the underlying construct and IIV over the course of the task would therefore be contaminated with changing levels of fatigue. It should be noted that such position effects may also occur at the beginning of a test. In fact, some of my research suggests that fatigue is a much less important aspect of performance than warm-up or learning, such that longer tests are actually more accurate indicators of the construct than shorter tests (Bowles, Wise, & Kingsbury, 2007). Future research should address the role of position effects on the assessment of IIV. This issue is not unique to long tests, however, as practice and period effects can affect the validity of conclusions about IIV when assessed across occasions.

The third challenge is collecting appropriate data. Although some specialized data collection methodologies have been proposed (e.g., measurement bursts; Nesselroade, 1991), measuring IIV inherently suffers from all the difficulties associated with longitudinal studies: high cost, sample attrition, etc. With ICIRMs, a large number of items are necessary, but they can be administered within a single measurement occasion. This would eliminate or sharply limit problems of attrition and reduce participant costs dramatically. However, it becomes necessary to develop a very large number of unique items to avoid repeating an item. Item development can be costly, and validating that the items are good indicators of the underlying construct can be even costlier. Lessening this concern is that many tasks typically used in studies of IIV have items that are easy to develop. For example, new items in the working memory task described in the example require only simple math problems and new permutations of to-be-remembered letters.

Another data collection challenge is that typical test protocols cannot be used for assessing IIV with ICIRMs. To identify IIV separately from changes in the items, the order of item administration must vary across participants. Typical versions of psychological tests have a fixed order, whether the test is paper-and-pencil or computerized. Varying the order of administration requires either programming adjustments or multiple forms. Archival data cannot generally be used.

11.5.2 Benefits

Despite the challenges inherent in this modeling technique, it offers some key benefits. First, it is the only extant model that allows for the assessment of IIV with nonrepeated items within a single measurement occasion. Intratask IIV is the closest approximation to instantaneous variability available from empirical research. The method presented in this chapter opens the door for the measurement of IIV at the shortest time frame possible for a much wider class of measurement instruments and psychological constructs.

Second, although a large number of item administrations may be necessary to achieve sufficiently precise estimates of IIV, this method provides a dramatic decrease in data collection costs. It is very expensive to repeatedly assess participants across enough experimental sessions to achieve reliable measurement of IIV (Estabrook et al., 2008). Adding additional item administrations within a single occasion is substantially less expensive. It may be possible to use a mixed data collection method: a smaller number of items assessed repeatedly over a small number of occasions. This type of data would still require an ICIRM with IIV, but may reduce the burden of long testing sessions with a modestly increased cost of multiple sessions.

Finally, it is important to note that this method may yield different results than the assessment of IIV across occasions. Although the magnitude of IIV at shorter time frames can affect the magnitude of IIV at longer time frames (Huxhold et al., 2007), they are conceptually and theoretically distinct. Thus, IIV in an intratask change framework can yield important and independent insights into the nature of human behavior.

11.5.3 Conclusion

ICIRMs provide a novel method for assessing IIV within a single measurement occasion by considering individual variability at the item level. Empirical and theoretical research has demonstrated the importance of IIV as a scientific endeavor despite the challenges encountered in its measurement. IIV occurring within a task is the closest approximation to the precise meaning of IIV inherent in theory, highlighting the need for assessing IIV with intratask change models. The model presented in this chapter is complex, difficult to estimate, and has large data requirements, but shows some potential in measuring IIV at the shortest time frame possible. Further effort is needed at developing more accurate estimation methods and identifying experimental characteristics that yield the most accurate and precise conclusions about IIV.

ACKNOWLEDGMENT

The author wishes to thank Martin Sliwinski and Jacquie Mogle for their assistance with collecting the data in the example.

REFERENCES

Andrich, D. (1978). A rating formulation for ordered response categories. *Psychometrika, 43*, 357–374.

Anstey, K. J. (1999). Sensorimotor variables and forced expiratory volume as correlates of speed, accuracy and variability in reaction time performance in late adulthood. *Aging, Neuropsychology, and Cognition, 6*, 84–95.

Baker, F. (2001). *The basics of item response theory.* College Park, MD: ERIC Clearinghouse on Assessment and Evaluation.

Bejar, I. I. (1983). Subject matter experts assessment of item statistics. *Applied Psychological Measurement, 7*, 303–310.

Birnbaum, A. (1968). Some latent trait models and their use in inferring an examinee's ability. In F. M. Lorg & M. R. Novick (Eds.), *Statistical theories of mental test scores*, (pp. 397–479). Reading, MA: Addison-Wesley.

Bowles, R. P. (2009). *Item response models for intratask change.* Manuscript in revision.

Bowles, R. P., Wise, S. L., & Kingsbury, G. G. (2008). *A report on position effects in the NCLEX RN examination.* Chicago: National Council of State Boards of Nursing.

Butler, A., Hokanson, J., & Flynn, H. (1994). A comparison of self-esteem lability and low trait self-esteem as vulnerability factors for depression. *Journal of Personality and Social Psychology, 66*, 166–177.

Cattell, R. B. (1988). The data box: Its ordering of total resources in terms of possible relational systems. In J. R. Nesselroade & R. B. Cattell (Eds.), *Handbook of multivariate experimental psychology: Perspectives on individual differences* (2nd ed.) (pp. 69–130). New York: Plenum.

Deary, I. J., & Der, G., (2005). Reaction time, age, and cognitive ability: Longitudinal findings from age 16 to 63 years in representative population samples. *Aging, Neuropsychology and Cognition, 12*, 187–215.

Eid, M., & Diener, E. (1999). Intraindividual variability in affect: Reliability, validity, and personality correlates. *Journal of Personality and Social Psychology, 76*, 662–676.

Eizenman, D., Nesselroade, J., Featherman, D., & Rowe, J. (1997). Intraindividual variability in perceived control in an older sample: The MacArthur successful aging studies. *Psychology and Aging, 12*, 489–502.

Embretson, S. E., & Reise, S. (2000). *Item response theory for psychologists.* Mahwah, NJ: Erlbaum.

Estabrook, R., Grimm, K. J., & Bowles, R. P. (2009). *A Monte Carlo simulation study assessment of the reliability of within-person variability.* Manuscript in revision.
Ferrer, E., Salthouse, T. A., Stewart, W. F., & Schwartz, B. S. (2004). Modeling age and retest processes in longitudinal studies of cognitive abilities. *Psychology and Aging, 19,* 243–259.
Fischer, G. H. (1973). The linear logistic test model as an instrument in educational research. *Acta Psychologica, 36,* 359–374.
Fiske, D. W., & Rice, L. (1955). Intra-individual response variability. *Psychological Bulletin, 57, 3,* 217–250.
Fox, N., & Porges, S. (1985). The relation between neonatal heart period patterns and developmental outcome. *Child Development, 56,* 28–37.
Fuentes, K., Hunter, M. A., Strauss, E., & Hultsch, D. F. (2001). Intraindividual variability in cognitive performance in person with chronic fatigue syndrome. *The Clinical Neuropsychologist, 15,* 210–227.
Geman, S., & Geman, D. (1984). Stochastic relaxation, Gibbs distributions, and the Bayesian restoration of images. *IEEE Transactions on Pattern Analysis and Machine Intelligence, 6,* 721–741.
Hale, S., Myerson, J., & Smith, G. A., (1988). Age, variability, and speed: Between-subjects diversity. *Psychology and Aging, 3,* 407–410.
Hultsch, D. F., & MacDonald, S. W. S. (2004). Intraindividual variability in performance as a theoretical window onto cognitive aging. In R. A. Dixon, L. Bäckman, & L.-G. Nilsson (Eds.), *New frontiers in cognitive aging* (pp. 65–88). Oxford: Oxford University Press.
Huxhold, O., Li, S.-C., Schmiedek, F., & Lindenberger, U. (2009). *Age differences of intra-individual processing fluctuations in postural control across trials and across days.* Manuscript in preparation.
Jensen, A. R. (1992). The importance of intraindividual variation in reaction time. *Personality and Individual Differences, 13,* 869–881.
Kagan, J. (1994). *Galen's prophecy.* New York: Basic Books.
Karpicke, J. D., & Roediger, H. L. (2007). Repeated retrieval during learning is the key to long-term retention. *Journal of Memory and Language, 57,* 151–162.
Klauer, K. C., & Sydow, H. (2001). Modeling learning in short-term learning tests. In A. Boomsma, M. A. J. van Duijn, & T. A. B. Snijders (Eds.), *Essays on item response theory.* New York: Springer.
Lenhart, A., Horrigan, J., Rainie, L., Allen, K., Boyce, A., Madden, M., & O'Grady, E. (2003). *The ever-shifting Internet population.* Retrieved May 1, 2006 from Pew Internet and American Life Project Web site: www.pewinternet.org/pdfs/PIP_Shifting_Net_Pop_Report.pdf
Masters, G. N. (1982). A Rasch model for partial credit scoring. *Psychometrika, 60,* 523–547.
Nesselroade, J. R. (1991). The warp and woof of the developmental fabric. In R. Downs, L. Liben, & D. Palermo (Eds.), *Visions of development, the environment, and aesthetics: The legacy of Joachim F. Wohlwill* (pp. 213–240). Hillsdale, NJ: Erlbaum.
Nesselroade, J. R., & Ford, D. H. (1985). P-technique comes of age: Multivariate, replicated, single-subject designs for research on older adults. *Research on Aging, 7,* 46–80.
Newell, K. M., Liu, Y. T., & Mayer-Kress, G. (2001). Time scales in motor learning and development. *Psychological Review, 108,* 57–82.
Pincus, S. M. (1991). Approximate entropy as a measure of system complexity. *Proceedings of the National Academy of Sciences, USA, 88,* 2297–2301.

Pincus, S. M., & Goldberger, A. L. (1994). Physiological time-series analysis: What does regularity quantify? *American Journal of Physiology (Heart Circulatory Physiology), 266*, H1643–H1656.

Ram, N., Rabbitt, P., Stollery, B., & Nesselroade, J. R. (2005). Cognitive performance inconsistency: Intraindividual change and variability. *Psychology and Aging, 20*, 623–633.

Rasch, G. (1980). *Probabilistic models for some intelligence and attainments tests* (expanded edition). Chicago: University of Chicago Press. (Original work published 1960).

Schretlen, D. J., Munro, C. A., Anthony, J. C., & Pearlson, G. D., (2003). Examining the range of normal intraindividual variability in neuropsychological test performance. *Journal of the International Neuropsychological Society, 9*, 864–870.

Slifkin, A. B., & Newell, K. M. (1998). Is variability in human performance a reflection of system noise? *Current Directions in Psychological Science, 7*, 170–177.

Slifkin, A. B., & Newell, K. M. (1999). Noise, information transmission, and force variability. *Journal of Experimental Psychology: Human Perception and Performance, 25*, 837–851.

Sosnoff, J. J., & Newell, K. M. (2006). The generalization of perceptual-motor intra-individual variability in young and old adults. *Journals of Gerontology: Psychological Science, 61*, P304–P310.

Sparapani, R., & Hayat, M. (2007). *SAS macros for BUGS* [computer software]. Retrieved December 12, 2007 from http://www.mcw.edu/pcor/bugs/.

Spiegelhalter, D. J., Thomas, A., Best, N. G., & Lunn, D. (2004). WinBUGS version 1.4.1 [Computer software]. London: Imperial College and MRC.

Tulving, E. (1967). The effects of presentation and recall of material in free recall learning. *Journal of Verbal Learning and Verbal Behavior, 6*, 175–184.

Turner, M. L., & Engle, R. W. (1989). Is working memory capacity task dependent? *Journal of Memory and Language, 28*, 127–154.

Unsworth, N., Heitz, R. P., Schrock, J. C., & Engle, R. W. (2005). An automated version of the operation span task. *Behavior Research Methods, 37*, 498–505.

Vega-Lopez, S., Ausman, L. M., Griffith, J. L., & Lichtenstein, A. H. (2007). Inter- and intra-individual variability in glycemic index values for white bread determined using standardized procedures. *Diabetes Care, 30*, 1412–1417.

Verhelst, N. D., & Glas, C. A. W. (1993). A dynamic generalization of the Rasch model. *Psychometrika, 58*, 395–425.

Verhaeghen, P., & Salthouse, T. A. (1997). Meta-analyses of age-cognition relations in adulthood: Estimates of linear and nonlinear age effects and structural models. *Psychological Bulletin, 122*, 231–249.

Verhelst, N. D., & Glas, C. A. W. (1995). Dynamic generalizations of the Rasch model. In G. H. Fischer & I. W. Molenaar (Eds.), *Rasch models: Foundations, recent developments, and applications* (pp. 181–201). New York: Springer.

Yen, W. M. (1993). Scaling performance assessments: Strategies for managing local item dependence. *Journal of Educational Measurement, 30*, 187–213.

Zhang, Z., McArdle, J. J., Wang, L., & Hamagami, F. (2008). A SAS interface for Bayesian analysis with WinBUGS. *Structural Equation Modeling, 15*, 705–728.

Part III

Modeling Interindividual Differences in Change and Interpersonal Dynamics

12

Developing a Random Coefficient Model for Nonlinear Repeated Measures Data

Robert Cudeck and Jeffrey R. Harring

12.1 INTRODUCTION

The random coefficient model has been applied extensively in many different research settings in recent years. In the social sciences, the model has proven to be especially valuable for the study of individual differences in repeated measures problems or longitudinal studies. The main appeal of the method is that the process of change is described for each individual, an approach that is especially natural in the study of behavior. At the same time, the model also represents average change in the population, and connects average change with the collection of developmental patterns for individuals. Characteristics of development can be further accounted by covariates such as demographic variables, achievement, or health status, which may be important in explaining individual differences in development.

Most actual uses of this method have been in solving problems where development or growth shows a relatively constant rate of change over time, and so a linear model is appropriate. There are situations, however, where the rate of change for the behavior under study is slower or faster in some time intervals than others. In these cases, a linear model is not adequate and a nonlinear function is preferable. The most common nonlinear model is a polynomial function such as the quadratic or cubic. These options are popular for two reasons. First, a low-order polynomial model often works well. Since goodness-of-fit is important, the ability of a polynomial to effectively summarize longitudinal data is not inconsequential. Second, because polynomial models are linear in the parameters of the function, they can be estimated relatively easily with standard software. In itself this practical advantage is a compelling reason for turning to a polynomial model when the change process is nonlinear in form.

On the other hand, polynomial functions have well-known liabilities for studying nonlinear change. In some cases, another nonlinear function can account for data even better than a polynomial, and may do so with fewer parameters. Thus, on the basis of parsimony and fit, a polynomial may not be the best choice among alternatives. Another consideration is that the coefficients of polynomial functions do not have a clear-cut and scientifically meaningful interpretation. It is extremely helpful if coefficients of a function give some information about the behavior that the function summarizes. This is especially important with random coefficients that may incorporate individual-level covariates to explain between-subject differences. Whenever possible it is desirable to take advantage of functions with interpretable parameters.

In complex longitudinal analyses, there are many choices to make about structure. It is a truism that each research problem has design and behavioral features that make the available data unique. When deciding on a function this means that informed scientific knowledge of the context is essential. A model chosen on the basis of theoretical considerations about behavior is preferable to other methods of model selection in which subject matter knowledge is secondary. This also implies that although there are functions that describe different kinds of data well, there is inevitably a need to tailor a model to fit a problem, or at least to search widely to find a structure that performs appropriately. Surveys of standard nonlinear functions, such as those reviewed by Lewis (1966), Bates and Watts (1988), or Seber and Wild (1989), are excellent sources for candidate models. Many of these can be adapted easily. The value of the process in the end is a structure that is particularly well suited to the characteristics of the data.

A reviewer of this chapter pointed out that exploratory statistical tools that fit a flexible function to data, such as the lowess smoother, can highlight important features of repeated measures not immediately apparent otherwise (see Diggle, Liang, & Zeger, 1994, Chapter 3.2; Fitzmaurice, Laird, &

Ware, 2004, Chapter 3.3). Although we do not pursue this topic, it is an extremely valuable exploratory process. An offsetting liability is that general smoothers do not always produce parsimonious functions with parameters that are associated with scientifically meaningful elements of the response. As the reviewer observed, by themselves "special functional parameters may trump other considerations" in the choice of a model. Our view is that functions that include parameters of this kind are so informative and helpful that their existence in a model is often reason enough to consider a function.

The goal of this chapter is to illustrate how a plausible random coefficient model is developed for repeated measures data when the pattern is nonlinear. Inasmuch as this general nonlinear model is not widely applied in the social sciences, a detailed example demonstrating the overall approach may be useful. The data we examine come from an interesting visual task in which participants read a set of standardized sentences to assess their visual acuity. The print size with which the sentences are displayed varies from large to quite small. Reading speed slows as print size decreases, but the decline in speed is more rapid for small print sizes than for large. This makes the overall pattern nonlinear in shape. The problem is to decide on a function that relates reading speed to print size. Although the analysis of these data is informative in its own right, it is the process of deciding on a particular model from among alternatives that illustrates the broader issue.

12.1.1 MNREAD Acuity Chart

The scientific focus of attention in this study is the assessment of visual acuity by means of the MNREAD acuity chart (Mansfield, Ahn, Legge, & Luebker, 1993). Participants ($N = 30$) were normal sighted adults. MNREAD is a continuous-text, reading-acuity chart consisting of 19 sentences. Each sentence has 60 characters displayed on three lines. Vocabulary on the stimuli is appropriate for third-grade readers. The first three sentences of one form of the chart are shown in Figure 12.1.

Print size, the independent variable in this analysis, is measured according to a standardized system. It is based on the logarithm of minimum angle of resolution (log MAR) with reference to the angle subtended by the height of the lower case letter x. The range of this measurement is -0.5 to 1.3 in steps of 0.1. The order of administration of the sentences is always from largest to smallest. The last sentence at log MAR $= -0.5$ is so small that

My father takes me
to school every day
in his big green car

Everyone wanted to
go outside when the
rain finally stopped

They were not able
to finish playing the
game before dinner

FIGURE 12.1 The first three sentences of the MNREAD chart. Each sentence has 60 characters displayed on three lines.

many participants with normal vision have difficulty making out the text. Reading speed was recorded for each sentence as words per minute (WPM) and calculated as the number of words read correctly divided by the time taken to read the sentence (measured to the nearest 0.1 s). A correction for errors was also applied.

The profiles of reading speeds for ten individuals are shown in Figure 12.2. Two features of the profiles are especially important scientifically and clinically in summarizing the data. As is evident in the figure, reading speed in terms of WPM is relatively constant across larger print sizes. The WPM rate that is not affected by increasing print size is called the *maximum reading speed*. It is essentially the average WPM across the larger of the print sizes. A complicating issue in calculating maximum reading speed is that the set of sentences that make up larger print sizes varies from one person to another. Second, at some point in reading sentences at smaller print size performance deteriorates and falls off rapidly as print size decreases. The WPM that marks the changepoint is another important variable called the *critical print size*. It is defined as the smallest print size that can be read with maximum reading speed. In the figure, maximum reading speeds vary between approximately 175 and 275 WPM; critical print sizes vary between approximately −0.1 to 0.1 log MAR. One purpose of describing these data with a function is to obtain a model-based estimate of both maximum reading speed and critical print size. Recently, Cheung, Kallie, Legge, and Cheong (2008) presented a preliminary report of these data, emphasizing results that are most relevant for vision research.

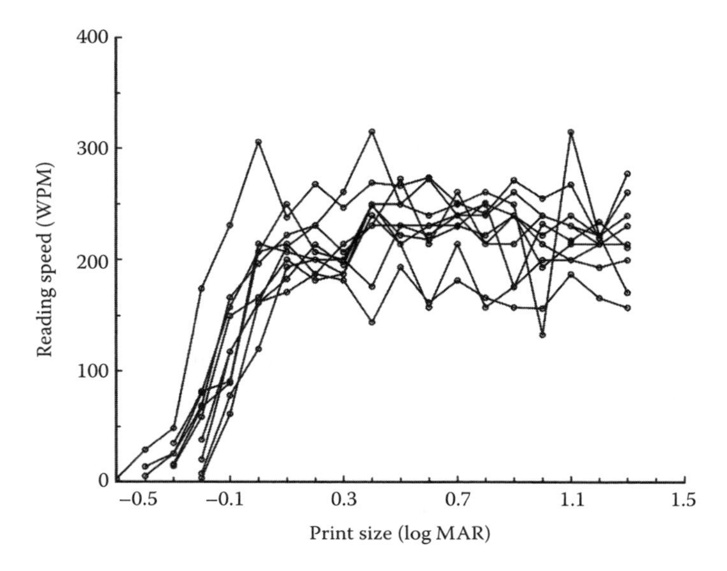

FIGURE 12.2 Reading speed (in WPM) across the MNREAD chart sentences for a random subset of individuals with normal vision. Maximum reading speed, between approximately 175 and 275 WPM for these cases, is the reading rate that does not improve if print size is increased. Critical print size, between approximately −0.1 to 0.1, is the point at which the print size negatively affects reading speed.

In contrast, this chapter is focussed more on statistical issues, especially on alternative response functions, of which there are many possibilities. We also describe completely the covariance structure of the random coefficient model, which was not reviewed at all by Cheung et al.

12.1.2 Evaluating a Model

In developing a model, the objective is to find a version that performs well and that produces information about the process being studied that is different from the measurements actually obtained. It is the model parameters that give new information. Optimally the model is designed so that parameters represent novel features of individual change that can be used to address questions that are difficult to answer without the model. We state here the criteria that a good model should exhibit, then illustrate them at some length subsequently.

First, the target function should fit well. To the extent possible, it is obviously essential that the function follow the data closely. When the within-subject variability is large, it is seldom possible to be dogmatic about the ultimate choice. Even when within-subject variability is zero, there generally are several possible prospects to consider. When two or more contenders fit similarly, the best that can be done is to review the relative merits of the alternatives and give reasons why one is preferable under the circumstances.

Second, the form of the curve should make sense for the major outcome variable in light of what is assumed to be appropriate for the context. Basically, appropriateness means that the function should exhibit a pattern of change across the predictor that captures the important and systematic fluctuations in the response. Evaluating this criterion requires experience in the scientific domain and often turns on subjective judgment.

Third, the parameters of a model should be interpretable and should give useful information about individual differences. Parameters of a function that simply define a curve but that have no special significance are undesirable. The criterion of clear, unambiguous meaning for all parameters of a function is important for understanding the behavior that the function describes. Interpretability is also important because in a random coefficient model the parameters are used as dependent variables in a level 2 model which account for the effects of covariates. For the level 2 model to make sense, it is essential that the coefficients at level 1 have a clear definition.

These three criteria—fit, appropriateness, and interpretability—are common standards when judging the success of mathematical models, and they are especially important when nonlinear processes are under investigation. It sometimes happens that two candidate functions fit data essentially in the same manner and more or less equally satisfactorily. If this occurs, then one model may be preferable because it is more appropriate than the other. In another situation, two functions may both have interpretable parameters and may be judged to be comparably appropriate. In this instance, goodness-of-fit of the two models can be used to decide which is preferable. Although all three components are important, the extent that the criteria are emphasized in an overall decision is again a matter of judgment. Most functions can be expressed in several equivalent ways, some of which are more helpful than others in terms of the information on the parameters. It is frequently the case that two experienced researchers working with the same data reach different conclusions as to the most appropriate model.

12.2 ALTERNATIVE MODELS FOR THE MNREAD DATA

In this section, we review several different functions for the MNREAD data. The general goal is to tailor the function to the repeated measures to find an effective representation of the profile of reading scores. The strategy is to examine the behavior of each candidate function with data from a typical individual, modifying and elaborating as needed so that the main features of the data are satisfactorily represented by the function. Toward this end, the reading speeds for one person are listed in Table 12.1. In the analysis of data from one individual, the approach used is simply nonlinear, least squares regression. This is obviously an exploratory exercise. Graphs are invaluable. When a function has been identified that appears to work well for a single person's data, the framework is extended to a nonlinear random coefficient model and applied to the data from an entire sample. Proceeding from a single case to the full sample provides a check on the model development phase, ensuring that the final function performs adequately for all individuals. Requiring that the function applies reasonably well to most individuals in the sample ensures that the preliminary analyses do not overfit a single profile of scores used in the exploratory phase.

In the model for a single individual, the jth repeated measurement, y_j, $j = 1, \ldots, n$, is assumed to be composed of a smooth functional component of model m, f_{jm}, plus residual, e_{jm}. The function depends on unknown parameters, $\theta_m = (\theta_1, \ldots, \theta_{q_m})'$, as well as the design value for the jth response, x_j, often the occasion of measurement or elapsed time from the beginning of the study. For the MNREAD data, the predictor is not occasion

TABLE 12.1

Reading Speed (WPM) and Print Size (log MAR) by One Individual on the 19 MNREAD Sentences

Sentence	19	18	17	16	15	14	13	12	11	10
WPM	m	10.8	111.1	142.9	176.5	176.5	200.0	200.0	206.9	206.9
log MAR	−0.5	−0.4	−0.3	−0.2	−0.1	0.0	0.1	0.2	0.3	0.4

Sentence	9	8	7	6	5	4	3	2	1
WPM	206.9	214.3	214.3	214.3	214.3	214.3	222.2	222.2	230.8
log MAR	0.5	0.6	0.7	0.8	0.9	1.0	1.1	1.2	1.3

Sentence 19 at the smallest print size, log MAR = −0.5, could not be read and is marked as missing (m).

or time but rather the print size of each sentence. The function is

$$f_{jm} = f_m(x_j, \theta_m).$$

To simplify notation, we often will exclude the arguments as well as subscript of the function. The general model has the familiar form

$$y_j = f_{jm} + e_{jm}.$$

In the model development stage, we ignore the problem of the variance structure and correlation pattern among e_{jm} for repeated measures and simply concentrate on selecting an adequate f_m.

For individuals with complete data on the MNREAD sentences, the number of measurements is $n = 19$. The subject whose data are shown in Table 12.1 was not able to read the sentence at the smallest print size—WPM is missing for y_{19}. This gives $n = 18$ measurements. In the sample of individuals examined subsequently, the smallest print size that was most frequently read was log MAR $= -0.4$. When results with a function are clear, we prefer to use the original stimulus measurements as predictor

$$x_j = \log \text{MAR}_j,$$

where log MAR_j is the print size of the jth sentence. With other functions, parameters are easiest to interpret if the predictor is

$$x_j^* = \log \text{MAR}_j + 0.4.$$

This shift transformation locates the y intercept at the sample modal minimum print size, which is convenient for all the functions that have a y intercept. Again, following the actual protocol used with the chart, the sentences are in order of decreasing size: $x_1 > x_2 > \cdots > x_{19}$.

12.2.1 Quadratic and Cubic Polynomials

The pattern of the data in Figure 12.2 is clearly nonlinear. A reasonable and very popular possibility for this situation is a low degree polynomial such as the quadratic or cubic. For many problems, these sometimes describe data well. On the other hand, polynomials are general-purpose tools that are appealing because of their familiarity and often satisfactory fit, not because they are obviously appropriate in all contexts. Irrespective of their other merits, polynomials can serve the useful purpose of defining a starting point from which to compare other alternatives.

The quadratic and cubic are, respectively,

$$f_{jq} = \beta_0 + \beta_1 x_j^* + \beta_2 x_j^{*2}, \quad f_{jc} = \beta_0 + \beta_1 x_j^* + \beta_2 x_j^{*2} + \beta_3 x_j^{*3}.$$

Figure 12.3 shows the least squares fitted function for f_c as the broken line. Table 12.2 gives two measures of model fit: the mean square residual and squared correlation between actual and fitted values of y. Using the cubic function as an example, the fit statistics are

$$\text{MSR}(y_j, \hat{f}_{jc}) = n^{-1} \sum (y_j - \hat{f}_{jc})^2, \quad r^2(y_j, \hat{f}_{jc}) = \text{corr}^2(y_j, \hat{f}_{jc}),$$

where the predicted value is $\hat{f}_{jc} = \hat{\beta}_0 + \hat{\beta}_1 x_j^* + \hat{\beta}_2 x_j^{*2} + \hat{\beta}_3 x_j^{*3}$, where $\hat{\beta}_k$, $k = 0, \ldots, 3$, are least squares estimates. Based on the indices of fit, the quadratic performs poorly, mostly because it overpredicts at smaller print sizes. It also fails to represent the sharp change in WPM that occurs for log MAR values in the range −0.2 to 0.1.

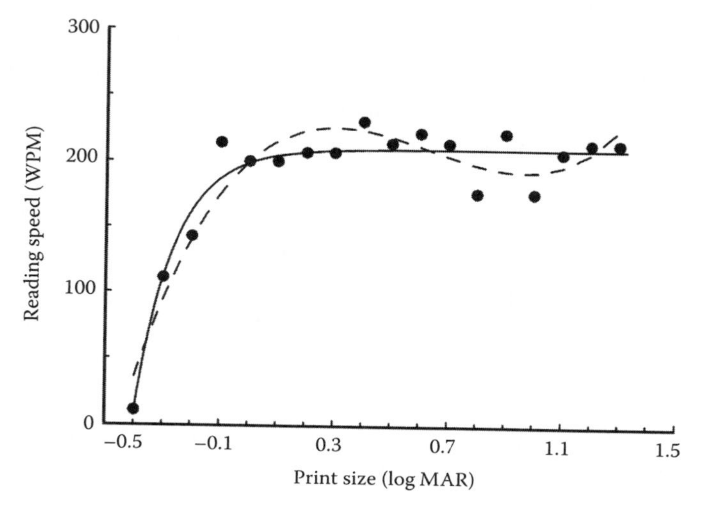

FIGURE 12.3 Fitted functions for the cubic polynomial (broken line) and exponential (solid line) models for one individual. Although the cubic fits relatively well, three of its four parameters are not interpretable. Furthermore, the cubic is curvilinear over the large print sizes where it is assumed that WPM is essentially constant. With the exponential, the transition from the smallest to larger print sizes is too gradual.

TABLE 12.2

Measures of Model Fit and Number of Parameters for Each Function

Model	MSR	r^2	Parameters
Quadratic	905.4	0.665	3
Cubic	302.0	0.888	4
Exponential	236.3	0.912	3
Linear–linear (Equation 12.4)	223.3	0.917	3
Linear–linear (Equation 12.2)	222.5	0.918	4
Quadratic–linear (Equation 12.9)	219.0	0.919	4
Linear–linear with smooth transition	223.7	0.917	3

The fit of the cubic is a great improvement over the quadratic: $\text{MSR}(y_j, \hat{f}_{jc}) = 302.1$, $r^2(y_j, \hat{f}_{jc}) = 0.888$. Although it is better than the quadratic in following the rapid change in reading speed between smaller and larger print sizes, it can be seen in Figure 12.3 that the transition is too gradual compared with the actual data. Another deficiency is that the function is of no help in locating the critical print size. And over the larger print sizes where it is assumed that reading speed is essentially constant, f_c is curvilinear. In summary, although the cubic is better than the quadratic, it still has several defects.

A further problem with both these models is that only one parameter of either function is interpretable. For each, β_0 is the y intercept, the predicted value of y when $x_j^* = 0$. The other coefficients, however, have no simple interpretation in terms of the protocol or the change process under investigation. For example, the parameter estimates from the cubic are $\hat{\theta}_c = (35.7, 656.1, -707.7, 227.9)'$. The intercept, $\hat{\beta}_0 = 35.7$, is not greatly discrepant compared with the corresponding WPM, $y_{18} = 10.8$. The second coefficient, $\hat{\beta}_1 = 656.1$, does not have a straightforward interpretation in terms of the profile of reading speeds. β_1 is called the coefficient of x_j and β_2 the coefficient of x_j^2. The coefficients determine the shape of the function, but have no direct scientific meaning that gives information about the process. The value of interpretable parameters is so great that functions whose coefficients do not have this property are often excluded from consideration whether the function fits well or not.

12.2.2 Exponential

The exponential function is frequently used where there is a rapid increase in response from a low starting value up to a plateau. This pattern is common to many kinds of growth and learning variables and can be tried in the present example as well. The exponential is

$$f_{je} = \alpha_1 - (\alpha_1 - \alpha_0)\exp(-\rho x_j^*), \quad \rho > 0. \tag{12.1}$$

It is noteworthy that the three parameters are interpretable. When $x_j^* = 0$, at the small 18th sentence, $f_{je} = \alpha_0$. So α_0 is the y intercept, the level of the response at the smallest print size that most participants could read. When x_j^* is very large, $f_{je} \rightarrow \alpha_1$. Therefore, α_1 is the maximum performance corresponding to large print sizes, a model-based estimate of maximum reading speed. The coefficient ρ controls how rapidly the function proceeds from α_0 to α_1 as x_j^* increases. For this reason, ρ is known as the rate parameter of the function.

It is worth emphasizing that all three parameters are summaries of the complete set of measurements. Thus α_1, for example, is not equal to any particular WPM, but instead is an estimate based on the entire collection, the slower WPM measurements as well as the faster. Because α_1 is a summary, it is assumed to be a more reliable indicator of maximum reading speed than any particular WPM for a large print size would be.

Indices of model fit for the exponential function are listed in Table 12.2. Least-squares estimates are given in the table below with standard errors in parentheses. Since this is a small data set, the standard errors are not small. Estimated WPM at $x_j^* = 0$ is $\hat{\alpha}_0 = 8.85$, and maximum reading speed, $\hat{\alpha}_1 = 209.8$, are reasonable given the data. The fitted function is shown in Figure 12.3 as the solid line. The exponential fits the data much better than the cubic, $\text{MSR}(y_j, \hat{f}_{je}) = 236.3$ and $r^2(y_j, \hat{f}_{je}) = 0.912$ versus $\text{MSR}(y_j, \hat{f}_{jc}) = 302.0$ and $r^2(y_j, \hat{f}_{jc}) = 0.888$, and does so with one fewer coefficient.

$\hat{\alpha}_0$	$\hat{\alpha}_1$	$\hat{\rho}$
8.85(16)	209.8(4.8)	7.22(1.3).

Another way to write the exponential is

$$f_{je} = \alpha_1 - (\alpha_1 - \alpha_0)2^{-x_j^*/\lambda}, \quad \lambda > 0,$$

where α_0 and α_1 are again initial and maximum reading speed. Here, $\lambda = \ln(2)/\rho$ is the print size that corresponds to half the improvement in reading speed between α_0 and α_1 . When $x^* = \lambda, f_{je} = \alpha_1 - \frac{1}{2}(\alpha_1 - \alpha_0)$. Although ρ in Equation 12.1 is understandable as an index that governs the rate of increase of the function, λ is even more concrete since it is an estimated print size. In fitting this version, $\hat{\alpha}_0$ and $\hat{\alpha}_1$ are the same, while $\hat{\lambda} = 0.096$, with $\text{se}(\hat{\lambda}) = 0.02$.

12.2.3 Two-Phase, Linear–Linear

One limitation of the exponential is that it gives no direct information about the critical print size. An interesting function that measures critical print size explicitly is the behavior of a piece-wise linear spline. General theory of two-phase models is reviewed by Seber and Wild (1989, Chapter 9). Multiphase models are flexible because each section can be specified to conform to a particular aspect of the overall change process. One of the most interesting features of a two-phase model is the knot or join point. The knot, a parameter to be estimated, is the x-value where the sections meet. The knot is especially interesting for the MNREAD data as the critical print size. In this way, the model uses the data to produce information not specifically available in the original set of measurements but which has special significance scientifically.

The most straightforward two-phase model is linear–linear. Once again we use $x_j = \log \text{MAR}_j$ because results are clearer with this version of the predictor. In its most general form, the linear–linear function is written as

$$f_j = \begin{cases} \alpha_0 + \alpha_1 x_j, & x_j \leq \tau, \\ \beta_0 + \beta_1 x_j, & x_j > \tau, \end{cases}$$

where the first segment is $\alpha_0 + \alpha_1 x_j$ and the second $\beta_0 + \beta_1 x_j$. The segments operate for values of x_j that are less than the knot τ or greater than τ. Nominally there are five coefficients: $(\alpha_0, \alpha_1, \beta_0, \beta_1, \tau)$. In many cases, however, the two phases join at $x_j = \tau$, which implies that at the knot, $\alpha_0 + \alpha_1\tau = \beta_0 + \beta_1\tau$. Because of this equality, one parameter is redundant and can be eliminated. It is convenient to define the intercept of the first phase in terms of the other coefficients by setting $\alpha_0 = \beta_0 + \beta_1\tau - \alpha_1\tau$. Then the function is

$$f_{jL} = \begin{cases} (\beta_0 + \beta_1\tau - \alpha_1\tau) + \alpha_1 x_j, & x_j \leq \tau, \\ \beta_0 + \beta_1 x_j, & x_j > \tau, \end{cases} \tag{12.2}$$

with coefficients $\theta_L = (\alpha_1, \beta_0, \beta_1, \tau)'$. These are the slope of phase 1, the intercept and slope of phase 2, and change point.

A more compact expression is convenient and emphasizes that the two segments make up a single function. It is written as

$$f_{jL} = \beta_0 + \beta_1 x_j + (\beta_1 - \alpha_1)(\tau - x_j)_+. \tag{12.3}$$

The last term is the truncation operator, defined as zero or the positive value of the argument, depending on its sign

$$u_+ = \begin{cases} u, & u \geq 0, \\ 0 & \text{otherwise.} \end{cases}$$

As examples, $(5.1 - 4)_+ = 1.1$, $(3 - 2.9)_+ = 0.1$, but $(-2)_+ = 0$ and $(1 - 5)_+ = 0$.

Another version is appropriate for the MNREAD data where reading speed is constant across larger print sizes. Because the rate of change in the second phase is assumed to be zero, one can set $\beta_1 = 0$ so that the model becomes

$$f_{jF} = \begin{cases} (\beta_0 - \alpha_1 \tau) + \alpha_1 x_j, & x_j \leq \tau, \\ \beta_0, & x_j > \tau. \end{cases} \tag{12.4}$$

Equivalently as a single expression, Equation 12.4 can be written as

$$f_{jF} = \beta_0 - \alpha_1(\tau - x_j)_+. \tag{12.5}$$

For the MNREAD data, α_1 is still the slope of the first phase; τ the critical print size; β_0 is directly interpreted as the maximum reading speed. As with τ, β_0 is then particularly meaningful for this context. It is a summary of all WPM measurements and produces a coefficient that is not directly assessed in the original data.

Most functions can be expressed in two or more equivalent ways. More than an algebraic exercise, a re-expression can be helpful scientifically if the parameters of one form give information that is directly related to the behavior in a manner than is more relevant than others. As an example using model 12.4, it might be of interest to re-write the function to obtain a different kind of information about individual differences in the first phase, still keeping the same linear–linear format. In the first phase, α_1 is the slope over smaller print sizes. As an alternative, consider a specific WPM set by the investigator. For example, it might be $w_0 = 35$. Define the print size, κ, that produces reading speed of w_0 WPM. That is, when $x = \kappa$, $f = w_0$, so that κ is an unknown parameter of the model. The model is still linear–linear, but α_1 in Equation 12.4 is replaced in an equivalent model that includes κ. This version is

$$f_{jF} = \begin{cases} w_0 + \dfrac{(\beta_0 - w_0)(x_j - \kappa)}{\tau - \kappa}, & x_j \leq \tau, \\ \beta_0, & x_j > \tau. \end{cases} \tag{12.6}$$

It can be seen that at $x = \kappa, f = w_0$, and as before, at $x = \tau, f = \beta_0$. The parameters are (κ, τ, β_0). Because Equations 12.4 and 12.6 are equivalent, the decision to use one or the other depends on the relative merits of the respective parameterizations in the opinion of the investigator.

As shown in Table 12.2 with the data in Table 12.1, functions 12.4 and 12.2 fit almost the same. Of course, Equations 12.4 and 12.6 fit the same exactly. Estimates from model Equations 12.2 or 12.3, the most general of the three because it does not assume $\beta_1 = 0$, are below

$$\begin{array}{cccc} \hat{\alpha}_1 & \hat{\beta}_0 & \hat{\beta}_1 & \hat{\tau} \\ 661(120) & 209(7.5) & -2.29(10) & -0.116(0.04). \end{array}$$

A graph of the fitted function is shown in Figure 12.4 as the broken line. The estimated knot, marked on the graph as the broken vertical line, is $\hat{\tau} = -0.116$. The interpretation of this value is that if many alternate forms of MNREAD sentences were administered to a person with many different sets of print sizes, $\hat{\tau}$ is the long-term or expected changepoint. The slope in the second phase is slightly negative: $\hat{\beta}_1 = -2.29$ but with a large standard error. If function 12.2 is taken as the final model, then there is no specific coefficient that gives information about maximum reading speed. If $\beta_1 \neq 0$ then performance on the response is either increasing or decreasing over x_j in the second phase. In this context, $\beta_1 \neq 0$ implies that there is no model-based maximum reading speed in the range of the log MAR values. When $\beta_1 > 0$, one could still make use of the two-phase model and define maximum reading speed as the maximum y_j in the interval $x_j > \tau$. On the other hand, when $\beta_1 < 0$ then maximum WPM occurs at the print size $x = \tau$, with the maximum equal to $\beta_0 + \beta_1\tau$.

Both versions of the piece-wise linear model have the property that in the first phase the rate of improvement of reading speed over increasing print size (α_1) changes instantly at $x = \tau$ to a very different rate in the

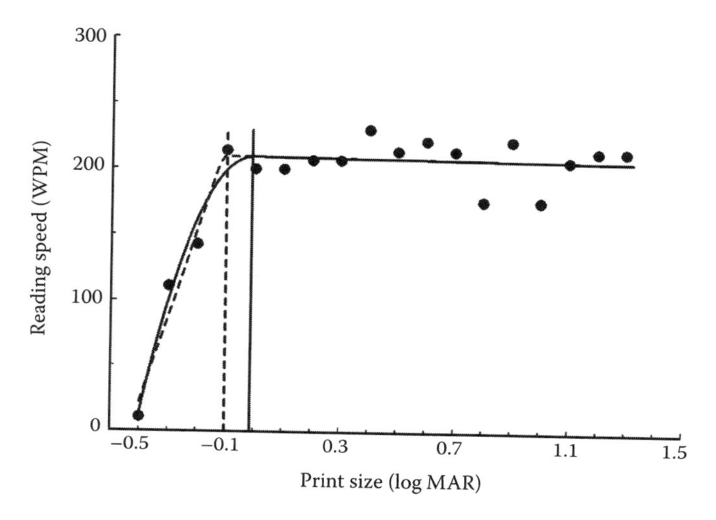

FIGURE 12.4 Two, two-phase models: linear–linear from Equation 12.3 (broken line) and quadratic–linear from Equation 12.9 (solid line). Both functions fit well. Estimated knots for each model (the vertical lines) differ by approximately 0.1 log MAR units.

second phase (β_1). A sudden change in rate at τ is not realistic if print size is viewed as a continuous variable, the implication being that two sentences differing only slightly in size are associated with distinctly different rates. A more plausible assumption is that the transition between phases is gradual and smooth. Several functions can be considered that display this type of process. It will turn out that the improvement in fit for models specifying a gradual transition is not dramatic and so the appeal of the modification is appropriateness scientifically. This assessment is subjective, but may be the reason to consider structures that are slightly more flexible than Equations 12.2 or 12.4.

12.2.4 Two-Phase, Quadratic–Linear

Another two-phase model consists of quadratic and linear components. Extending the linear–linear models in an obvious way, the quadratic–linear function is

$$f_j = \begin{cases} \alpha_0 + \alpha_1 x_j + \alpha_2 x_j^2, & x_j \leq \tau, \\ \beta_0 + \beta_1 x_j, & x_j > \tau. \end{cases} \tag{12.7}$$

It is often most reasonable if the segments join at $x = \tau$ with a smooth transition, giving the process shown as the solid line in Figure 12.4. As reviewed in Appendix 12.1, introducing these constraints imposes two restrictions on the parameters, one pair of which is

$$\alpha_1 = \beta_1 - 2\alpha_2\tau, \quad \alpha_0 = \beta_0 + \beta_1\tau - \alpha_1\tau - \alpha_2\tau^2.$$

Substituting these into Equation 12.7 produces a four-parameter model

$$f_j = \begin{cases} \beta_0 + \beta_1 x_j + \alpha_2(x_j - \tau)^2, & x_j \leq \tau, \\ \beta_0 + \beta_1 x_j, & x_j > \tau. \end{cases} \tag{12.8}$$

Or more compactly as a single expression

$$f_j = \beta_0 + \beta_1 x_j + \alpha_2(\tau - x_j)_+^2.$$

The final set of parameters is $(\alpha_2, \tau, \beta_0, \beta_1)$.

The meaning of β_0, β, and τ in model 12.8 is connected either to the profile of reading speeds or to the print size in a way that gives useful information about the data. However, α_2, the coefficient of the squared difference, $x_j - \tau$, is not related to the profile of scores in any obvious way. Other versions of the quadratic–linear function can be suggested. They have the same form as model 12.8; so there is no change in the general shape or loss of fit. We introduce these possibilities because they include parameters that are all interpretable.

A second version of the quadratic–linear model can be written as

$$f_{jI} = \begin{cases} c_1(x_j - \kappa) + c_2(x_j^2 - \kappa^2), & x_j < \tau, \\ \omega + \gamma(x_j - \tau), & x_j \geq \tau. \end{cases} \tag{12.9}$$

In this specification, γ is the slope of the second phase and τ the knot. κ, an estimated print size, is the x intercept of the first phase. At $x = \kappa, f_{iI} = 0$. Substantively for our problem, κ is interpreted as the print size at which an individual cannot make out any part of a sentence. The last parameter is ω, the WPM at the knot. When $x = \tau, f_{iI} = \omega$. If $\gamma \leq 0$, then ω is maximum reading speed. However, if $\gamma > 0$ then the maximum is the largest y_j in the region $x_j > \tau$. The constants of the first segment are

$$c_2 = \frac{\gamma(\tau - \kappa) - \omega}{(\tau - \kappa)^2}, \quad c_1 = \gamma - 2c_2\tau.$$

These are obtained, similar to the development in Appendix 12.1 for model 12.8, to satisfy the conditions that the segments join at the knot with a smooth transition between phases.

The parameters of Equation 12.9 are $\theta_I = (\kappa, \gamma, \tau, \omega)$. They are interesting components closely tied to the data and give useful information about the profile of MNREAD scores that is not directly measured. Both κ and τ are estimated values of the independent variable, x; ω is an estimated value pertaining to the response; γ is a slope, the rate of change in y per unit change in x in the second segment.

A third version of the same basic model will be introduced. In Equation 12.9, κ is the x intercept, the estimated print size corresponding to $y = 0$. A straightforward modification of the function replaces κ with the value of x that is associated with an arbitrary reading speed different from zero, as was carried out for model 12.6. Again, for example, reading speed can be set at $w_0 = 35$ WPM so that when $x = k$, $f = w_0$. To accommodate this change, the first segment includes the target WPM and the model becomes

$$f_{jC} = \begin{cases} w_0 + c_1(x - \kappa) + c_2(x^2 - \kappa^2), & x < \tau, \\ \omega + \gamma(x - \tau), & x \geq \tau. \end{cases} \quad (12.10)$$

Three of the parameters in Equation 12.10 have the same meaning as in Equation 12.9: τ, γ, and ω are the knot, the slope of the second segment, and WPM at the change point, respectively. As advertised, κ is the estimated x-value corresponding to $f_C = w_0$. The constants that satisfy the constraints for this version of the model are

$$c_2 = \frac{w_0 + \gamma(\tau - k) - \omega}{(\tau - k)^2}, \quad c_1 = \gamma - 2c_2\tau.$$

Obviously, Equation 12.9 is a special case of Equation 12.10 that occurs by taking $w_0 = 0$. Again, although the parameterizations of Equations 12.8 through 12.10 are different, the fit of the three forms to any single set of data is identical.

The measures of fit in Table 12.2 were obtained by applying model 12.9. It performs best among those examined so far, although only marginally so compared to Equations 12.3 and 12.5. Least squares estimates of parameters for Equation 12.9 are

$\hat{\kappa}$	$\hat{\gamma}$	$\hat{\tau}$	$\hat{\omega}$
−0.413(0.02)	−2.14(11)	−0.008(0.06)	209(8.4).

The fitted function is shown in Figure 12.4 as the solid line.

Several issues are worth noting. The first, and a potentially important difference between models 12.9 and 12.3, is in the estimated knots. For the former it is −0.116 while for the latter it is −0.008, a discrepancy of more than 0.10 in log MAR units. This is large enough to be scientifically meaningful. The estimate under function 12.9 seems too high given the observed data. Another issue is that for both models the estimated slope in phase 2 is slightly negative. Under model 12.2 or 12.3, $\hat{\beta}_1 = -2.29$; under model 12.9, $\hat{\gamma} = -2.14$. Although the standard error is large, this means the individual tends to read larger print sizes more slowly than smaller ones. Because the MNREAD sentences are always presented in the order of large to small, the negative slope should probably be interpreted as a practice effect, and that even as the sentences get smaller reading speed improves as he or she become accustomed to the task. Although practice effects are undesirable, it is valuable that based on this function the slight decline in phase 2 can be detected within the variability of measurements at the larger print sizes. It was noted earlier with the exponential model that the function is strictly increasing for all increases in print size. From a visual inspection of the data, the slight decline in WPM at large print sizes is appropriate. Consequently, the estimate of $\hat{\gamma} = -2.14$ under model 12.9 is more accurate than is the steady increase of WPM over increases in print sizes that is implied by function 12.1. Still another point is based on the estimate of $\hat{\kappa} = -0.413$. This subject was just able to read sentence 18 at log MAR $= -0.4$. The estimated print size at his or her visual threshold is slightly smaller.

12.2.5 Linear–Linear Model with Smooth Transition

Functions 12.2 through 12.6 give plausible estimates of maximum reading speed and critical print size. A liability of this model is that the transition between phases is abrupt. In contrast, the quadratic–linear model provides a smooth transition between phases; however, the critical print size seemed to occur too early, before the decrease in reading speed that is apparent in

Figure 12.4, for example. Several modifications to the linear–linear model have been suggested in which the shift between segments is gradual and smooth (Bacon & Watts, 1971; Griffiths & Miller, 1973). The resulting model has flavors of both the linear–linear and quadratic–linear models. Like function 12.2, the new model is analogous to a linear–linear process. And like (12.8) it has first- and second-order continuity between regimes. The form we review is adapted so that the slope of the second phase is approximately zero for large x:

$$f_{jS} = \beta_0 + \frac{\alpha_1}{2}\left(x_j - \tau - \sqrt{(x_j - \tau)^2 + \lambda}\right), \quad \lambda \geq 0. \tag{12.11}$$

Here, as in Equation 12.2, α_1 is approximately the slope of the first phase, τ the knot, and β_0 the maximum reading speed associated with large print sizes. Exactly at the knot $x = \tau$, WPM is $f_j = \beta_0 - \alpha_1\sqrt{\lambda}/2$. The parameter λ controls the transition between linear phases. Several versions of the function with different values of λ are shown in Figure 12.5. As $\lambda \to 0$, the function becomes the standard linear–linear model, and approaches model 12.5 from below. For $\lambda > 0$, the function rounds the corner increasingly gradually, approaching the intercept β_0 of the second segment. With small problems, as when fitting measurements from individuals, the data may be too sparse to estimate λ. An ad hoc procedure is

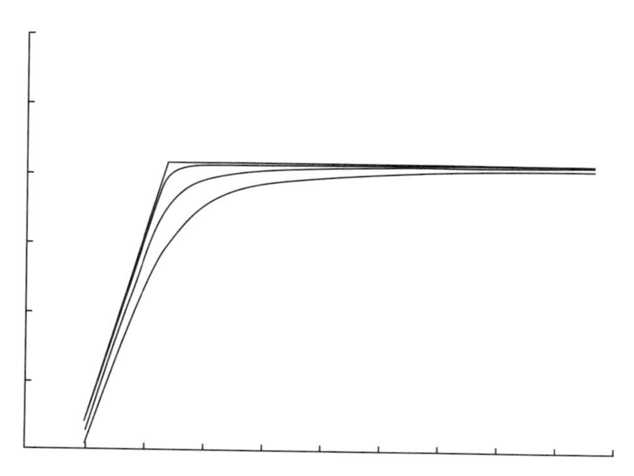

FIGURE 12.5 Function 12.11 with four different values of the smoothing parameter λ. The linear–linear model uses $\lambda = 0$. The other three versions are $\lambda = 0.001, 0.01$, and 0.03. These options produce curves between segments that are increasingly more gradual.

to set the parameter to a small value, such as $\lambda = 0.001$, which appears to work satisfactorily.

It is apparent from Equation 12.11 and the examples shown in Figure 12.5 that the slope of the second segment is not exactly zero but instead is slightly positive over larger print sizes. This is a feature of the model that follows from the behavior of this particular function. Since the sentences are administered from large to small, the slight slope implies a slow decrease in reading speed across smaller print sizes until the rapid decreases below the knot.

The last line of Table 12.2 has measures of fit for this model which, considering it requires only three parameters, are comparatively good. Estimates are

$$\begin{array}{ccc} \hat{\alpha}_1 & \hat{\beta}_0 & \hat{\tau} \\ 664(116) & 208(4.2) & -0.120(0.04). \end{array}$$

The fitted function is shown in Figure 12.6. The estimated knot, $\hat{\tau} = -0.120$, and maximum value, $\hat{\beta}_0 = 208.0$, are similar to the corresponding estimates based on function 12.2. The agreement suggests that

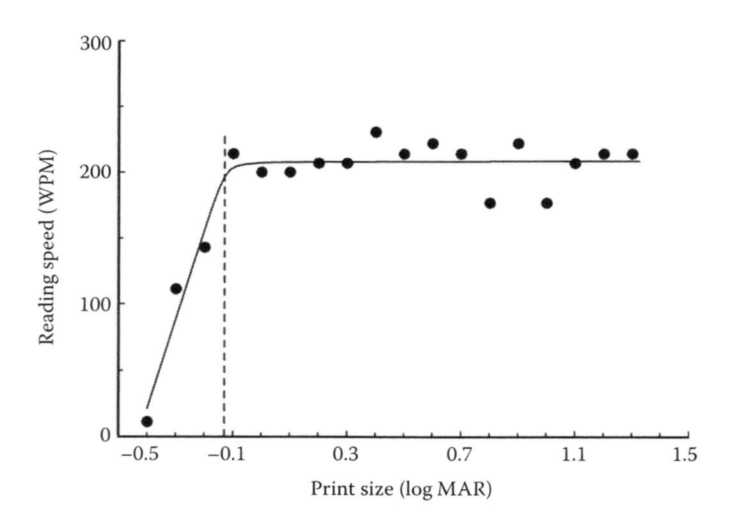

FIGURE 12.6 The linear–linear model with a smooth transition. The estimated knot with this function seems well placed according to the steady performance down to log MAR = −0.10 by this participant.

both β_0 and τ of Equation 12.11 are reasonable as ways to operationalize the two components, critical print size, and maximum reading speed.

12.2.6 Summary

The review of functions for these data has covered 10 alternatives, and the list is hardly exhaustive. As often happens, the choice of function is not clear-cut. The quadratic and cubic models can be eliminated from consideration on the basis of poor fit, and because they include parameters that are not interpretable. The exponential function fits relatively well and has coefficients that are understandable; however, our impression is that the transition between smaller and larger print sizes is too gradual and does not adequately represent the rapid shift in WPM that is evident in the graph of the data. Neither does the exponential provide information about critical print size.

Both types of two-phase model, linear–linear and quadratic–linear, perform well and nearly the same with these data. By their construction, the characteristic segments of the MNREAD profile are clearly reflected in two-phase models. For each of these functions, critical print size is a parameter. Moreover, for those models that specify a slope of zero in the second phase, these functions also include a parameter that corresponds directly to maximum reading speed.

Our preference with these data is function 12.11. It performs well, has understandable parameters, gives a sensible estimate of critical print size and maximum reading speed. The smooth transition between segments is an enhancement that we believe improves on the abrupt change of model 12.2 and its variants, or of the too gradual change of model 12.7 and its variants.

A reviewer of this chapter pointed out that in addition to the obvious ad hoc smoothing parameter, $\lambda = 0.001$, the utility of these features of Equation 12.11 is subjective and debatable. It is likely that other knowledgeable investigators working with the same data would end up with a different function and perhaps one that is more attractive scientifically. This assertion is inarguable. In any event, as has often been stated, the best that can be done is to be explicit about the selection and performance criteria that make one function preferable to others. The debate about functional form is always valuable. Also, it is generally preferable to select or adapt a function rather than to uncritically accept a familiar model simply because it is traditional.

12.3 A RANDOM COEFFICIENT MODEL FOR THE MNREAD DATA

The goal of this analysis is to identify a plausible response function for profiles of individual reading performance, and then to extend the function to a random coefficient model in order to describe individual differences (e.g., Morrell, Pearson, Carter, & Brant, 1995). The result is a straightforward two-level model, but one that is effective and parsimonious for describing the reading profiles exhibited in Figure 12.2. The random coefficient model is appealing because it does not assume a single process for all individuals, or that a description of the average profile in some way characterizes every person. It is rather a subject-specific model (Vonesh & Chinchilli, 1997, Section 7; Davidian & Giltinan, 1995, Chapter 4), which places primary emphasis on the explicit representation of individual repeated measures. An adequate description of the mean profile is less important in subject-specific models than is the accurate representation of individuals. This makes them especially attractive in the study behavior. We present a brief summary of the three components of the model and the various modifications leading up to the final structure.

12.3.1 Model 12.11 with Random Coefficients

Based upon Equation 12.11, with a minor change in notation, define the function for the ith individual on the jth stimulus as

$$y_{ij} = \beta_i + \frac{\alpha_i}{2}\left(x_{ij} - \tau_i - \sqrt{(x_{ij} - \tau_i)^2 + \lambda}\right) + e_{ij}, \tag{12.12}$$

where the set of print sizes and reading speeds are (x_{ij}, y_{ij}), $j = 1, \ldots, n_i$. The coefficients are also associated with the ith case, only in this development are the sum of fixed parameters and random effects

$$\beta_i = \beta + b_i, \quad \alpha_i = \alpha + a_i, \quad \tau_i = \tau + t_i, \tag{12.13}$$

where β, α, and τ are fixed population parameters and b_i, a_i, and t_i are random effects unique to individual i. In the review of response functions with one subject's data, properties of possible models were reviewed in detail. This gives some assurance that (12.12) is reasonable for other individuals as well. The response function is often the main focus of attention in a random coefficient model, but there are several other aspects of the full system that must be specified also.

First, it is assumed that the random effects are normal with zero means and covariance matrix $\mathbf{\Phi}$. This is a standard assumption but also plausible here. Second, the residuals are assumed to be normally distributed with zero expected values and covariance matrix $\mathbf{\Psi}_i$. Because the within-subject variability is not negligible, several submodels were considered for the residual variances, $\psi_j = \text{var}(e_{ij})$. The patterns we examined included exponential, power, and linear functions of the individual means, as well as basic patterns for different variances at different print sizes. After some exploratory analyses with these alternatives, it was found that a simple, homogeneous level 1 structure is adequate, $\mathbf{\Psi}_i = \sigma_e^2 \mathbf{I}_{n_i}$.

To summarize, the subject-specific response function for the random coefficient model is given in Equation 12.12, with individual coefficients (12.13). The within-subject covariance matrix is $\mathbf{\Psi}_i(n_i \times n_i)$, a function of a single parameter. The between-subject covariance matrix is $\mathbf{\Phi}$. It was not possible to estimate the coefficient of the transition function with data from a single individual only. Estimating λ is possible in the full model however. When estimating λ it was found that there was no improvement in the model's performance by making it a free parameter; so we retain the previous setup with fixed $\lambda = 0.001$. Altogether the structure requires ten parameters, $\beta, \alpha, \tau, \varphi_{11}, \varphi_{21}, \ldots, \varphi_{33}, \sigma_e^2$.

12.3.2 Fitting the Model

Random coefficient models can be fit with several computer programs. Perhaps the most accessible is NLMIXED in SAS (Wolfinger, 1999). It includes a flexible syntax for specifying the response function, a number of different distribution assumptions for the level 1 and level 2 random effects, several estimation options, and a very general framework for hypothesis tests. Prediction of the random effects and individual coefficients is a straightforward option.

After additional analyses, two modifications were made to the form of $\mathbf{\Phi}$, which most likely are the consequences of the small sample. It was found that the random effects on the individual slope coefficient were not needed. When this set of random effects was excluded, the fit of the reduced model was only slightly poorer than the original model with three random effects. The slope was fixed at a common value for all $\alpha_i = \alpha$. This decision eliminates three elements from $\mathbf{\Phi}$. The other modification was that the confidence interval for the covariance between b_i and t_i included zero. Assuming these random effects are uncorrelated; the level 2 covariance structure is simply

$$\mathbf{\Phi} = \mathrm{cov}(b_i, t_i) = \begin{pmatrix} \varphi_1 & \\ 0 & \varphi_2 \end{pmatrix}.$$

Empirical Bayes predictions of individual coefficients are obtained after the parameters are estimated. They have the appealing property that the estimates are optimal over the class of linear combinations of the data (Davidian & Giltinan, 1995, pp. 75–76). This means that even though the predicted coefficients $\hat{\beta}_i$ and $\hat{\tau}_i$ pertain to the ith individual, the estimates gain strength from information in the total sample.

12.3.3 Parameter Estimates and the Curve of Typical Values

Maximum likelihood estimates of the remaining six parameters based on $N = 30$ readers are as follows, with standard errors in parentheses

$\hat{\alpha}$	$\hat{\beta}$	$\hat{\tau}$	$\hat{\varphi}_1$	$\hat{\varphi}_2$	$\hat{\sigma}_e^2$
521.0(21)	210.0(5.8)	0.096(0.02)	949.6(258)	0.0086(0.002)	593.0(40.7).

The estimate of maximum reading speed is $\hat{\beta} = 210.0$ and the critical print size $\hat{\tau} = 0.096$. These are of considerable interest scientifically as a description of the population averages on these features of reading. The mean slope over smaller print sizes is $\hat{\alpha} = 521.0$; so there is a sizeable rate of improvement as print size increases. As stated earlier, when $x = \hat{\tau}$, the estimated reading speed is $f = \hat{\beta} - \hat{\alpha}\sqrt{10^{-3}}/2 = 201.76$. The parameter estimates of the function are called the typical values. They are interpreted as the values of the individual coefficients for a person whose scores on these variables are equal to the population means. The response function

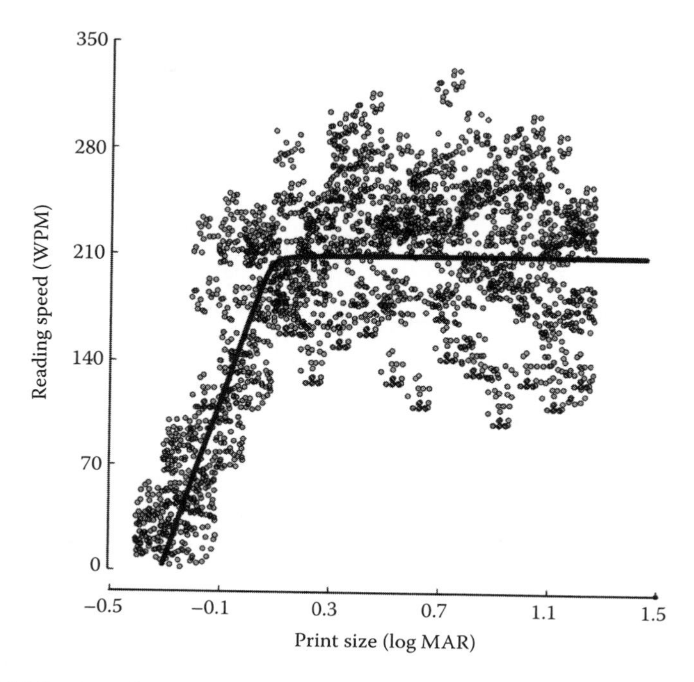

FIGURE 12.7 A random selection of 50% of the sample with the function evaluated at the parameter estimates. These are called the typical values because they are the scores of a person whose individual coefficients equal the parameters. The trajectory for the typical values gives a reasonable snapshot of performance on the MNREAD sentences for the "average" or typical individual.

evaluated at $\hat{\beta}$, $\hat{\alpha}$, and $\hat{\tau}$ is shown in Figure 12.7 with approximately 50% of the sample. To better see the data, the scores have been jittered. The function for the "average person" clearly tracks through the data swarm well.

12.3.4 Subject-Specific Functions

In a subject-specific model, information regarding individual differences is more important than the typical values. The estimated variance of β_i is large, $\hat{\varphi}_1 = 949.6$ (standard deviation $\sqrt{\hat{\varphi}_1} = 30.8$), and has a large standard error, $\text{se}(\hat{\varphi}_1) = 258$. The sample range on predicted values of $\hat{\beta}_i$ is (142.1–262.9). The estimated variance on the second set of coefficients is $\hat{\varphi}_2 = 0.0086$, and the sample range of $\hat{\tau}_i$ is (−0.067–0.283).

Of course, the main point of the analysis is the representation of individual reading profiles. The trellis display with 12 records in Figure 12.8

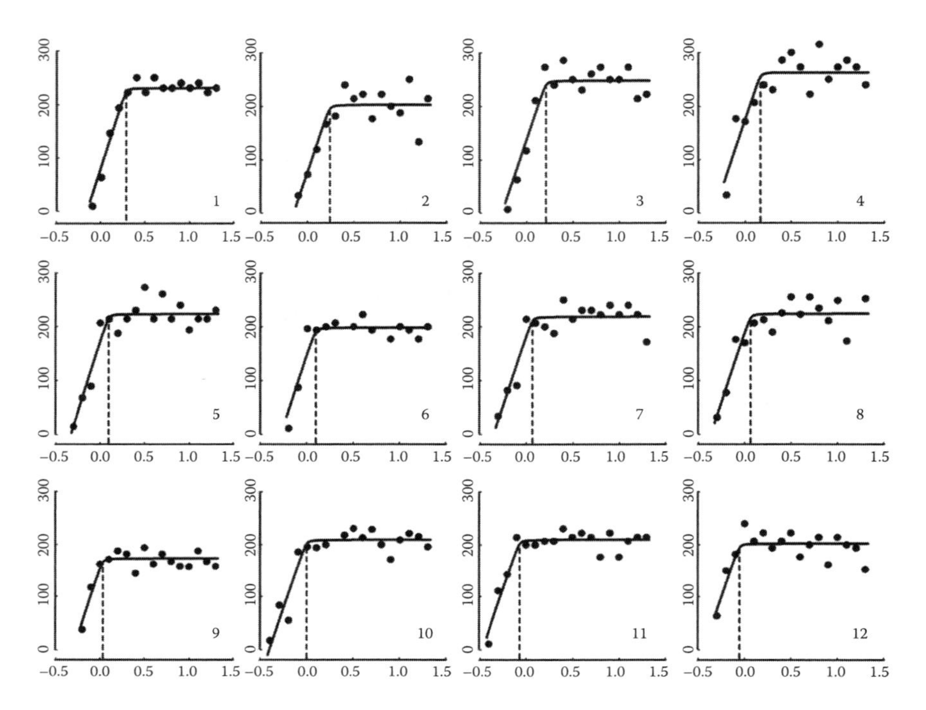

FIGURE 12.8 A trellis display of 12 sets of individual data with individual fitted functions. The graphs are ordered in terms of estimated $\hat{\tau}_i$ (vertical dashed line), with the largest in Graph 1 and lowest in Graph 12. Both $\hat{\tau}_i$ and $\hat{\beta}_i$ vary appreciably in this figure.

shows many interesting features. The plots are ordered by decreasing $\hat{\tau}_i$, from the upper-left corner to the lower right. Differences between persons on $\hat{\beta}_i$ are also evident. Compare, for example, Case 4—whose reading speed is fast—with Case 9 in the lower left, who reads much more slowly. The fact that $\text{cov}(\beta_i, \tau_i) = 0$ means that these two coefficients vary independently so that some individuals with high values of β_i also have high values on τ_i, while for others τ_i is low. This means that fast readers on large text sentences may show a decline in reading speed before others who read more slowly on large text. These differences in performance are described well by the models.

It is also clear in the plot that excluding random effects from the slope by fixing $\alpha_i = \alpha$, which was not anticipated before the analysis, is not unreasonable. All individuals shown in the display have identical slopes over smaller print sizes. The implication is that although $\hat{\beta}_i$ and $\hat{\tau}_i$ vary between persons, the rate of increase in performance over the small sentences is the same for all.

Qualitatively, individual models fit some persons much better than others. Case 2 is variable over the profile; Cases 1 and 6 are quite consistent. The reading speeds for Case 3 and especially for case 12 show a downward sloping trend from left to right over larger print sizes. As mentioned earlier, this probably indicates an order effect related to presentation of the sentences. Even with these signs of individual variability, the subject-specific function works well for the most part.

Both critical print size and maximum reading speed are latent variables that are estimated under the model. Judging from the figure, it appears that the predicted values for $\hat{\beta}_i$ are reasonable in all the cases, and that the fitted function over the large print sizes is effective. On the other hand, with respect to $\hat{\tau}_i$ the ability of the function to cleanly distinguish between print sizes associated with maximum reading speed and those that are not is often successful, but not always. Judging by eye, $\hat{\tau}_i$ appears too large for Cases 5, 6, 7, and 10. This judgment is subjective, however. At the least $\hat{\tau}_i$ provides a respectable initial estimate.

An important extension of the basic random coefficient model is incorporating covariates to explain the observed variability on the individual coefficients. Both $\hat{\beta}_i$ and $\hat{\tau}_i$ describe interesting features of the reading profiles. It is informative to identify covariates such as health indicators, educational attainment, or demographic variables to understand how the individual differences arise. Unfortunately, additional covariates are unavailable in this example; so further study along these lines is precluded. However, the search for effective covariates is in many ways the most valuable part of a successful application.

To summarize results, the fit of the model to individuals is generally good. The coefficients β_i, τ_i, and α_i of the two-phase model are interpretable summaries of the profiles of reading scores. Both within- and between-subjects variability are represented effectively. The performances of the individual functions and also the function of the typical values are adequate. Taken as a whole, function 12.11 and the hierarchical model seem to work well.

12.4 DISCUSSION

The random coefficient model is a subject-specific model, designed to account for individual sets of repeated measures with individual response functions. It also accounts for within-subject variability—to describe lack of fit of the individual function—and between-subject variation—to describe the extent to which individuals differ on the individual coefficients. In this example, the level 1 covariance structure was simple. For the between-subject variation, two coefficients showed substantial differences in the sample while one was constant. This type of a result is an extremely useful characteristic of the general model.

Nonlinear patterns in repeated measures data are not uncommon in the behavioral sciences. By far the most popular alternative for this circumstance is the simple quadratic function. Although it is hard to criticize a popular model, a number of alternative functions for the MNREAD data are attractive and fit data well. More important, these functions give information that is directly relevant to the data. Tailoring the function to the context, so that the information produced is as useful as possible, is invaluable.

Two-phase models have a distinguished record of service in many disciplines. Generally they fit well. They can be parameterized so that coefficients are interpretable. They take many forms, linear–linear and quadratic–linear being especially simple. They work well in various scientific domains because behavior that develops in recognizable regimes, such as before and after an intervention or before and during a developmental stage, are so common. We have attempted to show in this chapter that several versions can be effective in summarizing these data in the hope that similar functions might be useful in others.

APPENDIX 12.1 THE QUADRATIC–LINEAR MODEL WITH A SMOOTH TRANSITION BETWEEN PHASES

The two segments of the quadratic–linear function in Equation 12.7 need not join at the knot. The model is appropriate for situations where in moving from one phase to the other there is a discontinuity at $x = \tau$. Although there are behavioral processes with discontinuities, for the MNREAD data it makes sense to consider a single smooth function over the print sizes and that is smooth at the knot. Algebraically, this means that at $x = \tau$ the segments must be equal and also that first derivatives be equal.

From the first condition, $\alpha_0 + \alpha_1\tau + \alpha_2\tau^2 = \beta_0 + \beta_1\tau$. Because of this equality, one of the six coefficients is redundant and can be eliminated. There is more than one way to handle this situation. The intercept of the first phase is not especially informative, so we have chosen to define α_0 in terms of the others as $\alpha_0 = \beta_0 + \beta_1\tau - \alpha_1\tau - \alpha_2\tau^2$. The number of independent coefficients is reduced from six to five.

The second condition is

$$\frac{d}{dx}(\alpha_0 + \alpha_1 x_j + \alpha_2 x_j^2)\bigg|_{x=\tau} = \frac{d}{dx}(\beta_0 + \beta_1 x_j)\bigg|_{x=\tau},$$

so that

$$\alpha_1 + 2\alpha_2\tau = \beta_1.$$

This equality means that one other coefficient is redundant. It is simplest to define α_1 in terms of the others: $\alpha_1 = \beta_1 - 2\alpha_2\tau$. The two constrained coefficients are then

$$\begin{aligned}
\alpha_1 &= \beta_1 - 2\alpha_2\tau \\
\alpha_0 &= \beta_0 + \beta_1\tau - \alpha_1\tau - \alpha_2\tau^2 \\
&= \beta_0 + \beta_1\tau - (\beta_1 - 2\alpha_2\tau)\tau - \alpha_2\tau^2 \\
&= \beta_0 + \alpha_2\tau^2
\end{aligned}$$

Substituting these definitions into Equation 12.7 gives the function in Equation 12.8. The final number of coefficients is four.

REFERENCES

Bacon, D. W., & Watts, D. G. (1971). Estimating the transition between two intersecting straight lines. *Biometrika, 58*, 525–534.

Bates, D. M., & Watts, D. G. (1988). *Nonlinear regression analysis and its applications.* New York: Wiley.

Cheung, S.-H., Kallie, C. S., Legge, G. E., & Cheong, A. M. Y. (2008). Nonlinear mixed-effects modeling of MNREAD data. *Investigative Ophthalmology and Visual Science, 49*, 828–835.

Davidian, M., & Giltinan, D. M. (1995). *Nonlinear models for repeated measurement data.* London: Chapman & Hall.

Diggle, P. J., Liang, K.Y., & Zeger, S. L. (1994). *Analysis of longitudinal data.* Oxford: Oxford University Press.

Fitzmaurice, G. M., Laird, N. M., & Ware, J. H. (2004). *Applied longitudinal analysis.* New York: Wiley.

Griffiths, D. A., & Miller, A. J. (1973). Hyperbolic regression—a model based on two-phase piecewise linear regression with a smooth transition between regimes. *Communications in Statistics, 2*, 561–569.

Lewis, D. (1966). *Quantitative methods in psychology.* Iowa City, IA: University of Iowa Press.

Mansfield, J. S., Ahn, S. J., Legge, G. E., & Luebker, A. (1993). A new reading acuity chart for normal and low vision. *Ophthalmic and Visual Optics/Noninvasive Assessment of the Visual System Technical Digest, 3*, 232–235.

Morrell, C. H., Pearson, J. D., Carter, H. B., & Brant, L. J. (1995). Estimating unknown transition times using a piecewise nonlinear mixed-effects model in men with prostate cancer. *Journal of the American Statistical Association, 90*, 45–53.

Seber, G. A. F., & Wild, C. J. (1989). *Nonlinear regression.* New York: Wiley.

Vonesh, E. F., & Chinchilli, V. M. (1997). *Linear and nonlinear models for the analysis of repeated measurements.* New York: Dekker.

Wolfinger, R.D. (1999). Fitting nonlinear mixed models with the new NLMIXED procedure. *Proceedings of the 24th Annual SAS Users Group International Conference (SUGI 24),* 287-24.

13

A Bayesian Discrete Dynamic System by Latent Difference Score Structural Equations Models for Multivariate Repeated Measures Data

Fumiaki Hamagami, Zhiyong Johnny Zhang, and John J. McArdle

Longitudinal analyses by latent curves methods have become useful to model a general trajectory of behavioral responses (Rao, 1958; McArdle & Epstein, 1987; McArdle & Hamagami, 1991, 1992; Meredith & Tisak, 1990). As a methodological alternative to longitudinal data analyses, the dynamic system approach by means of difference or differential equations allows an investigation of both inter- and intravariable cause–effect relationships on the time dimension (Arminger, 1986; Beddington, Free, & Lawton, 1975; Coleman, 1968; Goldberg, 1986; McArdle, 1988; Molenaar, 1985; Nesselroade, McArdle, Aggen, & Meyers, 2001; Nesselroade & Molenaar, 1999; Tuma & Hanna, 1986; Sheinerman, 1996). In a similar vein, McArdle and Nesselroade (1994) introduced the use of latent difference scores on longitudinal factor scores derived from the multivariate longitudinal structural equation modeling (SEM) (see also McArdle, 1988). In subsequent works, McArdle and Hamagami (1995, 2001) expanded the use of difference equations applied to multiple occasions, which structurally allows dynamic interpretations. Structural latent difference score models are specifically designed to accommodate interindividual variability of initial conditions and the rate of change of the dynamic system model among different people (Nesselroade, 1991). Hamagami and McArdle (2001) demonstrated that dynamical parameters of structured latent difference score models were accurately recovered by traditional SEM under a variety of missing data situations by Monte Carlo simulations (Little & Rubin, 1987; McArdle, 1994; Schafer, 1997). Both deterministic and stochastic parameters of the dynamics system were correctly recovered using full information maximum likelihood estimation (Lange, Westlake, & Spence, 1976) using Mx program (Neale, Boker, Xie, & Maes, 2003).

In several researches mainly in quantitative social science, the Bayesian method (BE) was used to investigate multivariate latent variable models. Several investigations of Bayesian factor analyses were initially reported (Martin & McDonald, 1975; Bartholomew, 1981, 1991; Press & Shigematu, 1989). More prior researches also adopted the Bayesian approach to analyze the confirmatory factor model and robust factor models (Ansari & Jedidi, 2000; Ansari, Jedidi, & Dube, 2002; Hayashi & Sen, 2002; Hayashi & Yuan, 2003; Lee & Press, 1998).

Several previous researches on new computational algorithms have demonstrated how BEs could be used to investigate complex statistical models (Gelman, Carlin, Stern, & Rubin, 1996; Gilks, Richardson, & Spiegelhalter, 1996; Congdon, 2001, 2003). In the BE, derivation of the posterior distribution of model parameters is necessarily of utmost concern. For a simple model such as the simple regression model, it is feasible to analytically derive posterior parameter distributions (see Silva, 1996). However, analytical derivation of posterior distribution of highly complex models (e.g., Zeger & Karim, 1991) involving multiple model parameters is practically intractable due to the fact that it mathematically involves high-dimensional multiple integrals. The Gibbs sampling algorithm was introduced to circumvent this difficulty (Geman & Geman, 1984). Congdon (2001, 2003) demonstrated that Bayesian analyses are no longer limited to only simple statistical models by means of the newly developed Bayesian algorithm.

Also, the general focus of Bayesian researches was shifted to structural equation models that involve multivariate structures, latent variables, and simultaneous equations (see Arminger & Muthén, 1998; Fornell & Rust, 1989; Jedidi & Ansari, 2001; Jedidi, Ramaswamy, & DeSarbo, 1996; Lee & Song, 2003, 2004; Lee, Song, & Poon, 2004; Rupp, Dey, & Zumbo, 2004;

Scheines, Hoijtink, & Boomsma, 1999; Song & Lee, 2004). Also, the Gibbs sampling algorithm allows complex nonlinear structural equation models (see Arminger et al., 1998; Lee et al., 2003, 2004).

A detailed discussion of the latent difference score model and the bivariate latent difference score model was presented in McArdle (2001) and McArdle et al. (2001). As a synopsis, we provide only a basic definition of these models. Here we focus on the Bayesian estimation (BE) to analyze these models since these models have been previously investigated by the SEM approach only. In the first part of this chapter, we apply both the Bayesian approach and traditional SEM to univariate longitudinal repeated measures data. This portion of the presentation includes univariate analyses of longitudinal data from a published example on the Wechsler Intelligence Scale for Children (McArdle & Epstein, 1987). We also employ Monte Carlo simulations to examine aspects of both estimation techniques, and we compare the results obtained by these two different estimation methods. In the second part, we examine the same problems for the more complex case of bivariate discrete dynamic systems using latent difference scores.

13.1 BE METHODS

For the estimation of the latent difference score model, the previous studies used an SEM-based approach (McArdle et al., 2001, 2004; McArdle, 2001). The estimation of the model parameters can be achieved using the standard SEM software (e.g., LISREL, Mplus, Mx). We propose the BE method to estimate dynamic parameters for the latent difference score model. The Bayesian method is an approach for statistical inference in which all the uncertain parameters are interpreted in terms of Bayesian subjective probability as opposed to Fisherian or frequentist's logical (or objective epistemic) probability. The Bayesian approach starts with the formulation of a model (M) that represents our research interests. Then we characterize a *prior distribution* $p(\theta)$ to the unknown parameters of the model, which represents our beliefs, or already established prior information about the parameters before collecting data. After conducting a study and obtaining empirical data $(y \mid \theta; M)$, we apply the Bayes rule to derive the posterior distribution ($p(\theta \mid y; M)$), for these unknown model parameters, which updates the degree of belief in the light of new empirical data. Let information from the data be expressed as $f(y \mid \theta; M)$, which is also the likelihood function in terms of the traditional SEM approach. Then the posterior of the unknown parameters can be expressed as probability density functions of the prior multiplied by the likelihood functions given by empirical data and model parameters. Mathematically, the posterior distribution function is expressed as

$$p(\theta \mid y; M) = \frac{p(\theta) f(y \mid \theta; M)}{\int f(y \mid \theta; M) d\theta} \propto p(\theta) f(y\theta; M).$$

Although in theory the prior distribution can be any form of density distributions, we will choose a conjugate prior distribution for inferential convenience. Conjugate distributions mean that the prior and the posterior distributions come from the same family of density distributions, usually the exponential family (Lee, 2004; Silva, 1996). If we had no prior information or we do not want to include the prior information by choice, we could specify a noninformative prior like a normal distribution with a large variance (e.g., 10e + 6).

All the inferences of the parameters are based on the posterior distribution. For example, the point estimation of θ is obtained as the average of all instances of parameter estimates, that is,

$$\hat{\theta} = E(\theta) = \int \theta \, p(\theta \mid y; M) d\theta.$$

With the increase of the number of the parameters, the analytical solution of the integration above would become impractical. The Gibbs sampling can circumvent this difficulty. Gibbs sampling is an algorithm to generate a sequence of samples from the joint distribution of two or more variables (or model parameters). The purpose of such a sequence is to approximate the multidimensional joint distribution, or to sequentially solve the formulaic complexity of multiple integrals so as to derive expected values of model parameters. The Gibbs sampling is an example of a Markov chain Monte Carlo (MCMC) algorithm. The Gibbs sampling is applicable when the joint distribution of a group of parameters cannot be expressed explicitly, but the conditional distribution of each parameter is known. The Gibbs sampling algorithm is a piecemeal process to generate an instance from the distribution of each parameter, conditional on the algorithmically updated values of the other parameters. Geman and Geman (1984) showed that the joint and marginal distributions that were derived from the MCMC sequences would converge at an exponential rate to the posterior joint and marginal distributions of parameters. The Gibbs sampling is particularly well adapted to sampling the posterior distribution of a Bayesian network, since Bayesian networks are typically specified as a collection of conditional distributions (see Gelman et al., 1995; Gilks et al., 1996; Congdon, 2003).

For the latent difference score model, we choose a noninformative prior for each parameter and estimate the model parameters using the program WinBUGS (Spiegelhalter, Thomas, & Best, 1999). We have divided the following section into two parts. The first part includes analyses of the univariate difference score models, and the second part includes analyses of the bivariate difference score models. Within each univariate and bivariate modeling framework, first we conduct a Monte Carlo simulation study in order to evaluate the performance of the BE method. Data based on both the univariate and the bivariate models are generated according to a set of preset population parameters. These parameters are means and variances of level and slope scores, residual variances, self-feedback parameters, coupling parameters, and covariances among latent level and slope scores. We set the sample size to 200, which is comparable to the size of the Wechsler Intelligence Scale for Children (WISC) data that sampled 204 children (Osborne & Suddick, 1972). Six repeated observations are generated for each subject. For each model, 50 samples are generated. The parameter estimations from the 50 samples are used to evaluate the empirical distribution of the parameters.

We also evaluate the ability of estimation methods to analyze the truncated data, which by design removes a portion of data reflecting missing measurement occasions. For the generated data, we insert the missing occasions by deleting all the observations for the third and fifth occasions. The pattern of missing occasions corresponds to the empirical WISC data (Osborne et al., 1972). The incomplete data are analyzed by both SEM and Bayesian methods.

Second, as an application to empirical data, the WISC data that were used in McArdle (1987, 2001) are applied to both the Gibbs sampling and the SEM estimation methods to examine whether or not Bayesian and SEM methods produce the same conclusions.

13.2 PART I: FITTING A UNIVARIATE LATENT DIFFERENCE SCORE MODEL

13.2.1 Univariate LDS Model

Let us assume that variable Y is repeatedly observed over time ($t = 1$ to T) on a sample of subjects ($n = 1$ to N). Also, we assume that a manifest score ($Y[t]_n$) is the sum of a true score ($g[t]_n$) and an unaccounted score such as measurement errors ($ey[t]_n$):

$$Y[t]_n = g[t]_n + ey[t]_n. \tag{13.1}$$

We next define change scores as

$$\Delta g[t]_n = g[t]_n - g[t-1]_n \quad \text{and} \quad g[t]_n = g[t-1]_n + \Delta g[t]_n. \tag{13.2}$$

This means that $\Delta g[t]$ is a *latent difference score* between two successive occasions. We apply a specific definition to a latent difference score at time t as

$$\Delta g[t]_n = g_{sn} + \beta g[t-1]_n. \tag{13.3}$$

This representation simply means that a difference score between time t and time $t - 1(\Delta g[t]_n)$ is determined as the sum of two terms: a self-feedback effect ($\beta g[t-1]_n$), and a linear constant effect (g_{sn}). We then algebraically manipulate a difference equation, a current true score, and a preceding true score. As a result, we express a system that has current true scores as dependent variables and immediate past scores as predictors,

$$\begin{aligned} g[t]_n &= g[t-1]_n + \Delta g[t]_n. \\ &= (1+\beta)g[t-1]_n + g_{sn}. \end{aligned} \tag{13.4}$$

This true score dynamical model is then perturbed by a residual term. Thus, observed scores are described as

$$\begin{aligned} Y[t]_n &= g[t]_n + ey[t]_n \\ &= g[t-1]_n + \Delta g[t]_n + ey[t]_n \\ &= (1+\beta)g[t-1]_n + g_{sn} + ey[t]_n. \end{aligned} \tag{13.5}$$

In order to account for sources of interindividual differences (i.e., Nesselroade, 1991) on Y, the level and linear slope components are defined at a second level as

$$g_{0,n} = \mu_{y0} + d_{g0,n},$$
$$g_{s,n} = \mu_{ys} + d_{gs,n}, \tag{13.6}$$

where μ_{y0} and μ_{ys} are the means of latent level and slope variables, while $d_{g0,n}$ and $d_{gs,n}$ are individuals' deviation scores from the means of latent level and slope scores.

These two latent variables are distributed as multivariate normal; that is,

$$\begin{pmatrix} g_s \\ g_0 \end{pmatrix} \sim MN\left[\begin{pmatrix} \mu_{gs} \\ \mu_{g0} \end{pmatrix}, \begin{pmatrix} \phi^2_{gs} & \\ \phi_{gsg0} & \phi^2_{g0} \end{pmatrix}\right]. \tag{13.7}$$

The path diagram in Figure 13.1 represents this model. In this path diagram, squares represent observed variables, while circles represent

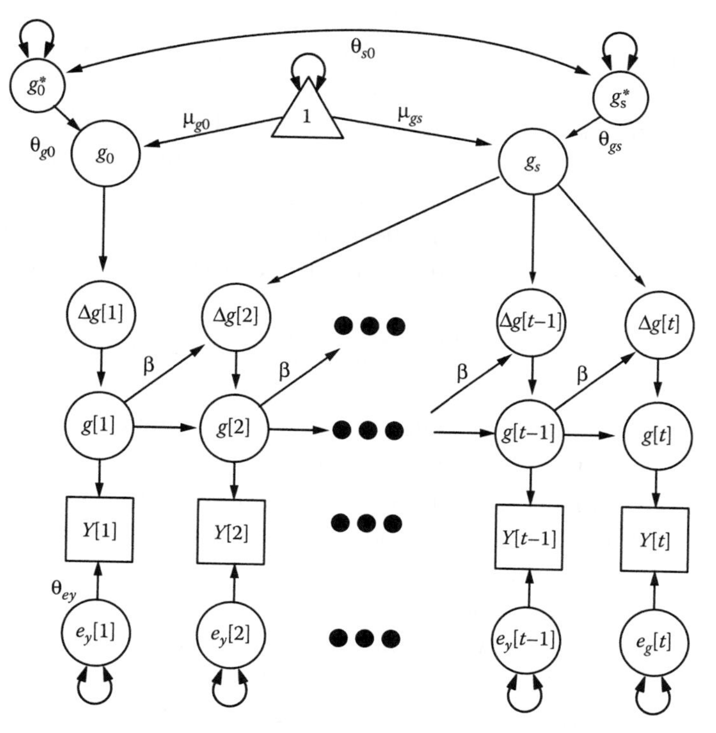

FIGURE 13.1 A univariate latent difference score model for longitudinal data.

latent variables. Single-headed arrows are deterministic parameters such as regression coefficients, or factor loadings, while a double-headed arrow represents stochastic parameters such as variance and covariance. A triangle represents a constant. Any arrow originating from the triangle represents an intercept or mean of variables pointed by the arrow. A circle labeled by $g[.]$ is a true score, a circle labeled by $\Delta g[.]$ is a latent change score, a circle labeled by g_0 is a latent level variable, and a circle labeled by g_s is a latent slope variable. A path from $g[t-1]$ to $\Delta g[t]$ is an effect of the previous true score on a current change score, which is termed as self-feedback (β). A square $Y[2]$ is pointed by $e_y[2]$ and $g[2]$. This means that $Y[2] = g[2] + ey[2]$. Similarly, $g[2]$ is pointed by $g[1]$ and $\Delta g[2]$, which is translated to $g[2] = g[1] + \Delta g[2]$. Also, $\Delta g[2]$ is pointed by $g[1]$ with a factor of β and by gs. This part of the path diagram tells us that $\Delta g[2] = \beta g[1] + g_s$.

13.2.2 Monte Carlo Results for the Univariate Model

The univariate results of Monte Carlo simulation analyses from the SEM and BE methods are summarized in Table 13.1. Table 13.1 shows the average of parameter estimates along with differences between the true values and average estimates for the univariate model based on 50 simulated samples for both complete data ($N = 200$ and six repeated measures) and incomplete data without the third and fifth measurement occasions. Table 13.2 shows the Monte Carlo standard deviations (SD_θ) and the average standard errors (MSE_θ) based on the 50 samples. These two values were calculated as

$$\mathrm{SD}_\theta = \frac{\sum_{B=1}^{50} (\theta_B - \mu_\theta)^2}{49} \quad \text{and} \quad \mathrm{MSE}_\theta = \frac{\sum_{B=1}^{50} \mathrm{SE}_{\theta,B}}{50}, \tag{13.8}$$

where θ_B is a parameter estimate at a Monte Carlo sample, μ_θ is the average of parameter estimates over 50 samples indexed by B, and $\mathrm{SE}_{\theta,B}$ is the standard error of a parameter estimate at each Monte Carlo run.

Both SEM and Bayesian methods can accurately recover parameters of the simulated univariate model very well. When we deliberately truncated the data, overall, the parameter estimations were not as precise as those from complete data. However, the estimations were still very close to the true values. From the results, we concluded that both the SEM method and the Bayesian method equally and accurately recovered model parameters of the univariate latent difference score model.

TABLE 13.1

Average of the Estimates for Univariate Latent Difference Score Model from 50 Simulated Samples

		Complete Data				Incomplete Data			
		SEM		BE		SEM		BE	
	True	Mean	Dev.	Mean	Dev.	Mean	Dev.	Mean	Dev.
β	0.10	0.10	0	0.10	0	0.10	0	0.11	−0.01
θ^2	9.00	8.96	0.04	9.05	−0.05	9.08	−0.08	9.30	−0.30
μ_{ys}	3.00	2.97	0.03	3.05	−0.05	2.95	0.05	2.71	0.29
μ_{y0}	20.00	19.97	0.03	19.94	0.06	19.96	0.04	20.02	−0.02
ϕ_s^2	1.00	1.02	−0.02	1.05	−0.05	1.02	−0.02	0.94	0.06
ϕ_{s0}	2.00	1.99	0.01	2.13	−0.13	2.02	−0.02	1.92	0.08
ϕ_0^2	20.00	20.01	−0.01	19.98	0.02	19.81	0.19	19.81	0.19

Note: BE refers to the Bayesian estimation method; SEM refers to the structural equation modeling method; "True" indicates population parameter values; "Mean" indicates the mean of parameter estimates over 50 Monte Carlo samples; "Dev." indicates a difference between true and average estimates; for the model parameters, β refers to a self-feedback parameter of the model; θ^2 is residual variance; μ_{ys} is the mean of the linear slope; μ_{y0} is the mean of the latent level; ϕ_s^2 is variance of the latent slope; ϕ_{s0} is covariance between the latent slope and level; and ϕ_0^2 is variance of the latent level.

TABLE 13.2

Comparisons of Empirical Standard Deviation and Mean Standard Errors for the Simulated Univariate Latent Difference Score Model

	Complete				Incomplete			
	SEM		BE		SEM		BE	
	SD	MSE	SD	MSE	SD	MSE	SD	MSE
β	0.01	0.01	0.01	0.01	0.01	0.02	0.01	0.01
θ^2	0.46	0.45	0.47	0.46	0.69	0.64	0.72	0.67
μ_{ys}	0.34	0.39	0.34	0.30	0.43	0.46	0.44	0.38
μ_{y0}	0.38	0.37	0.37	0.36	0.37	0.37	0.38	0.36
ϕ_s^2	0.23	0.20	0.23	0.19	0.23	0.22	0.22	0.20
ϕ_{s0}	0.56	0.56	0.58	0.53	0.62	0.61	0.63	0.58
ϕ_0^2	2.50	2.45	2.54	2.46	2.70	2.52	2.76	2.58

Note: BE: Bayesian estimation method; SEM: structural equation modeling method. SD is computed as standard deviation of parameter estimates over 50 Monte Carlo simulations; MSE is computed as average of standard errors of parameter estimates over 50 simulation samples; for the latent difference score model, β refers to a self-feedback parameter of the model; θ^2 is residual variance; μ_{ys} is the mean of the linear slope; μ_{y0} is the mean of the latent level; ϕ_s^2 is variance of the latent slope; ϕ_{s0} is covariance between the latent slope and level; and ϕ_0^2 is variance of the latent level.

TABLE 13.3

Univariate Analysis of the WISC Data Verbal Variable

		SEM		BE	
		Estimate	SE	Estimate	SE
Self-feed parameter ($v[t-1] \rightarrow v[t]$)	β	0.07	0.03	0.10	0.02
Uniqueness variance	θ^2	12.59	1.25	12.47	0.91
Mean of the slope	μ_{ys}	2.83	0.87	1.78	0.59
Mean of the level	μ_{y0}	20.15	0.55	20.39	0.39
Variance of the slope	ϕ_s^2	1.10	0.39	0.76	0.20
Covariance of the level and slope	ϕ_{s0}	1.67	1.07	0.63	0.74
Variance of the level	ϕ_0^2	20.45	3.94	20.55	2.81

Note: BE refers to the Bayesian estimation method; SEM refers to the structural equation modeling method.

Furthermore, from the SDs calculated from the estimates of parameters (SD) and the average standard errors (MSE) in Table 13.3, we could conclude: (1) overall, the MSEs were smaller than SDs, which means that the standard errors were underestimated for both methods, no matter whether missing data were present or not; (2) generally, the SEM method and the BE method could estimate the parameters with the same degree of accuracy; and; (3) when data were incomplete, the estimates were slightly less accurate than when data were complete. However, even with truncated data, all parameters were accurately estimated.

The points above can be easily grasped by inspecting the empirical density plots of the self-feedback parameter and slope mean (refer to Figure 13.2). For example, density distributions of the self-feedback parameter (β) based on the complete data showed more leptokurtic shape than that based on the incomplete data. Under both complete and incomplete simulated data, shapes of density distributions were morphometrically similar between the BE and SEM. This implies that Bayesian and SEM estimates of each simulation run are numerically similar to each other.

13.2.3 Results of the Analysis of the WISC Data

As mentioned earlier, the data structure of the WISC data included four measurement occasions only (ages 6, 7, 9, and 11 in years). Since a latent difference score model requires an equidistance between adjacent occasions, all subjects were considered as having missed the third occasion (age

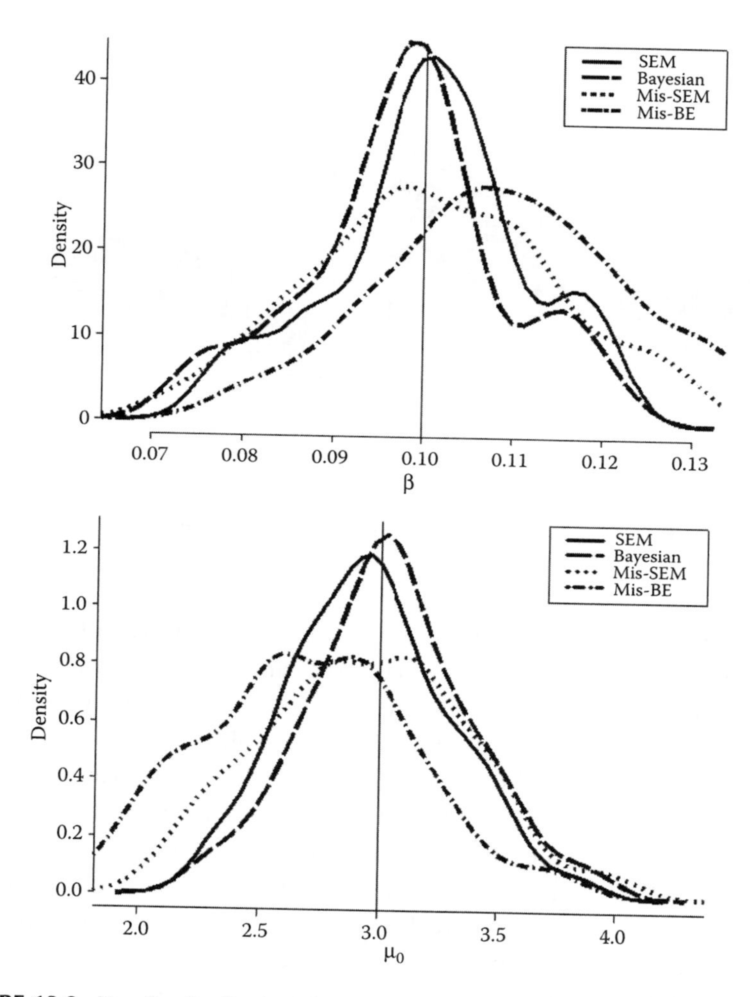

FIGURE 13.2 Density distribution plots for the posterior self-feedback parameters and the posterior slope mean based on 50 Monte Carlo samples.

8) and the fifth occasion (age 10) of six repeated measures. In terms of the path diagram representation, the third and fifth occasions were filled with phantom latent variables as fillers. There were no missing values in either the verbal or performance scores for $N = 204$ subjects. For the analysis of the WISC data, the results for the univariate analysis of Verbal variable are presented in Table 13.3. We observed some numerical differences between the SEM and Bayesian estimates. However, given the standard errors of estimates, the SEM estimates were within the credibility region of Bayesian

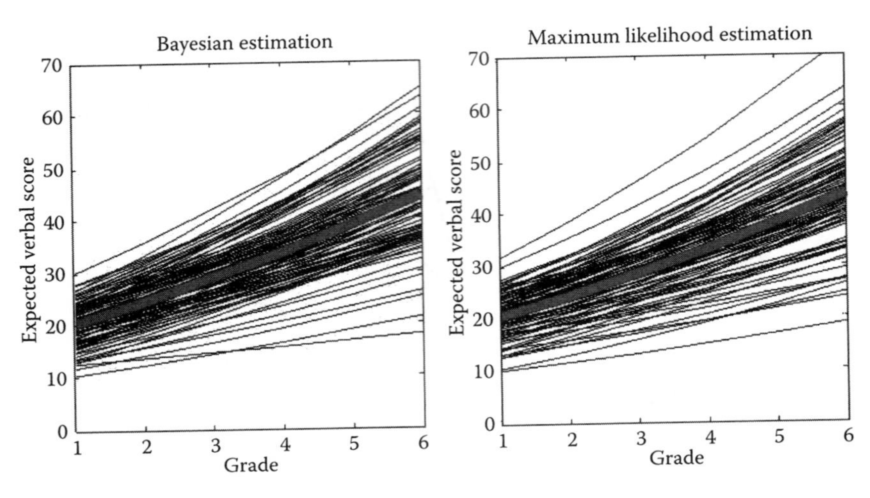

FIGURE 13.3 Expected verbal scores based on the univariate latent difference score model for the WISC verbal scores.

estimates and vice versa. Therefore, all the estimates were not statistically different when comparing between the SEM and Bayesian results. Based on the numerical results, the change scores for the verbal score were positive ($\Delta v[t] = 0.07v[t-1] + 2.83$ for BE, while $\Delta v[t] = 0.10v[t-1] + 1.79$ for SEM estimation). This implies that the higher the previous score, the higher the change score. For example, using Bayesian estimates, if the previous score was 50, then the change score would be 6.33. If the previous score was 80, the change score would be inflated to 8.43. Expected trajectories were produced in Figure 13.3. A curve in the heavy solid line was the average curve, while other curves were expected trajectories based on variance and covariance of the latent level and slope scores.

13.3 PART II: FITTING A BIVARIATE DIFFERENCE SCORE MODEL

In bivariate dynamic systems, we are interested in examining how two change processes proceed and react concurrently, and so longitudinal causal inter-relations between two change processes can be examined. A dynamic effect of one variable on a change score of another variable is coined a *coupling* effect. In an algebraic form, a bivariate difference score model is expressed as

$$\Delta g[t]_n = \beta_g g[t-1]_n + g_{sn} + \gamma_{gf} f[t-1]_n \tag{13.9}$$

for the g process, and

$$\Delta f[t]_n = \beta_f f[t-1]_n + f_{sn} + \gamma_{fg} g[t-1]_n \tag{13.10}$$

for the f process. Most importantly, γ_{gf} is a coupling effect from f to Δg, and γ_{fg} is a coupling effect from g to Δf. So what do these simultaneous change scores tell us? Change scores of one variable are influenced not only by the previous score of its own variable but also by the previous score of another variable in addition to a linear slope score. These six elements concurrently feed into characteristics of growth and trajectories of two parallel processes.

By algebraically manipulating these change scores and the fundamental equations ($f[t]_n = f[t-1]n + \Delta f[t]_n$ and $g[t]_n = g[t-1]_n + \Delta g[t]_n$), we can express the true score as a dependent variable. When an error term is added to each process, we derive simultaneous equations of the observed scores for two parallel processes, that is,

$$Y[t]_n = (1 + \beta_g) g[t-1]_n + g_{sn} + \gamma_{gf} f[t-1]_n + ey[t]_n \tag{13.11}$$

for the Y process, and

$$X[t]_n = (1 + \beta_f) f[t-1]_n + f_{sn} + \gamma_{fg} g[t-1]_n + ex[t]_n \tag{13.12}$$

for the X process. Latent level (initial conditions, g_0 and f_0) and slope scores for the g and f processes are assumed to evince interindividual variability. Therefore,

$$\begin{aligned} g_{0,n} &= \mu_{g0} + d_{g0,n}, \\ g_{s,n} &= \mu_{gs} + d_{gs,n}, \\ f_{0,n} &= \mu_{f0} + d_{f0,n}, \\ f_{s,n} &= \mu_{fs} + d_{fs,n}. \end{aligned} \tag{13.13}$$

Equation 13.10 shows that latent level and slope scores are defined by their mean (μ_{g0}, μ_{gs}, μ_{f0}, and μ_{fs}) and deviations from respective means

(d_{g0}, d_{gs}, d_{f0}, and d_{fs}). These four latent variables are distributed as multivariate-normal, that is,

$$\begin{pmatrix} g_0 \\ g_s \\ f_0 \\ f_s \end{pmatrix} \sim MN \left[\begin{pmatrix} \mu_{g0} \\ \mu_{gs} \\ \mu_{f0} \\ \mu_{fs} \end{pmatrix}, \begin{pmatrix} \phi_{g0}^2 & & \text{symmetric} & \\ \phi_{g0gs} & \phi_{gs}^2 & & \\ \phi_{g0f0} & \phi_{gsf0} & \phi_{f0}^2 & \\ \phi_{g0fs} & \phi_{gsfs} & \phi_{f0fs} & \phi_{fs}^2 \end{pmatrix} \right]. \quad (13.14)$$

In the above symmetric matrix, variance and covariance terms among the level and slope variables are represented by ϕ. The path diagram for the bivariate difference score model is shown in Figure 13.4. In this path diagram, a path from a circle representing a true score ($g[.]$ and $f[.]$) point to a circle representing a latent change variable ($\Delta f[.]$ and $\Delta g[.]$) is a dynamical parameter of interest. Specifically, a structural path originating from a circle labeled by $g[.]$ to a circle labeled by $\Delta f[.]$ represents a dynamical coupling from g to a latent change in f, while that from $f[.]$ to $\Delta g[.]$ represents a coupling from f to a latent change in g. Similarly, a path originating from a circle labeled by $g[.]$ to a circle labeled by $\Delta g[.]$ represents a self-feedback of the g process. All self-feedback parameters within a variable are equal

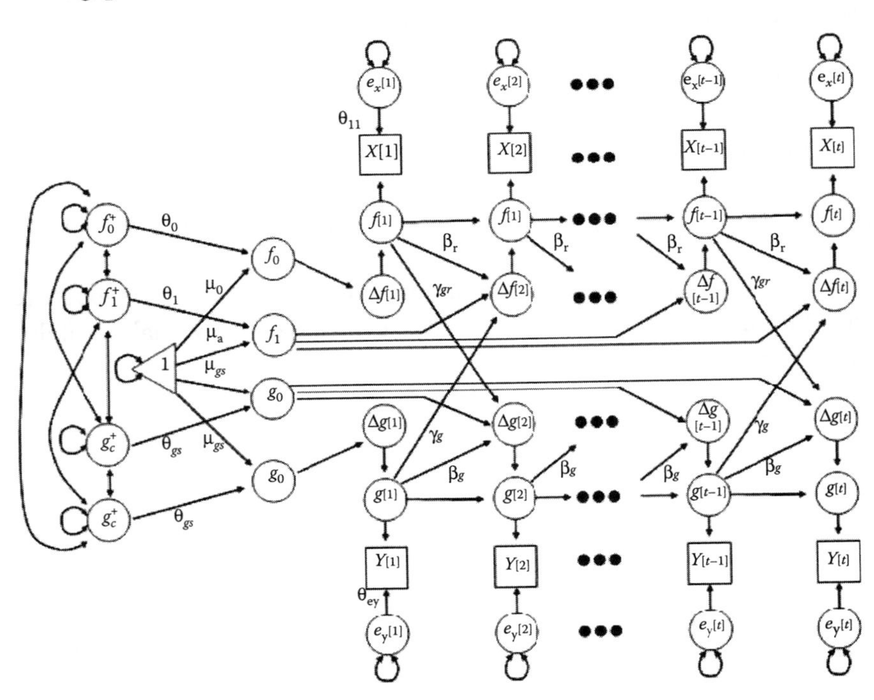

FIGURE 13.4 Path diagram for a bivariate latent difference score model.

over time. Also, we set equality constraints on coupling parameters over time within a variable. Thus, we only estimate four separate dynamical parameters, that is, two self-feedback and two coupling parameters.

13.3.1 Monte Carlo Results for the Bivariate Model

The parameter estimates for the bivariate difference score model based on SEM and the MCMC method are summarized in Table 13.4. The average standard errors and the SD of the estimated parameters summarized over 50 Monte Carlo samples are given in Table 13.5. Parallel to findings from the univariate longitudinal analyses, both the SEM and the Bayesian methods demonstrated consensus in accuracy of recovering preset parameters. Most critical dynamic parameters (i.e., $\beta_g = -0.5$, $\gamma_{gf} = -0.25$, $\beta_f = -0.5$, $\gamma_{fg} = 0.25$, $\mu_{gs} = 47.5$, and $\mu_{gs} = 32.5$) were recovered with high accuracy for both SEM and Bayesian approaches. For example, average dynamic systems based on the complete simulation data were estimated as

$$\begin{cases} \Delta g[t] = -0.5g[t-1] - 0.25f[t-1] + 47.55 \\ \Delta f[t] = -0.5f[t-1] - 0.25g[t-1] + 32.39 \end{cases} \tag{13.15}$$

based on the SEM approach, and

$$\begin{cases} \Delta g[t] = -0.5g[t-1] - 0.25f[t-1] + 47.40 \\ \Delta f[t] = -0.5f[t-1] - 0.25g[t-1] + 32.33 \end{cases} \tag{13.16}$$

based on BE.

These derived difference equations were very close to the preset dynamics system. This indicates that both Bayesian and SEM analyses were able to recover the eigen system that uniquely characterizes multivariate dynamics. For the incomplete data analyses, both SEM and Gibbs sampling methods recovered the true dynamics and numerically the average dynamic systems were obtained as

$$\begin{cases} \Delta g[t] = -0.52g[t-1] - 0.24f[t-1] + 47.59 \\ \Delta f[t] = -0.51f[t-1] - 0.27g[t-1] + 32.30 \end{cases} \tag{13.17}$$

based on the SEM method, and

$$\begin{cases} \Delta g[t] = -0.5g[t-1] - 0.25f[t-1] + 47.47 \\ \Delta f[t] = -0.5f[t-1] - 0.25g[t-1] + 32.29 \end{cases} \tag{13.18}$$

based on the Gibbs sampling method.

TABLE 13.4

Parameter Estimates for the Bivariate Latent Difference Score Model

		Complete Data				Incomplete Data			
		SEM		BE		SEM		BE	
Parameter	True	Mean	Dev.	Mean	Dev.	Mean	Dev.	Mean	Dev.
β_g	−0.50	−0.50	0	−0.50	0	−0.52	0.02	−0.50	0
γ_{gf}	−0.25	−0.25	0	−0.25	0	−0.24	−0.01	−0.25	0
β_f	−0.50	−0.50	0	−0.50	0	−0.51	0.01	−0.50	0
γ_{fg}	0.25	0.25	0	0.25	0	0.27	−0.02	0.25	0
μ_{gs}	47.50	47.55	−0.05	47.40	0.10	47.59	−0.09	47.47	0.03
μ_{g0}	5.00	5.04	−0.04	5.12	−0.12	5.05	−0.05	5.10	−0.10
μ_{fs}	32.50	32.39	0.11	32.33	0.17	32.30	0.20	32.29	0.21
μ_{f0}	5.00	5.00	0	5.04	−0.04	5.02	−0.02	5.04	−0.04
θ^2_{ey}	25.00	25.09	−0.09	25.66	−0.66	25.37	−0.37	26.19	−1.19
θ^2_{ex}	25.00	24.95	0.05	25.62	−0.62	24.58	0.42	25.75	−0.75
ϕ^2_{gs}	6.25	5.92	0.33	5.77	0.48	6.44	−0.19	5.67	0.58
ϕ_{gsg0}	6.25	6.20	0.05	6.36	−0.11	6.53	−0.28	6.35	−0.10
ϕ^2_{g0}	25.00	25.22	−0.22	23.14	1.86	24.92	0.08	23.25	1.75
ϕ_{gsfs}	−1.25	−1.16	−0.09	−1.08	−0.17	−1.78	0.53	−1.06	−0.19
ϕ_{g0fs}	2.50	2.33	0.17	2.32	0.18	1.93	0.57	2.19	0.31
ϕ^2_{fs}	6.25	6.25	0	6.31	−0.06	7.05	−0.80	6.24	0.01
ϕ_{gsf0}	2.50	2.22	0.28	1.95	0.55	2.10	0.40	1.85	0.65
ϕ_{g0f0}	−5.00	−4.95	−0.05	−5.19	0.19	−5.09	0.09	−4.81	−0.19
ϕ_{fsf0}	6.25	6.32	−0.07	6.66	−0.41	6.75	−0.50	6.80	−0.55
ϕ^2_{f0}	25.00	25.16	−0.16	23.00	2.00	25.37	−0.37	22.84	2.16

Note: BE: Bayesian estimation method; SEM: structural equation modeling method. "True" indicates population parameter values; "Mean" indicates the mean of parameter estimates over 50 Monte Carlo samples; "Dev." indicates a difference between true and average estimates. β_g is self-feedback of the verbal score; γ_{gf} is a coupling from the performance to the verbal score; β_f is a self-feedback of the performance score; γ_{fg} is a coupling from the verbal to performance scores; μ_{gs} is the mean of the verbal slope; μ_{g0} is the mean of the verbal level; μ_{fs} is the mean of the performance slope; μ_{g0} is the mean of the performance level; θ^2_{ey} is the uniqueness of the verbal scores; θ^2_{ex} is the uniqueness of the performance scores; $\phi^2_{..}$ is variance of either level or slope, while $\phi_{..}$ is covariance of level and slope components, where a subscript ".." represents either gs (the verbal slope), $g0$ (the verbal level), fs (the performance slope), or f_0 (the performance level).

Parallel to the findings from univariate analyses, results based on the complete data exhibited smaller average standard errors and SD of parameter estimates over 50 Monte Carlo simulations than those based on the incomplete data.

TABLE 13.5

Comparisons of Empirical Standard Deviation and Mean Standard Errors for the Simulated Bivariate Latent Difference Score Model

	Complete				Incomplete			
	SEM		BE		SEM		BE	
	SD	MSE	SD	MSE	SD	MSE	SD	MSE
β_g	0.02	0.02	0.02	0.02	0.13	0.02	0.02	0.02
γ_{gf}	0.01	0.01	0.01	0.01	0.07	0.01	0.01	0.01
β_f	0.01	0.01	0.01	0.01	0.07	0.01	0.01	0.02
γ_{fg}	0.02	0.02	0.02	0.02	0.15	0.03	0.02	0.02
μ_{gs}	0.42	0.45	0.43	0.46	0.64	0.50	0.50	0.51
μ_{g0}	0.51	0.50	0.51	0.49	0.51	0.50	0.51	0.50
μ_{fs}	0.51	0.45	0.50	0.46	0.62	0.51	0.51	0.47
μ_0	0.57	0.50	0.59	0.49	0.60	0.50	0.60	0.49
θ^2_{ey}	1.24	1.25	1.21	1.27	3.04	1.77	2.20	1.83
θ^2_{ex}	1.04	1.24	1.08	1.26	1.28	1.73	1.31	1.74
ϕ^2_{gs}	0.81	0.86	0.80	0.85	3.88	1.23	1.00	1.04
ϕ_{gsg0}	1.72	1.40	1.46	1.39	2.48	1.60	1.47	1.48
ϕ^2_{g0}	4.32	4.58	4.34	4.34	5.07	4.73	4.99	4.48
ϕ_{gsfs}	0.63	0.63	0.61	0.62	4.39	0.96	0.65	0.75
ϕ_{g0fs}	1.42	1.40	1.37	1.36	2.95	1.64	1.57	1.48
ϕ^2_{fs}	0.91	0.91	0.89	0.95	4.69	1.33	1.01	1.08
ϕ_{gsf0}	1.21	1.39	1.20	1.37	2.24	1.56	1.37	1.53
ϕ_{g0f0}	3.48	3.19	3.61	3.10	3.45	3.22	3.67	3.17
ϕ_{fsf0}	1.60	1.43	1.32	1.42	2.12	1.62	1.43	1.52
ϕ^2_{f0}	4.25	4.55	4.49	4.47	4.40	4.72	4.78	4.68

Note: See note for Table 13.2.

The density plots of the coupling parameters (γ_{gf} and γ_{fg}) and self-feedback parameters (β_g and β_f) were depicted in Figures 13.5 and 13.6, respectively. For the bivariate models, the sampling distribution of parameter estimates exhibited similar shapes between the SEM and Gibbs sampling methods regardless of whether data were complete or not.

13.3.2 Results for the Bivariate WISC

For the bivariate analysis of Verbal and Nonverbal scores, the model comparisons are summarized in Table 13.6. The results for the full difference

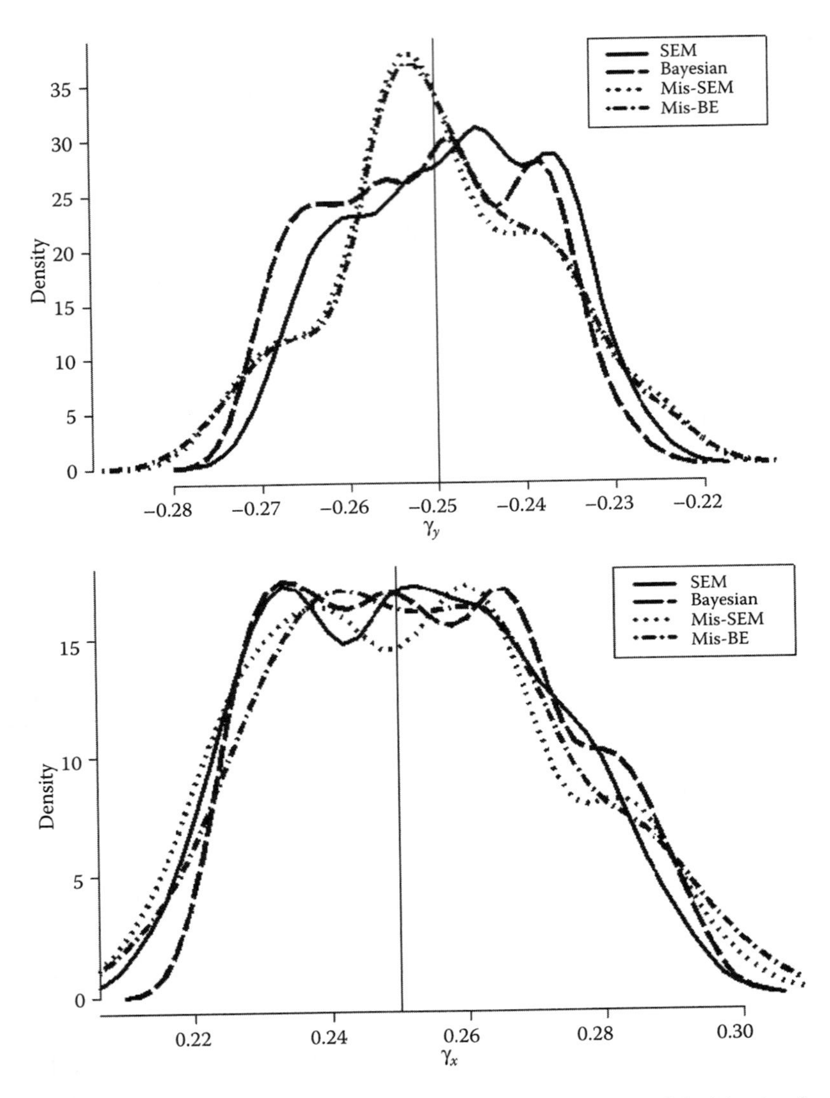

FIGURE 13.5 Density plots for the posterior coupling parameters of the bivariate latent difference score model based on 50 Monte Carlo samples.

score model are given in Table 13.7 (verbal is g and performance is f). We fitted four alternative bivariate models to the WISC data. Fit comparisons among these four models were used to examine whether one variable influenced a change in the other, or vice versa. The first model was the full model with both coupling parameters in the dynamic system. The second

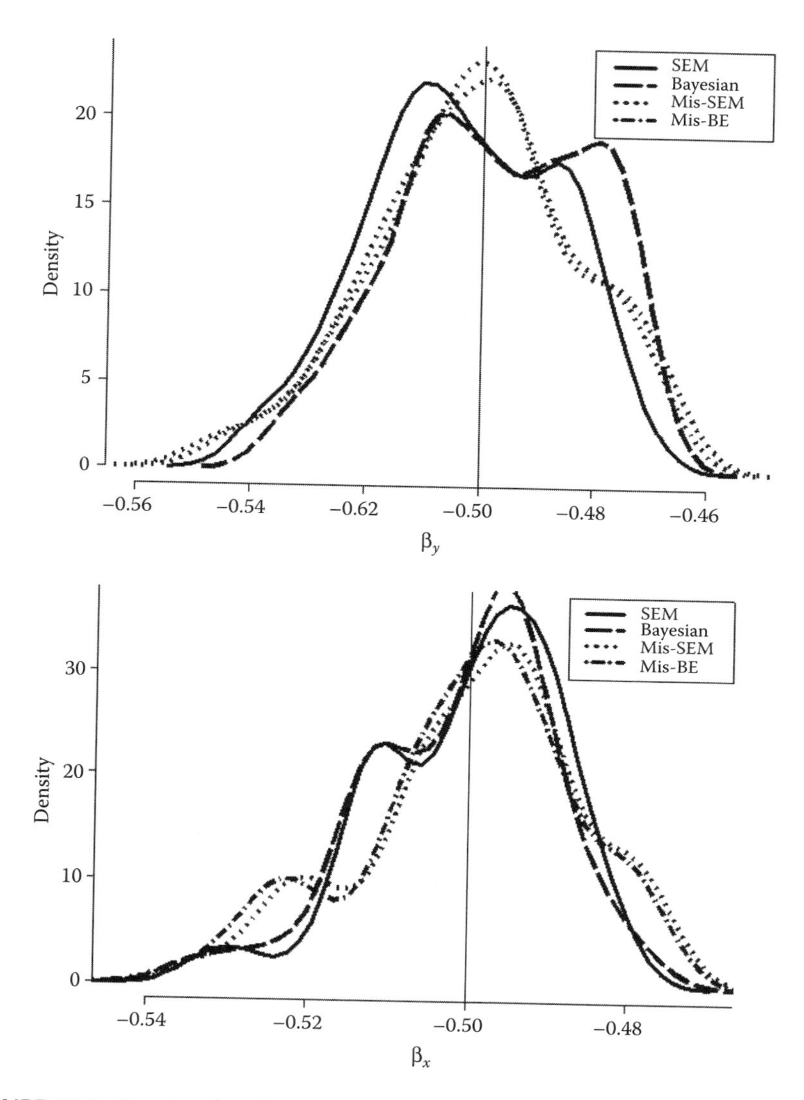

FIGURE 13.6 Density plots for the posterior self-feedback parameters of the bivariate latent difference score model based on 50 Monte Carlo samples.

model removed the coupling parameter from the Verbal to the Nonverbal, while the third model removed the coupling parameter from the Nonverbal to the Verbal. The last model removed both coupling effects from the system. For Bayesian analyses the deviance information criterion (DIC) was used to compare alternative models. A DIC difference of greater than 10 signals a substantial fit difference in which the lower valued DIC indicates a

TABLE 13.6

Model Fit Statistics

	SEM				WinBUGS	
	χ^2	AIC	BIC	RMSEA	pD	DIC
Full model	56	5200	5248	0.12	469	9665*
No nonverb on verb	65	5201	5251	0.13	477	9665*
No verb on nonverb	82	5219	5267	0.15	458	9692
No coupling	86	5220	5267	0.15	461	9699

Note: *The DIC for the full model is slightly smaller than that for the no nonverb on verb model; $\chi^2 = N^* - 2^* \log(L)$, where L refers to a likelihood function value based on ML estimation and N is the sample size; $\text{AIC} = -2^* \log(L) + 2^*p$, where p is the number of model parameters; $\text{BIC} = -2^* \log(L) + p^* \log(N)$; $\text{RMSEA} = \sqrt{\max\left[\left(\frac{2^*L}{\text{df}} - \frac{1}{N}\right), 0\right]}$ is a root mean square error of approximation. In this equation, df refers to degree of freedom; $pD = E[D(\theta)] - D[E(\theta)]$, where $D(\theta) = -2\log(L(y \mid \theta))$, a deviance index at parameter θ given by data y, and $E[]$ is an expectation operator; pD is called the effective number of parameters of the model. It is defined as the difference between the expected value of deviance ($E[D(\theta)]$) and a deviance value at the expected value of model parameters ($D[E(\theta)]$); $\text{DIC} = pd + E[D(\theta)]$ is deviance information criterion. Smaller DIC indicates better fit to data.

better fit. Based on BE, the model with a coupling effect from Nonverbal to Verbal removed was the best fit model, whereas SEM estimation indicated that the full model was the best fitted to the WISC data. A difference in χ^2 between the full model and any other model was statistically significant. Based on the parameter estimates of the bivariate full difference score model where both coupling parameters were assumed to exist, the derived dynamic system was described as

$$\begin{cases} \Delta v[t] = 0.44v[t-1] - 0.25p[t-1] + 0.27 \\ \Delta p[t] = -0.37p[t-1] + 0.32v[t-1] + 9.11 \end{cases} \quad \text{for SEM approach,} \tag{13.19}$$

$$\begin{cases} \Delta v[t] = 0.40v[t-1] - 0.20p[t-1] - 0.02 \\ \Delta p[t] = -0.31p[t-1] + 0.27v[t-1] + 9.01 \end{cases} \quad \text{for the BE.} \tag{13.20}$$

There were numerical differences in parameter estimates between the SEM and Gibbs sampling methods. However, each parameter estimate obtained via the SEM approach was located within the Bayesian credibility interval of an estimate obtained by the Gibbs sampling method. The mean of the slope factor of the Verbal process ($\mu_{gs} = 0.27$ by SEM and $\mu_{gs} = -0.02$ by BE) was seemingly numerically different. However, in

TABLE 13.7

Parameter Estimation for the Bivariate Model of WISC Data (Fixing the Variances of Slopes)

Parameters of the Model		SEM Est.	SEM SE	BE Est.	BE SE
Self-feedback of the verbal	β_g	0.44	0.07	0.39	0.04
Coupling from the performance to the verbal	γ_{gf}	−0.25	0.04	−0.20	0.03
Self-feedback of the performance	β_f	−0.37	0.06	−0.31	0.06
Coupling from the verb to performance	γ_{fg}	0.32	0.09	0.27	0.08
Mean of the slope of the verbal score	μ_{gs}	0.27	1.13	−0.02	0.59
Mean of the level of the verbal score	μ_{g0}	20.05	0.55	20.20	0.40
Mean of the slope of the performance	μ_{fs}	9.11	1.25	9.01	0.91
Mean of the level of the performance	μ_{f0}	18.07	0.81	18.22	0.62
Uniqueness of the verbal score	θ^2_{ey}	11.89	1.17	11.71	0.83
Uniqueness of the performance	θ^2_{ex}	22.70	2.21	22.41	1.43
Variance of the verbal slope	ϕ^2_{gs}	2.31	0.00	2.31	0.58
Covariance of the *v* level and *v* slope	ϕ_{gsg0}	−0.99	1.40	−1.80	1.01
Variance of the verbal level	ϕ^2_{g0}	21.54	3.81	22.93	2.89
Covariance of the *v* slope and *p* slope	ϕ_{gsfs}	3.63	0.38	3.62	0.83
Covariance of the *v* level and *p* slope	ϕ_{g0fs}	3.43	2.14	1.85	1.55
Variance of the performance slope	ϕ^2_{fs}	7.99	0.00	7.99	1.91
Covariance of the *v* slope and *p* level	ϕ_{gsf0}	4.80	2.00	3.84	1.60
Covariance of the *v* level and *p* level	ϕ_{g0f0}	24.90	4.82	28.61	3.83
Covariance of the *p* slope and *p* level	ϕ_{fsf0}	14.58	2.70	14.25	2.39
Variance of the performance level	ϕ^2_{f0}	46.39	8.83	55.97	7.13

both cases, they were found to be statistically not significant. Figure 13.7 shows expected latent curves of both Verbal and Nonverbal scores based on the full bivariate latent difference score model for $N = 100$. Two subfigures in the upper row are the expected latent curves derived from the Bayesian parameter estimates; the other two subfigures in the lower row were the expected curves based on SEM parameter estimates. By a visual inspection, there was similarity in the average latent curves of both Verbal and Nonverbal scores between BE and SEM estimations.

13.4 DISCUSSION

Previously, several researches demonstrated that the Bayesian technique could be used for analyses of a latent variable model such as static factor

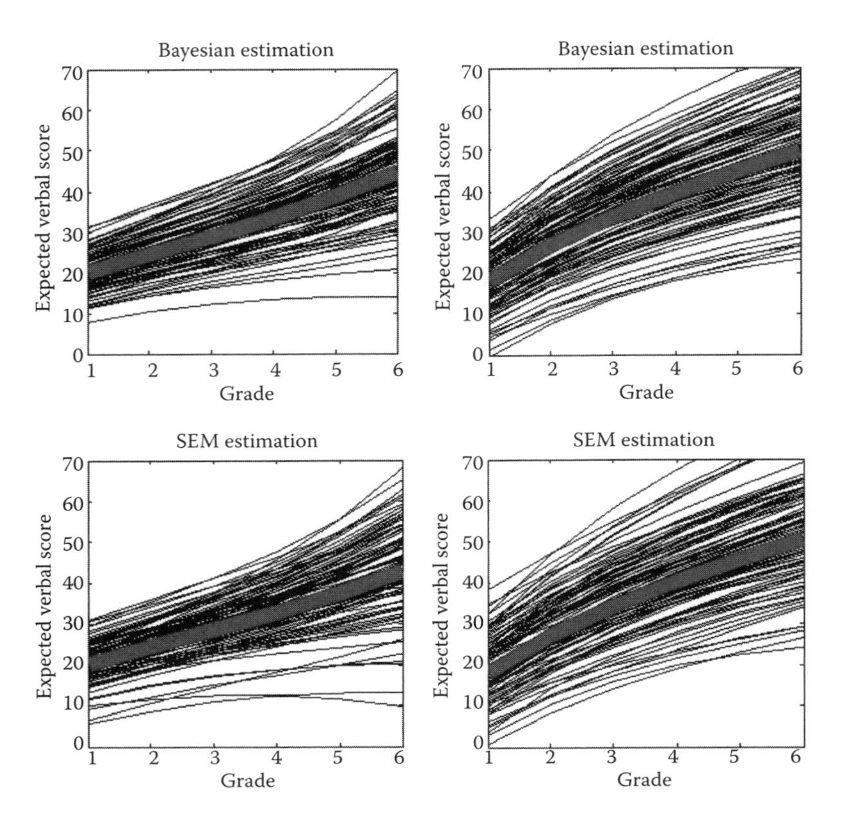

FIGURE 13.7 Expected verbal and performance latent growth curves based on the bivariate latent difference score models for the WISC verbal and performance scores.

models (e.g., Ansari et al., 2002; Bartholomew, 1981). One aspect of our research was focused on a longitudinal structural equation model using multivariate repeated measures. In particular, our research focused on comparison of the SEM and BE methods to numerically identify the discrete dynamic system models involving multiple subjects, multivariate repeated measures with interindividual and intraindividual variability of key latent variables. For this purpose, we adopted latent difference score models (McArdle, 2001; McArdle et al., 2001) as a dynamic system example. With the use of the Monte Carlo simulation study, we demonstrated that both SEM and BE methods were viable alternatives to numerically identify a system of latent difference score equations. Even with six repeated measures data format, both the SEM and the Bayesian approaches were able to accurately recover the population parameters for the preset dynamics system. In addition, we also demonstrated that even deliberately removing one-third of data from the simulation data, we were still able to correctly identify the dynamic system using both the SEM and the Gibbs sampling methods.

Our research justifies the use of the Gibbs sampling to estimate parameters for the complex latent variable longitudinal structural equation models where the number of latent variables far exceeds the number of observed variables in the model. Basically we concur with Arminger et al. (1998), Jedidi et al. (2001), and Lee et al. (2003, 2004) that the BE is a useful technique to model structural equation models. Prior to this research project, we used the Gibbs sampling method to investigate latent growth curves (Zhang, Hamagami, Wang, Nessleroade, & Grimm, 2007). We found that both SEM and Gibbs sampling produced almost identical results when non-informative priors were chosen. The findings of this study were consistent with previous findings on SEM and BE—the Bayesian algorithms and MLE-based SEM algorithms will yield the same numerical conclusions in cases where no prior information for parameters is provided. However, under Bayesian theory, if prior information is available and it is weighted heavily, the Bayesian approach can provide parameter estimates and goodness-of-fit indices that are more appropriate than standard MLE-based SEM estimates. With WinBUGS program (Spiegelhalter et al., 1999), it is now possible to analyze a variety of complex structured latent models, including the multilevel SEM models described as multiple group SEM by McArdle and Hamagami (1996). Recent books by Congdon (2001, 2003) and Gilks et al. (1996) illustrate that the Gibbs sampling method using WinBUGS program can be applied to models including categorical variable models, multilevel models, factor models, and SEM as examples for data analyses. One asset of WinBUGS is a script syntax that eliminates repetitive model statements that usually have to be spelled out in the traditional SEM software. As the number of repeated measures increases, repetitive statements make SEM programming laborious and tedious, while script syntaxes of WinBUGS simplify programming.

With interfacing the WinBUGS and SAS programs, BEs are now easily performed within the SAS computational environment. This interface allows reformat of SAS data into WinBUGS-readable forms as well as generation of initial values of the model parameters to be used for the WinBUGS. After the MCMC estimation algorithm stabilizes Bayes estimates, results are read back into the SAS environment to further examine the results.

Details of the procedures are described in Zhang, McArdle, Wang, and Hamagami (2008).

Finally, we recognize an ongoing controversy between Fisherian and Bayesian interpretation of statistical probability. This research is neither intended to advocate one method over the other, nor is this paper intended to resolve such a complex controversial issue. Instead, we can report an interesting finding about the issue of when the Bayesian approach could be beneficial or could become problematic.

13.4.1 When does Bayesian Modeling Work?

There are several factors to consider when it comes to the effectiveness of BE. One factor is whether or not the prior knowledge about the causal relationship is correct. Another factor is whether or not the study collects data from the true population. If the sample does not represent the target population, any estimation method, Bayesian or not, would not help reach the correct conclusion about the causal relationship. To answer the question of when BE helps, simulation analyses were conducted for the simple regression model. The model represents a simple regression in which a criterion variable, Y is predicted by a stimulus X. There are three parameters: (1) an intercept, (2) a regression coefficient, and (3) a residual variance. The study manipulated (1) the sample size ranging from $N = 20$ to $N = 1000$, (2) the status of the prior information, correct or incorrect, and (3) the characteristics of the sample, representing the true or false population. Numerical details of the Monte Carlo simulation are not presented here since this is not a primary focus of our paper. Instead, the major findings are presented.

13.4.2 Scenario 1: Using Noninformative Prior and the Sample from the Correct Population

Since the prior is noninformative, the data from the sample predominantly determines estimation of parameters. If the data were sampled from the correct population, the parameter estimates could be close to the population parameters. Generally the noninformative prior would lead to correct estimation of the population parameter. The larger the sample size, the more precise the estimation of the population parameters. This is the case that both Bayesian and non-Bayesian would come to the congruent conclusion where the inference about a conclusion is totally data dependent.

13.4.3 Scenario 2: Using Noninformative Prior and the Sample from the False Population

When the sample comes from the wrong population and the noninformative prior is used for BE, parameter estimates on average would converge near the parameters that are true to the false population. Therefore, this scenario would lead to a wrong inference about the causal relationship. The wrong sample is detrimental to any causal study. This is the case that both Bayesian and non-Bayesian would come to the wrong conclusion about the causal relationship. The wrong conclusion is totally manufactured by the wrong data.

13.4.4 Scenario 3: Using the Wrong Prior but the Sample from the Correct Population

When the sample is drawn from the true population but the wrong informative prior is used for BE, the parameter estimates are generally incorrect and lead to a wrong inference about a causal relationship. In this case, even the sample size over $N = 500$ will not help resolve an inaccurate conclusion about the causal relationship. This is the case that maximum likelihood estimation would result in the correct conclusion.

13.4.5 Scenario 4: Using the Strong Wrong Prior and the Sample from the False Population

When the sample is drawn from the wrong population and the wrong informative prior is used, parameter estimates are way off from the true parameters. This scenario would lead to a wrong inference about a causal relationship. It is apparent that the wrong sample and wrong prior knowledge exacerbate inaccuracy in the inference of a causal relationship. This is the case that we would not want to face since BE does not help.

13.4.6 Scenario 5: Using the Correct Prior and the Sample from the True Population

When the sample is drawn from the true population and the strong informative prior is set at the exact parameter value for the correct population, parameter estimates are generally trusted even with the small sample. This is the ideal scenario where subjective belief and sampling process mutually support each other and inference about the causal relationship from this situation is reliable. This is the case that we the audience would want to face since BE would augment the prior knowledge and subjective belief about the causal inference with the updated information.

13.4.7 Scenario 6: Using the Strong Correct Prior and the Sample from the False Population

When the sample is drawn from the wrong population but the informative prior is tapping the correct parameters expressive of the true population, inference about a causal relationship depends on the sample size. With the small sample sizes, that is, weak influence of the empirical data, the correct prior information on the target parameter will help in tapping the correct value and Bayesian estimates are in the neighborhood of the correct parameter values. With the large sample from the wrong population, the influence of the large amount of wrong data will dominate over the influence of the correct prior. Thus, this situation leads to a wrong inference on a causal relationship.

In conclusion, our main goal of this paper was to show that Bayesian and SEM could be used to fit data to a longitudinal structural equation model of dynamical nature. Deriving a final conclusion about a causal relationship is an extremely complicated process since the final decision is influenced by so many factors such as model misspecification, missampling from a wrong population, nonrandom sampling, nontrustworthy prior knowledge and misinformation about the causal relationship, timing of observations where critical time of the growth process might be completely missed, amount of empirical observations, and other unpreventable circumstances. All these factors are likely to contribute to generating biases in parameter estimates to some degree whether or not either Bayesian or SEM estimation is opted. For this reason, this paper was not intended to show our predilection of one methodology over the other. Any quantitative method conducive to making a correct decision about a causal relationship should be employed for furthering any scientific knowledge.

REFERENCES

Ansari, A., & Jedidi, K. (2000). Bayesian factor analysis for multilevel binary observations. *Psychometrika, 65,* 475–496.

Ansari, A., Jedidi, K., & Dube, L. (2002). Heterogeneous factor analysis models: A Bayesian approach. *Psychometrika, 67,* 49–78.

Arminger, G., & Muthén, B.O. (1998). A Bayesian approach to nonlinear latent variable models using the Gibbs sampler and the Metropolis–Hastings algorithm. *Psychometrika, 63,* 271–300.

Arminger, G. (1986). Linear stochastic differential equation models for panel data with unobserved variables. In N. Tuma (Ed.), *Sociological methodology* (pp. 187–212). San Francisco: Jossey-Bass.

Bartholomew, D. J. (1981). Posterior analysis of the factor model. *British Journal of Mathematical and Statistical Psychology, 34,* 93–99.

Bartholomew, D. J. (1994). Bayes' theorem in latent variable modelling. In P. R. Freeman & A. F. Smith (Eds.), *Aspects of uncertainty* (pp. 41–50). New York: Wiley.

Beddington, J. R., Free, C. A., & Lawton, J. H. (1975). Dynamic complexity in predator–prey models framed in difference equations. *Nature, 255(5503),* 58–60.

Coleman, J. S. (1968). The mathematical study of change. In H. M. Blalock & A. B. Blalock (Eds.), *Methodology in social research* (pp. 428–475). New York: McGraw-Hill.

Congdon, P. (2001). *Bayesian statistical modelling.* New York: Wiley.

Congdon, P. (2003). *Applied Bayesian modelling.* New York: Wiley.

Geman, S., & Geman, D. (1984). Stochastic relaxation, Gibbs distributions, and the Bayesian restoration of images. *IEEE Transactions on Pattern Analysis and Machine Intelligence,* 6, 721–741.

Gelman, A., Carlin, J. B., Stern, H. S., & Rubin, D. B. (1995). *Bayesian data analysis.* New York: Chapman & Hall.

Gilks, W. R., Richardson, S., & Spiegelhalter, D. J. (1996). *Markov chain Monte Carlo in practice.* New York: Chapman & Hall.

Goldberg, S. (1986). *Introduction to difference equation.* New York: Dover.

Fornell, C., & Rust, R. T. (1989). Incorporating prior theory in convariance structure analysis: A Bayesian approach. *Psychometrika, 54,* 249–59.

Hamagami, F., & McArdle, J. J. (2001). Advanced studies of individual differences linear dynamic models for longitudinal data analysis. In G. Marcoulides & R. Schumacker (Eds.), *Advanced structural equation modeling: New developments and techniques* (pp. 203–246). Mahwah, NJ: Erlbaum.

Hayashi, K., & Sen, P. K. (2002). Bias-corrected estimator of factor loadings in Bayesian factor analysis. *Educational and Psychological Measurement, 62,* 944–959.

Hayashi, K., & Yuan, K. H. (2003). Robust Bayesian factor analyses. *Structural Equation Modeling, 10(4),* 525–533.

Jedidi, K., & Ansari, A. (2001). Bayesian structural equation models for multilevel data. In G. A. Marcoulides & R. E. Schumacker (Eds.), *New developments and techniques in structural equation modeling* (pp. 129–157). Mahwah, NJ: Lawrence Erlbaum Associates.

Jedidi, K., Ramaswamy, V., & DeSarbo, W. S. (1996). On estimating finite mixtures of multivariate regression and simutaneous equation models. *Structural Equation Modeling, 3(3)*, 266–289.

Lee, P. M. (2004). *Bayesian statistics: An introduction*. New York: Arnold Publishers.

Lee, S. E., & Press, S. J. (1998). Robustness of Bayesian factor analysis estimates. *Communications in Statistics—Theory and Methods, 27*, 1871–1893.

Lee, S. Y. (1981). A Bayesian approach to confirmatory factor analysis. *Psychometrika, 46*, 153–160.

Lee, S. Y., & Song, X. Y. (2004). Evaluation of the Bayesian and maximum likelihood approaches in analyzing structural equation models with small sample sizes. *Multivariate Behavioral Research, 39*, 653–686.

Lee, S. Y., & Song, X. Y. (2003). Model comparison of nonlinear structural equation models with fixed covariates. *Psychometrika, 68*, 27-47.

Lee, S. Y., & Song, X. Y. (2004). Bayesian model comparison of nonlinear latent variable models with missing continuous and ordinal categorical data. *British Journal of Mathematical and Statistical Psychology, 57*, 131–150.

Lee, S. Y., Song, X. Y., & Poon, W. Y. (2004). Comparison of approaches in estimating interaction and quadratic effects of latent variables. *Multivariate Behavioral Research, 39(1)*, 37–67.

Little, R., & Rubin, D. (1987). *Statistical analysis with missing data*. New York: Wiley.

Martin, J. K., & McDonald, R. P. (1975). Bayesian estimation in unrestricted factor analysis: A treatment for Heywood cases. *Psychometrika, 40*, 505–517.

McArdle, J. J. (1988). Dynamic but structural equation modeling of repeated measures data. In J. R. Nesselroade, & R. B. Cattell (Eds.), *The handbook of multivariate experimental psychology* (Vol. 2, pp. 561–614). New York: Plenum Press.

McArdle, J. J. (1994). Structural factor analysis experiments with incomplete data. *Multivariate Behavioral Research, 29*, 409-454.

McArdle, J. J. (2001). A latent difference score approach to longitudinal dynamic structural analyses. In R. Cudeck, S. du Toit, & D. Sorbom (Eds.). *Structural equation modeling: Present and future* (pp. 342–380). Lincolnwood, IL: Scientific Software International.

McArdle, J. J., & Epstein, D. (1987). Latent growth curves within developmental structural equation models. *Child Development, 58*, 110-133.

McArdle, J. J., & Hamagami, F. (1991). Modeling incomplete longitudinal data using latent growth structural equation models. In L. Collins & J. L. Horn (Eds.), *Best methods for the analysis of change* (pp. 276–304). Washington, DC: American Psychological Association.

McArdle, J. J., & Hamagami, F. (1992). Modeling incomplete longitudinal data using latent growth structural models. *Experimental Aging Research, 18*, 145–166.

McArdle, J. J., & Hamagami, F. (1995). *A dynamic structural equation modeling analysis of theory of fluid and crystallized intelligence*. Paper presented a the annual meeing of the American Psychological Society and the European Congress of Psychology, Athens, Greece.

McArdle, J. J., & Hamagami, F. (1996). Multilevel models from a multiple group structural equation perspective. In G. Marcoulides & R. Schumacker (Eds.), *Advanced structural equation modeling techniques* (pp. 89–124). Hillsdale, NJ: Lawrence Erlbaum Associates.

McArdle, J. J., & Hamagami, F. (2001). Latent difference score stuructural models for linear dynamic analyses with incomplete longitudinal data. In L. Collins & A. Sayer (Eds.). *New methods for the analysis of change* (pp. 139–175). Washington, DC: APA Press.

McArdle, J. J., & Hamagami, F. (2004). Methods for dynamic change hypotheses. In K. van Montfort, J. Oud, & A. Satorra (Eds.). *Recent developments on structural equation models* (pp. 295–335). Dordrecht: Kluwer Academic Publishers.

McArdle, J. J., & Nesselroade, J. R. (1994). Structuring data to study development and change. In S. H. Cohen & H. W. Reese (Eds.), *Life-span developmental psychology: Methodological innovations* (pp. 223–267). Hillsdale, NJ: Lawrence Erlbaum Associates.

Meredith, W., & Tisak, J. (1990). Latent curve analysis. *Psychometrika, 55,* 107–122.

Molenaar, P. C. M. (1985). A dynamic factor model for the analysis of multivariate time series. *Psychometrika, 50,* 181-202.

Neale M. C., Boker, S. M., Xie, G., & Maes, H. H. (2003). *Mx: Statistical modeling* (6th Ed.). VCU, Richmond, VA: Department of Psychiatry.

Nesselroade, J. R. (1991). Interindividual differences in intraindividual changes. In J. L. Horn & L. Collins (Eds.), *Best methods for studying change* (pp. 92–105). Washington, DC: American Psychological Association.

Nesselroade, J. R., McArdle, J. J., Aggen, S. H., & Meyers, J. M. (2001). Alternative dynamic factor models for multivariate time-series analyses. In D. M. Moscowitz & S. L. Hershberger (Eds.), *Modelling intra-individual variability with repeated measures data: Advances and techniques.* Mahwah, NJ: Lawrence Erlbaum Associates.

Nesselroade, J. R., & Molenaar, P. C. (1999). Pooling lagged covariance structures based on short, multivariate time-series for dynamic factor analysis. In R.H. Hoyle (Ed.), *Statistical strategies for small sample research.* Newbury Park, CA: Sage Publications.

Osborne, R. T., & Suddick, D. E. (1972). A longitudinal investigation of the intellectual differentiation hypothesis. *Journal of Genetic Psychology, 121,* 83–89.

Press, S. J., & Shigemasu, K. (1989). Bayesian inference in factor analysis. In L. Gleser, M. Perleman, S. J. Press, & A. Sampson (Eds.), *Contributions to probability and statistics* (pp. 271–287). New York: Springer-Verlag.

Rao, C. R. (1958). Some statistical methods for the comparison of growth curves. *Biometrics, 14,* 1–17.

Rupp, A. A., Dey, D. K., & Zumbo, B. D. (2004). To Bayes or not to Bayes, from whether to when: Applications of Bayesian methodology to modeling. *Structural Equation Modeling, 11,* 424-451.

Schafer, J. L. (1997). *Analysis of incomplete multivariate data.* London: Chapman.

Scheinerman, E. R. (1996). *Invitation to dynamical systems.* Upper Saddle River, NJ: Prentice-Hall.

Scheines, R., Hoijtink, H., & Boomsma, A. (1999). Bayesian estimation and testing of structural equation models. *Psychometrika, 64,* 37–52.

Silva, D. S. (1996). *Data analysis: A Bayesian tutorial.* London: Oxford University Press.

Song, X. Y., & Lee, S. Y. (2001). Bayesian estimation and test for factor analysis model with continuous and polytomous data in several populations. *British Journal of Mathematical and Statistical Psychology*, 54, 237–263.

Song, X. Y., & Lee, S. Y. (2004). Bayesian analysis of two-level nonlinear structural equation models with continuous and polytomous data. *British Journal of Mathematical and Statistical Psychology*, 57, 29–52.

Spiegelhalter, D. J., Thomas, A., & Best, N. G. (1999). *WinBUGS Version 1.2 user manual.* Cambridge, UK: MRC Biostatistics Unit, Institute for Public Health, Available at www.mrcbsu.cam.ac.uk/bugs

Tucker, I. R. (1958). Determination of parameters of a functional relation by factor analysis. *Psychometrika, 23*, 19–23.

Tuma, N., & Hannan, M. (1984). *Social dynamics.* New York: Academic Press.

Zeger, S. L., & Karim, M. R. (1991). Generalized linear models with random effects: A Gibbs sampling approach. *Journal of American Statistical Association, 86*, 79–86.

Zhang, Z, Hamagami, F., Wang, L., Nesselroade, J. R., & Grimm, K. J. (2007). Bayesian analysis of longitudinal data using growth curve models. *International Journal of Behavioral Development, 31*, 374–383.

Zhang, Z., McArdle, J. J., Wang, L., & Hamagami, F. (2008). A SAS interface for Bayesian analysis with WinBUGS. *Structural Equation Modeling, 15*, 705–728.

14

Longitudinal Mediation Analysis of Training Intervention Effects

Lijuan Wang, Zhiyong Zhang, and Ryne Estabrook

14.1 INTRODUCTION

Intervention research constitutes a broad research category, encompassing a large number of experimental, psychological, and medical research designs. While this type of research can build on rather simple designs and few variables, multivariate longitudinal designs allow for tests of more complex treatment assignments and models, as well as mediation. The focus of this chapter is on models and methods for evaluating longitudinal intervention effects in the presence of mediation: that is, the methods for analyzing the longitudinal impact of an intervention or treatment when that impact is mediated by one or more other variables.

We explore the concept of mediation and its application to longitudinal intervention research. First, we review the history and basic ideas of mediation analysis, including developments in longitudinal mediation analysis. Second, we present a variation of the longitudinal mediation model (Cole & Maxwell, 2003) for intervention and training research, highlighting the features of the nonrepeated training interventions, the repeatedly measured mediation and output variables, and the estimation methods of the model. Finally, we apply this new model to data from the Advanced Cognitive Training for Independent and Vital Elderly (ACTIVE) study (Jobe et al., 2001) to demonstrate the capabilities of the model.

14.2 MEDIATION ANALYSIS

Mediation analysis has been widely used in psychological research to develop theories on whether there exists a third variable that accounts for the relationship between an input variable and an output variable (Baron & Kenny, 1986; Cole & Maxwell, 2003; Judd & Kenny, 1981a, 1981b; MacKinnon, Fairchild, & Fritz, 2007; Shrout & Bolger, 2002). For example, Salthouse (1996, p. 403) developed the theory that "increased age in adulthood is associated with a decrease in the speed with which many processing operations can be executed and that this reduction in speed leads to impairments in cognitive functioning" (see also, Salthouse, 1991, 1993).

The simplest and most widely used mediation model is the three-variable model or the single-mediator model portrayed in Figure 14.1. For the purpose of simplification, here we only look at the covariance structure without the means. In Figure 14.1, Y, X, and M represent the dependent or output variable, the independent or input variable, and the mediation variable, respectively. e_M and e_Y are residuals or measurement errors with variances σ^2_{eM} and σ^2_{eY}. The mediation models can be expressed by two regression equations,

$$\begin{aligned} M &= aX + e_M, \\ Y &= c'X + bM + e_Y, \end{aligned} \tag{14.1}$$

where a, c', and b are regression coefficients. Thus, a represents the relation between X and M. c' represents the relation between X and Y adjusted for M and b represents the relation between M and Y adjusted for X. c' is also called the direct effect of X on Y and ab is called the indirect effect of

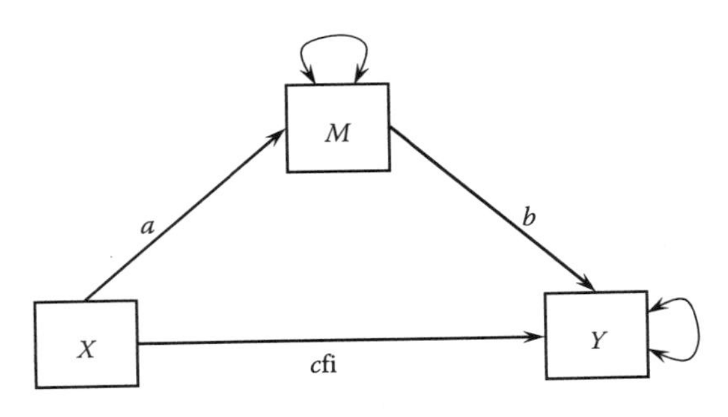

FIGURE 14.1 Path diagram of a single mediator model.

X on Y through mediation of M. The implied model without mediation effects is $Y = cX + e_Y$. When mediation effects have occurred, the indirect effect, ab, or the difference in the direct effect, $c' - c$, should be significantly different from 0 (e.g., Baron & Kenny, 1986; MacKinnon & Dwyer, 1993; Shrout & Bolger, 2002; Sobel, 1982).

Statistical approaches to estimating and testing mediation effects for the single mediator model have been discussed extensively in the psychological literature (e.g., Baron & Kenny, 1986; Bollen & Stine, 1990; MacKinnon et al., 2007; MacKinnon, Lockwood, Hoffman, West, & Sheets, 2002; Shrout & Bolger, 2002). There are two common ways of testing mediation effects. The first and perhaps most widely used method is the approach outlined in Baron and Kenny's (1986) work, where the mediation parameters are tested in a regression framework. This single sample method (named after MacKinnon et al., 2002) is based on a large-sample normal approximation test provided by Sobel (1982, 1986), which is easy to implement and understand but may have low statistical power in some situations such as studies with small sample sizes (e.g., MacKinnon et al., 2002). The second approach may be called the resampling method, which is based on the bootstrap resampling procedure (e.g., Bollen & Stine, 1990; Efron, 1979, 1987; Preacher & Hayes, 2004; Zhang & Wang, 2008). The resampling method does not require the large sample size assumption and could be more accurate and more powerful than the single sample method under certain conditions such as studies with small size and/or skewed outcome problems (e.g., MacKinnon et al., 2007; Shrout & Bolger, 2002; Zhang & Wang, 2008).

Although the single mediator model is widely used, many complex extensions have been developed (see the review by MacKinnon et al., 2007). For example, models with multiple mediators have been investigated and used (e.g., Cheung, 2007; MacKinnon, 2000; Rutter & Hine, 2005). Multilevel mediation models have also been developed and used to accommodate dependent observations that are nested within groups (e.g., Bauer, Preacher, & Gil, 2006; Kenny, Bolger, & Korchmaros, 2003; Krull & MacKinnon, 1999, 2001). Another important extension is the development of longitudinal mediation models (e.g., Cheong, MacKinnon, & Khoo, 2003; Cole & Maxwell, 2003; Collins, Graham, & Flaherty, 1998).

The application of longitudinal mediation models is an important conceptual development. Collins et al. (1998) defined the mediated process as a reaction chain in which the input variable first affects the mediator, which, in turn, affects the output variable over time. This definition is different from the one given by Baron and Kenny (1986), which focuses on whether the relation between the input variable and the output variable can be explained by means of a mediator. For Baron and Kenny (1986), the data from the input variable, the mediator, and the output variable can be collected at the same time when the mediation effects are tested. To operate the method in Collins et al. (1998), one needs to obtain the input variable, the mediator, and the output variable at different occasions such as $X_{t-2} \rightarrow M_{t-1} \rightarrow Y_t$. Most modern definitions of mediation are more in line with Collins et al. (1998). And the Collins' definition can be operated in a longitudinal study conveniently. However, it is possible that sometimes the mediation occurs so quickly that the concurrent relationship among the input, mediator, and output variances might be observed. In this case, the definition of Baron and Kenny (1986) can still operate in a meaningful way.

Figure 14.2 portrays the path diagram for a longitudinal mediation model discussed by Cole and Maxwell (2003). In this model, the input variable, the mediator, and the output variable are measured multiple times. One form of this model can be written as

$$\begin{aligned} X_t &= \beta_X X_{t-1} + e_{X_t}, \\ M_t &= \beta_M M_{t-1} + aX_{t-1} + e_{M_t}, \quad t = 3, \ldots, T, \\ Y_t &= \beta_Y Y_{t-1} + bM_{t-1} + cX_{t-2} + e_{Y_t}, \end{aligned} \tag{14.2}$$

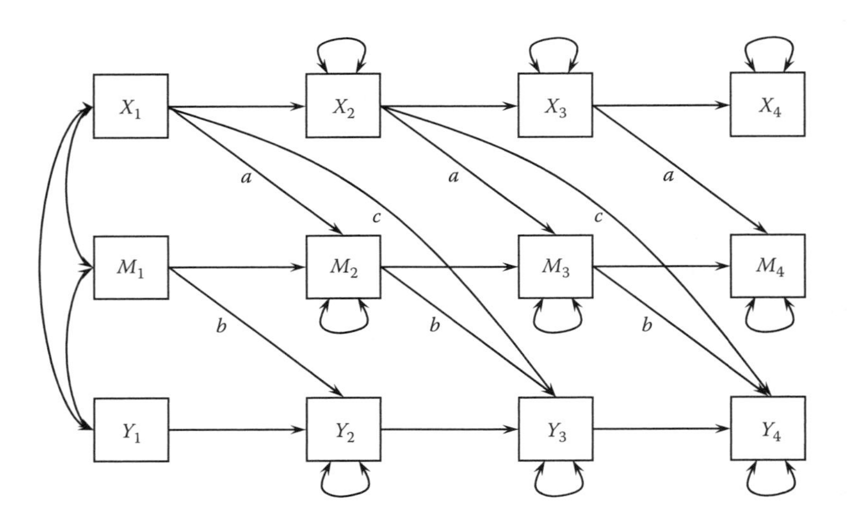

FIGURE 14.2 Path diagram of a longitudinal mediation model (see also Cole & Maxwell, 2003).

where X_t, M_t, and Y_t represent the observed data for X, M, and Y at time t, respectively; and e represents residual errors for each regression equation at time t. Notice that, in investigating mediation effects, M_{t-1} is first controlled before predicting M_t and Y_{t-1} is also controlled before predicting Y_t. This is because they are confounds and without controlling them, one may obtain spuriously inflated estimates of mediation effects (Cole & Maxwell, 2003). This model also implies that the unknown coefficients are invariant across time.

The model discussed by Cole and Maxwell (2003) is only one variety of longitudinal mediation models. This model is also called the autoregressive mediation model and a similar idea has been previously discussed by Gollob and Reichardt (1991), Judd and Kenny (1981b), and MacKinnon (1994). Cheong et al. (2003) proposed to use the latent growth curve models to analyze mediation effects where an input variable affects the growth (e.g., change from time 1 to time T) of the output variable through its influence on the growth (e.g., change from time 1 to time T) of the mediator. The autoregressive mediation model and the mediation model in the growth curve modeling framework have very different emphases. The former focuses more on the time-related relationship between the input and the output variables through a mediator variable, while the latter focuses on the effects of an input variable on the change of an output variable through the change of a mediator variable. Therefore, the former can be more easily applied to analyze lag effects and predict long-term effects. In this chapter, the autoregressive mediation approach is used.

14.3 METHODS FOR THE ANALYSIS OF TRAINING INTERVENTION WITH MEDIATION EFFECTS

Before introducing the methods for analyzing training intervention with mediation effects, let us consider a typical training intervention scenario. Suppose we have $T (T \geq 4)$ occasions of measures on mediation and output variables and one training intervention (a single measure). The training intervention happens between the first measurement occasion (baseline occasion) and the second measurement occasion. The research questions are whether there is a training intervention effect on the output variable, whether the training effect is mediated by the mediation variable, and how long the training effect would last.

For this training intervention example, the training interventions could be modeled as the X variable in Figure 14.2. However, there are no repeated measures on the training intervention itself. Instead, the training intervention can be considered as a shock to the mediation and output variable system. Therefore, the longitudinal mediation models described in Figure 14.2 may not fit the data structure of training intervention exactly. Furthermore, there are multiple occasions of data on mediation and output variables which could make the cross-sectional mediation method less sufficient to analyze the data. Therefore, it is necessary to develop a model to accommodate the data structure of the training intervention with mediation effects.

A prospective model for the analysis of training intervention with mediation effects is portrayed in Figure 14.3. M_t and Y_t represent the mediation variable and the outcome variable, respectively, for occasion t, $t = 1, 2, \ldots, T$. I represents the training intervention variable. The lowercase letters in the path diagram represent the unknown path coefficients. Certainly, there are different alternatives to this model. For instance, there could be a concurrent relationship between the mediation variable and the output variable instead of the lagged relationship described in Figure 14.3. Here we use this model [a similar idea has been discussed in MacKinnon (1994)], which can also be viewed as a variation of the longitudinal mediation model (Cole & Maxwell, 2003), as an example to illustrate the general idea of training intervention data analysis with mediation effects.

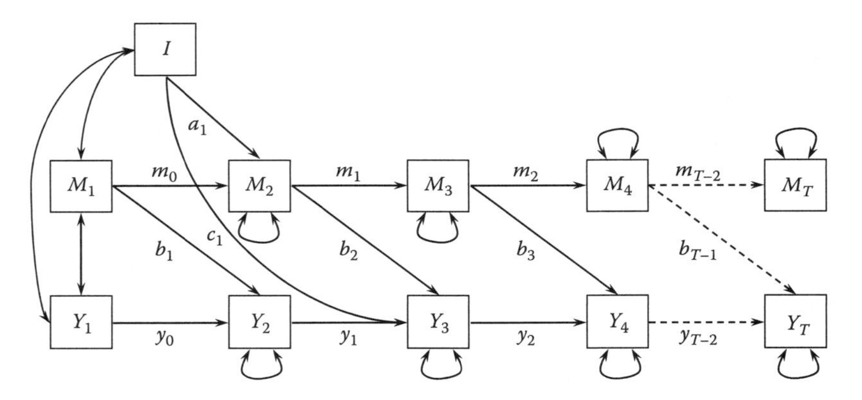

FIGURE 14.3 A model for analyzing training intervention with mediation effects.

In this model, training intervention has both direct effect and indirect effect through the mediator variable on the output variable. The direct effect of training intervention on Y_3 is c_1 and the indirect effect is a_1b_2. The total effect of training intervention on Y_3 is $c_1 + a_1b_2$. We can also calculate the total effect of training intervention on Y_4 by summarizing all paths from the training variable I to Y_4, $(c_1 + a_1b_2)y_2 + a_1m_1b_3$. Similarly, the training effect on Y_T can also be calculated. An underlying assumption of this model is that those who receive training change over time in the same way as those who do not receive training. However, this assumption can be relaxed by either adding an interaction term into the model or analyzing the data in the multiple group analysis framework.

14.3.1 Evaluating Training Effects

The whole sample of an intervention study can usually be divided into multiple groups based on the study design. For instance, there could be two groups in the study: a control group and a training group. To analyze the training effect, we need to estimate the unknown path coefficients. The model in Figure 14.3 implies that for the control group ($I = 0$), we have $Y_3 = b_2M_2 + y_1Y_2 + e_{Y_3}$. For the group receiving the training intervention ($I = 1$), we have $Y_3 = b_2M_2 + c_1 + y_1Y_2 + e_{Y_3}$. Thus, b_2 and y_1 are the same for both groups. Therefore, it is important to notice the underlying assumption that the coefficients, especially for *ms*, *bs*, and *ys*, are the same for both the control group and the training group. However, it could be also reasonable to believe that b_2 may be different for the two groups.

From a developmental perspective, the purpose of training intervention can be viewed as improving the performance/skills and/or preventing the decline of a targeted ability so that the targeted ability can maintain a high level of performance over time. There are different ways to achieve this goal. First, training may increase the level of performance of a targeted ability immediately after training. Thus, the level of performance will be at a higher level than otherwise without training in the future (see Figure 14.4a). Second, training may reduce the rate of decline of performance. Thus, the level of performance after training will also be at a higher level than otherwise without training as shown in Figure 14.4b. Third, the ideal outcome of training is an increased level of performance and a reduced rate of decline as portrayed in Figure 14.4c. These three patterns of training effects can be related to the following models.

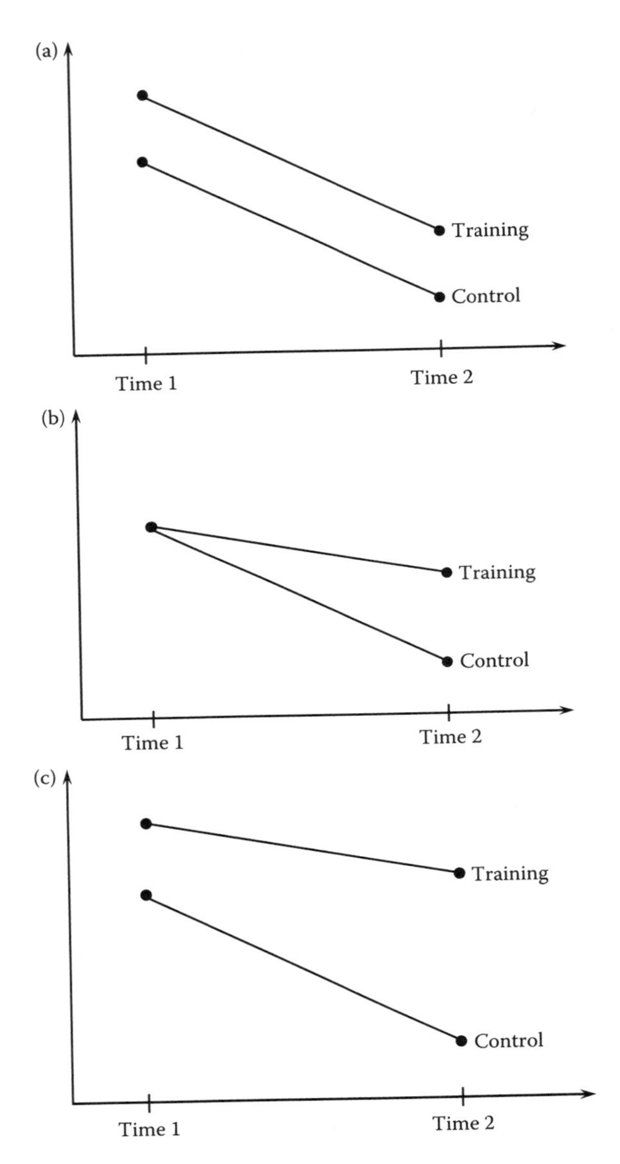

FIGURE 14.4 Three possible outcomes of training effects, (a) level only, (b) slope only, and (c) both level and slope.

In terms of the training intervention study, we may expect $Y_3 = b_2^* M_2 + c_1 + y_1^* Y_2 + e_{Y_3}$ with $b_2^* > b_2$ for the training group, which means that training could also influence the path coefficients. There are two methods for analyzing the influences of training effects on the path coefficients, which we dub the "interaction method" and the "multiple group method." For the interaction method, we can analyze the data from both the control group and the training group together by fitting a model with interactions to the raw data as

$$Y_3 = i + b_2 M_2 + c_1 I + y_1 Y_2 + d_1 M_2 I + d_2 Y_2 I + e_{Y_3}, \tag{14.3}$$

where i represents the intercept of the control group and d_1 and d_2 are coefficients for the interaction terms. Thus, for the control group ($I = 0$), $Y_3 = i + b_2 M_2 + y_1 Y_2 + e_{Y_3}$ and for the training group, $Y_3 = i + c_1 + (b_2 + d_1) M_2 + (y_1 + d_2) Y_2 + e_{Y_3}$.

For the multiple group method, we can fit separate models to the control and training groups,

$$Y_3 = i^{(j)} + b_2^{(j)} M_2 + y_1^{(j)} Y_2 + e_{Y_3}, \quad j = 0, 1, \tag{14.4}$$

where $j = 0$ for the control group and $j = 1$ for the training group. $i^{(j)}$ represents the intercept for the jth group. It can be shown that $b_2^{(0)} = b_2$, $y_1^{(0)} = y_1$, $b_2^{(1)} = b_2 + d_1$, $y_1^{(1)} = y_1 + d_2$, and $i^{(1)} - i^{(0)} = c_1$ with the parameters on the left side from the multiple group method and the parameters on the right side from the interaction method.

We can relate the models with the three patterns of training effects in Figure 14.4. If c_1 is significant and neither d_1 nor d_2 is significant, the pattern in Figure 14.4a is plausible. If only d_1 or d_2 or both are significant but c_1 is not significant, we could have the pattern in Figure 14.4b. If both c_1 and at least one of d_1 and d_2 are significant, the last pattern in Figure 14.4c could be detected.

Similarly, a_1 in Figure 14.3 can be estimated using either method. For example, with the multiple group method, we can first fit a model,

$$M_2 = i_M^{(j)} + m_0^{(j)} M_1 + e_{M_1}, \quad j = 0, 1, \tag{14.5}$$

to the control group ($j = 0$) and the training group ($j = 1$), separately. Then, $a_1 = i_M^{(1)} - i_M^{(0)}$. The training effect on Y_3 is $c_1 + a_1(b_2 + d_1)$ from the interaction method and $i^{(1)} - i^{(0)} + (i_M^{(1)} - i_M^{(0)}) b_2^{(1)}$ from the multiple group method. Furthermore, we have $c_1 + a_1(b_2 + d_1) = i^{(1)} - i^{(0)} + (i_M^{(1)} - i_M^{(0)}) b_2^{(1)}$ for the total effect.

There are advantages and disadvantages to either method. The interaction method is able to estimate all parameters in one step, but this procedure will become complex and difficult to interpret and implement as the number of parameters grows. The multiple group method is easier to implement, interpret, and is more flexible, which has the ability to deal with different variances due to treatment. In the current research, the multiple group method will be used for the data analysis. To summarize, the following steps can be applied to obtain the model parameter estimates. In the first step, the model described as below can be fit to each group separately,

$$
\begin{aligned}
M_t &= i_{M_t}^{(j)} + m_{t-2}^{(j)} M_{t-1} + e_{M_t}, \\
Y_t &= i_{Y_t}^{(j)} + b_{t-1}^{(j)} M_{t-1} + y_{t-1}^{(j)} Y_{t-1} + e_{Y_t},
\end{aligned}
\tag{14.6}
$$

where $i_{M_t}^{(j)}$ denotes the intercept of M_t for jth group, the superscript $^{(j)}$ denotes the jth group, $j = 0, 1$ represent the control group and the training group, respectively. In the second step, we can calculate a_1 by $a_1 = i_{M_2}^{(1)} - i_{M_2}^{(0)}$. In addition, we can calculate c_1 by $c_1 = i_{Y_3}^{(1)} - i_{Y_3}^{(0)}$. In the third step, we can calculate the training effects based on the estimated parameters. For example, the training effect on Y_3 is $c_1 + a_1 b_2^{(1)}$.

14.3.2 Evaluating Training Effects over Time

Predicting training effects beyond the observed occasions is of interest to researchers from both methodological and substantive perspectives. Methodologically, Cole and Maxwell (2003) have shown that the time interval was important for evaluating the indirect effects and the time interval may affect the estimated effects. By evaluating the training effects over time, the evolvement of the training effects could be captured and the training effects may be portrayed in a more accurate way. For example, training may only demonstrate its effects after a certain amount of time. Without estimating the training effects after this amount of time, one may not be able to observe the significance of training effects.

There are also many substantive studies on the long-term effects of training in different study areas. For example, Willis and Nesselroade (1990) examined the effects of multiple phases of cognitive training on older adults' intellectual performance over a 7-year period. Willis et al. (2006) found that cognitive training resulted in improved cognitive abilities specific to the abilities trained even 5 years after the initiation of the intervention. Schlaug, Norton, Overy, and Winner (2005) demonstrated that music training in children results in long-term enhancement of visual, spatial, verbal, and mathematical performance.

To predict the training effects beyond the observed occasions, stationarity needs to be tested and/or assumed. Stationarity has many different definitions under different contexts. For instance, in mathematical statistics, stationarity is observed when the probability distribution of a process at a fixed time is the same for all times. Kenny (1979, p. 287) defined stationarity as "an unchanging causal structure." Cole and Maxwell (2003, p. 560) interpreted Kenny's definition as "the degree to which one set of variables produces change in another set that remains the same over time." In the current research, Kenny's definition is used. We acknowledge that this is a rather weak adaption of the stationarity concept because only the regression coefficients are required to be invariant over time. And we do not require the residual variances to be invariant over time.

For the model portrayed in Figure 14.3, if it is stationary for the control group, one would expect that $m_0^{(0)} = m_1^{(0)} = m_2^{(0)} = \cdots = m_{T-2}^{(0)} \equiv m^{(0)}$, $b_1^{(0)} = b_2^{(0)} = b_3^{(0)} = \cdots = b_{T-1}^{(0)} \equiv b^{(0)}$, and $y_0^{(0)} = y_1^{(0)} = y_2^{(0)} = \cdots = y_{T-2}^{(0)} \equiv y^{(0)}$. For the training group, one would expect that $m_1^{(1)} = m_2^{(1)} = \cdots = m_{T-2}^{(1)} \equiv m^{(1)}$, $b_2^{(1)} = b_3^{(1)} = \cdots = b_{T-1}^{(1)} \equiv b^{(1)}$, and $y_2^{(1)} = \cdots = y_{T-2}^{(1)} \equiv y^{(1)}$. Here, the model parameters are invariant over time after the intervention treatment time-point.

To test the stationarity of the model, the chi-square difference test (likelihood ratio test) can be used. For example, to test $m_0^{(0)} = m_1^{(0)} = m_2^{(0)} = \cdots = m_{T-2}^{(0)}$, a model with freely estimated parameters can be first estimated to obtain the chi-square fit value χ_1^2 with degrees of freedom df_1. Then, we can constrain the parameters to be equal and estimate the model again and get χ_2^2 with df_2. Finally, we compare the chi-square difference $\Delta\chi^2 = \chi_2^2 - \chi_1^2$ with the critical value c_α from the chi-square distribution with degree of freedom $\text{df}_2 - \text{df}_1$. If $\Delta\chi^2 < c_\alpha$, we cannot reject the stationarity of the model. More tests, such as $m_0^{(0)} = m_1^{(0)} = m_2^{(0)} = \cdots = m_{T-2}^{(0)}$ versus $m_0^{(0)} = m_1^{(0)} = \ldots = m_{T-3}^{(0)} \neq m_{T-2}^{(0)}$ can be performed to test stationarity for all possible comparisons.

Note that we cannot test stationarity beyond the observed data. For example, although we can conclude that $m_0^{(0)} = m_1^{(0)} = \cdots = m_{T-2}^{(0)}$, we cannot say that $m_0^{(0)} = m_1^{(0)} = \cdots = m_{T-2}^{(0)} = m_{T-1}^{(0)}$ without collecting more data. However, if we assume that $m_0^{(0)} = m_1^{(0)} = \cdots = m_{T-2}^{(0)} = m_{t-1}^{(0)}$ for $t \geq T - 1$, we can make inference beyond observed data, such as inference on the training effects beyond the Tth occasion.

After obtaining the model parameters and satisfying the stationarity test, we can predict the training effects over time in a more parsimonious model. Because the training intervention happens between the first occasion and the second occasion and there is a lagged relationship between the mediation variable and the output variable, there are no training effects on the first occasion and the second occasion such as $I(1) = I(2) = 0$ with $I(t)$ representing the training effect at time t. At occasion 3, $I(3) = c_1 + a_1 b^{(1)}$. At occasion T, we have $I(T) = I(T-1)y^{(1)} + a_1[m^{(1)}]^{T-3}b^{(1)}$. With the stationarity, although we did not observe data from the occasion $T + 1$ and above, we can predict the training effect by using $I(t) = I(t-1)y^{(1)} + a_1[m^{(1)}]^{t-3}b^{(1)}, t > T$.

14.3.3 Multiple Training Interventions

In some studies, there could be more than one training intervention. For example, besides the training intervention between the first and the second measurement occasions, there could be another training intervention (we can call it "booster training intervention") for some of the participants between the second measurement occasion and the third measurement occasion (see Figure 14.5). In this case, the overall sample can be divided into three groups: a control group, an initial training group with only the first training intervention, and a booster training group with both the first training intervention and the second training intervention. The second training intervention has also both a direct effect and an indirect effect through the mediator variable on the output variable for the booster training group. The direct effect of the second training intervention on Y_4 is c_2 and the indirect effect is $a_2 b_3$. The total effect of the second training intervention on Y_4 is $c_2 + a_2 b_3$. Similarly, we can evaluate the second training effect over time, $B(1) = B(2) = B(3) = 0, B(4) = c_2 + a_2 b^{(2)}$, and $B(t) = B(t-1)y^{(2)} + a_2[m^{(2)}]^{t-4}b^{(2)}, t = 5, 6, \ldots$ with $B(t)$ representing the second training effect at time t and the superscript $^{(2)}$ denoting the

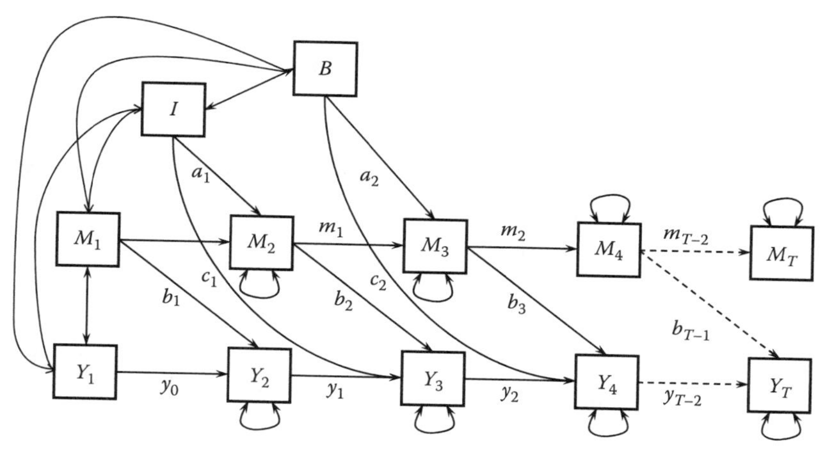

FIGURE 14.5 A model for analyzing two training interventions with mediation effects.

parameters from the booster training group. The overall training effects of the first training effect and the second training effect $O(t)$ at time t can then be calculated by $O(t) = I(t) + B(t)$.

14.3.4 Model Estimation and Confidence Intervals

For a mediation model, such as the one in Figure 14.5, different methods can be used to estimate the unknown parameters. The popular structural equation modeling (SEM) methods can usually be used to estimate the parameters for both the training effects parameters and other parameters simultaneously in SEM software. Furthermore, some SEM software, such as Mplus (Muthén & Muthén, 1998–2007), can also produce the standard errors for the training effects. In the current study, we program the estimation procedure in R (R Development Core Team, 2005), a free statistical program, based on the multiple group method outlined in a previous subsection. The procedure is based on the least squares method and cannot directly produce the standard error estimates for the unknown parameters. To estimate the standard errors, an additional bootstrap step can be used. The technical details of bootstrap methods can be found elsewhere (e.g., Efron, 1979, 1987; Efron & Tibshirani, 1993). Here, we focus only on the bootstrap procedure for the current study.

In the first step, we sample data from the original data set with replacement. For the training intervention data, there could be multiple groups, for example, the control group ($N = n_1$), the initial training group ($N = n_2$), and the booster training group ($N = n_3$). To keep the data structure, we first sample data from each group and then combine the sampled data together. More specifically, we first sample a data set with $N = n_1$ from the control group with replacement, sample a data set with $N = n_2$ with replacement from the initial training group, and then sample a data set with $N = n_3$ with replacement from the booster training group. After obtaining a sampled data set for each group, we can combine the three data sets together into one sample with $N = n_1 + n_2 + n_3$.

In the second step, we estimate the unknown parameters θ^* (denoting all the unknown parameters) and the training effects $I(t)^*$, $B(t)^*$, and $O(t)^*$ with $*$ denoting the results from the bootstrap sampling data. By repeating steps 1 and 2 for a number of times, denoting B, we can obtain a series of results for the unknown parameters θ_b^* and the training effects, $I(t)_b^*$, $B(t)_b^*$, and $O(t)_b^*$ with $b = 1, \ldots, B$. The confidence intervals for the unknown parameters and the training effects are then constructed using the quantiles of the bootstrap estimates of the unknown parameters and the training effects. For example, the $100(1 - \alpha)\%$ confidence interval can be constructed using the $\alpha/2$ and $1 - \alpha/2$ quantiles. An example of the R codes for the parameter estimation and confidence interval construction is provided in the CD.

14.4 EMPIRICAL DATA ANALYSIS

In the previous section, methods for analyzing training interventions with mediation effects have been introduced and discussed. In this section, the methods will be applied to an empirical study to illustrate the data analysis procedure.

The empirical data examined in this study is from the ACTIVE study (Jobe et al. 2001; Tennstedt, 2001). The ACTIVE study is a randomized and controlled study designed to determine whether cognitive training interventions can affect cognitively based measures of daily functioning. The cognitive training interventions included training in reasoning, memory, and speed. In the current study, we will investigate whether and how the training in reasoning ability affects the cognitively demanding everyday functioning.

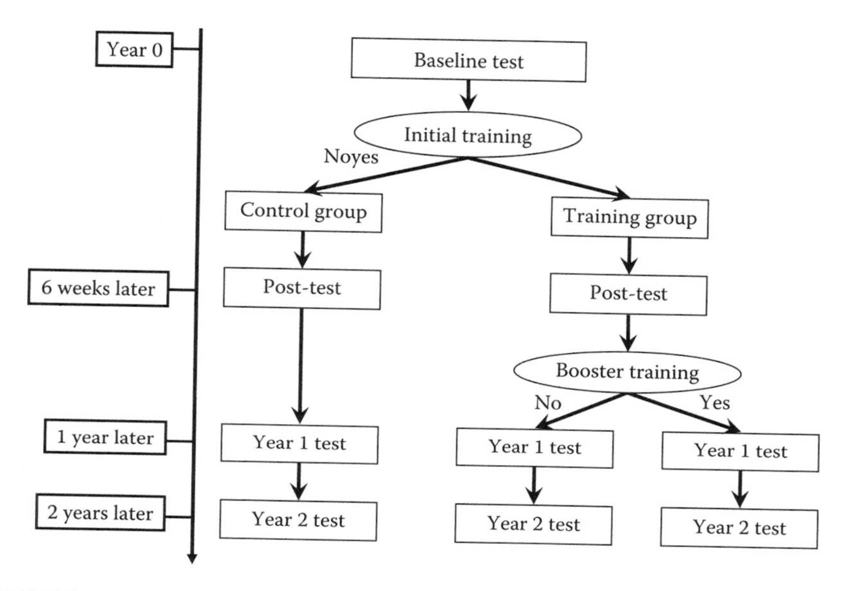

FIGURE 14.6 The ACTIVE reasoning training study design.

14.4.1 ACTIVE Study Design

The overall design of the ACTIVE study is given in Figure 14.6.* The procedure outlined below applies to training in each of three cognitive abilities: only the data from the reasoning ability training and control groups will be used in this study. All the participants ($N = 828$) examined in the current study were first given the baseline test. Participants were then randomly divided into the control group ($N = 414$) and the reasoning training group ($N = 414$). The reasoning training group was given the initial training on reasoning ability during a period of less than 6 weeks. Right after the initial training, participants in both the control and reasoning training groups were administered the post-test. Then the reasoning training group was divided into two groups randomly. One group ($N = 245$) was given a second or "booster" training course, mirroring the first training, about 11 months after the post-test. All participants were tested at the first and second years following the post-test.

* For a complete account of the research design of the ACTIVE study, refer to Jobe et al. (2001). The public data can be downloaded from http://www.icpsr.umich.edu/cocoon/ICPSR/STUDY/04248.xml.

14.4.2 Training Interventions

14.4.2.1 Initial Training Intervention

Initial training interventions were provided to participants in ten 60- to 75-min sessions through small groups with three to five participants. The training involved teaching strategies for finding the pattern in a letter or word series (e.g., a c e g i . . .) and identifying the next item in the series (Willis, 1987). Training sessions focused on applying these strategies to solve everyday problems (e.g., mnemonic strategies to remember a grocery list and reasoning strategies to understand the pattern in a bus schedule). Most participants received all 10 training sessions in a specified order within a 6-week interval with a small number of participants finishing training in less than 6 weeks. Participants who attended at least 80% of the training sessions (8 out of 10) were used in the current study. The initial training was conducted between May 1998 and December 1999 (Jobe et al. 2001).

14.4.2.2 Booster Training Intervention

The booster training was provided to a subset of participants who had received the initial training approximately 11 months after the end of the initial training. The booster training was delivered in four 75-min sessions over a 3-week period. The structure and content of the sessions were similar to those used in the initial training. The goal was to help participants maintain the gains made from the initial training. The booster training was conducted from May 1999 through December 2000 (Jobe et al., 2001).

14.4.3 Assessments

Both proximal and primary outcomes were measured. Proximal outcomes refer to the direct outcome measures of training interventions and primary outcomes refer to the outcome measures of cognitively demanding daily activities related to living independently (Jobe et al., 2001).

Three direct proximal outcomes were assessed: Word Series, Letter Series, and Letter Sets. These measures were standardized, timed, paper-and-pencil assessments, and were administered at each testing occasion. The Word Series (Gonda & Schaie, 1985) test consisted of 30 items. For each item, participants were presented a series of words and were required to choose the next word from five possible answers. The Letter Series

(Thurstone & Thurstone, 1949) test also consisted of 30 items. Instead of words, for each item, participants were presented a series of letters and were required to choose the next possible letter. The Letter Sets (Ekstrom, French, Harman, & Derman, 1976) test consisted of 14 items and participants were asked to select the set of letters that did not belong with the others. For each test, scores represented the total number of correct answers.

The primary outcome, the everyday problem-solving ability, was measured by the Everyday Problems Test (Willis & Marsiske, 1993). Participants were presented with 14 everyday stimuli, such as medication labels, transportation schedules, telephone rate charts, and Medicare benefit charts, and were asked to answer two questions about each stimulus. Scores represented the number of correct answers generated (Jobe et al., 2001).

14.4.4 Research Questions

Previous studies have shown that reasoning ability and everyday problem-solving ability are strongly related constructs, and that the reasoning ability can predict subsequent performance on cognitively demanding tasks of daily living, such as comprehension of medication labels, utilization of emergency telephone information, and understanding of transportation schedules (Diehl, Willis, & Schaie, 1995; Willis, 1996; Willis, Jay, Diehl, & Marsiske, 1992). In this study, we have two empirical research questions. The first research question is whether training interventions improve the proximal outcomes, which in turn improve the primary outcome. More specifically, we hypothesize that training interventions, both the initial and booster training, on reasoning improve reasoning ability, which in turn improves everyday problem-solving ability. The second question is how long the training effects would last.

14.4.5 Descriptive Statistics

To measure reasoning ability, a composite score was formed from the three measures—Word Series, Letter Series, and Letter Sets in the data analysis. First, the z scores for each test by pooling data from all four occasions were obtained and then the average of the z scores of the three tests, as the measure of reasoning ability, was calculated. The everyday problem test was also converted to z score in the analysis.

TABLE 14.1

Descriptive Statistics of the ACTIVE Sample

	Control		Initial		Booster		Overall	
	M	sd	*M*	sd	*M*	sd	*M*	sd
N	414		169		245		818	
Age	73.65	5.74	73.18	5.47	72.77	5.34	73.30	5.58
Gender	0.72	0.45	0.79	0.41	0.76	0.43	0.74	0.44
Education	13.57	2.59	13.69	2.54	13.58	2.71	13.60	2.61
R1	−0.31	0.83	−0.22	0.81	−0.28	0.82	−0.28	0.83
R2	−0.07	0.87	0.44	0.90	0.40	0.90	0.17	0.92
R3	−0.14	0.87	0.17	0.87	0.35	0.90	0.07	0.90
R4	−0.11	0.87	0.13	0.91	0.22	0.91	0.04	0.90
E1	−0.03	0.98	−0.03	0.96	−0.02	1.03	−0.03	0.99
E2	0.05	0.96	0.11	0.97	0.07	1.01	0.07	0.98
E3	0.01	1.00	0.00	1.02	0.00	1.01	0.00	1.01
E4	−0.03	1.00	−0.04	0.98	−0.08	1.10	−0.04	1.03

Note: *M*: mean; sd: standard deviation. R_t and E_t represent the reasoning ability and everyday problem test score at occasion *t*.

The descriptive statistics are summarized in Table 14.1 and the trajectories for both reasoning ability and everyday problem test are displayed in Figure 14.7. The average age of the whole sample was 73.3 (sd = 5.58) and the average education level was about 13.60 (sd = 2.61) years. Seventy-four

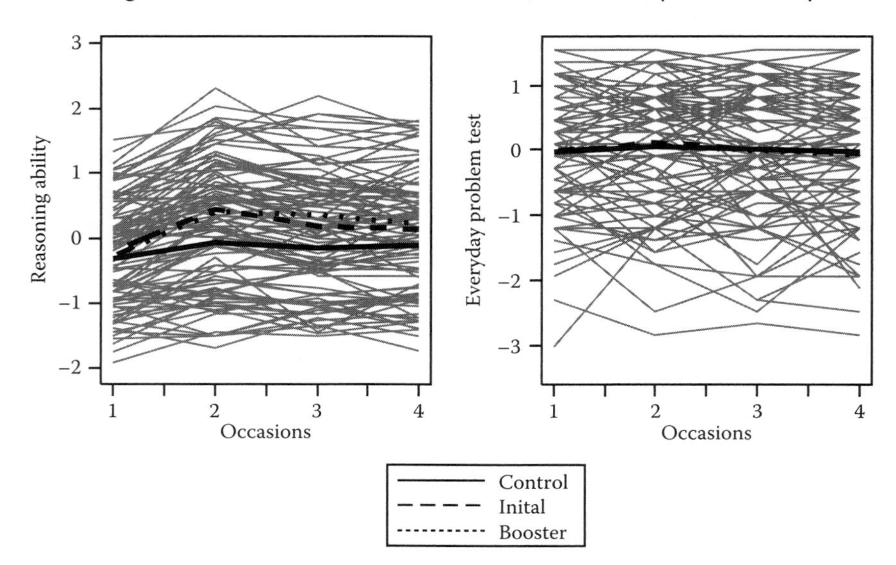

FIGURE 14.7 The trajectory plots of a subset of the ACTIVE data for the reasoning ability and the everyday problem-solving ability. The thick lines represent the mean trajectories from the three groups.

percent of the sample was female. There was no significant difference ($F = 2.22, p = 0.11$) in these demographic features (age, education level, and gender) among the three groups based on a multivariate analysis of variance (MANOVA) analysis. From both the trajectory plot and the descriptive statistics, reasoning ability and everyday problem-solving ability seemed to increase right after the training interventions. The deviations due to the initial training and booster training are reflected at time 2 and time 3, respectively, in Figure 14.7. However, we would like to emphasize that modeling the shape of the trajectories is not the focus of this study.

14.4.6 Model Selection

Before conducting the mediation analysis, an appropriate model needs to be selected to describe the relationship between the mediation variable and the output variable. In this section, we sought to first validate the nature of the mediation relationship between reasoning and everyday problem solving before the intervention effects are incorporated into the models as are shown in Figures 14.3 and 14.5.

Three possible models (see Figure 14.8) are considered for the ACTIVE data. Model 1 (Figure 14.8a) hypothesizes that there is a lag relationship between reasoning ability and everyday problem-solving ability (paths from R_t to E_{t+1}), and there is no concurrent relationship from R_t to E_t. This model implies that training first improves the reasoning ability and the reasoning ability at current occasion, and then in turn improves everyday problem solving ability at a later occasion. In other words, the influence of reasoning ability on everyday problem solving is conditional on the passage of time. This model directly reflects the ideas of longitudinal mediation analysis as in Figure 14.2.

Model 2 (Figure 14.8b) hypothesizes that there is a concurrent relationship between reasoning ability and everyday problem-solving ability from R_t to E_t, and there is no lag relationship between the two variables (paths from R_t to E_{t+1}). This model implies that the improvement in reasoning ability can immediately reflect on the improvement of everyday problem-solving ability. The time required for the conversion of reasoning-ability improvement to everyday problem-solving-ability improvement can be neglected or is much shorter than the time interval between measurement occasions.

Model 3 (Figure 14.8c) combines the ideas from both Model 1 and Model 2. The reasoning ability has both instantaneous and lag influences

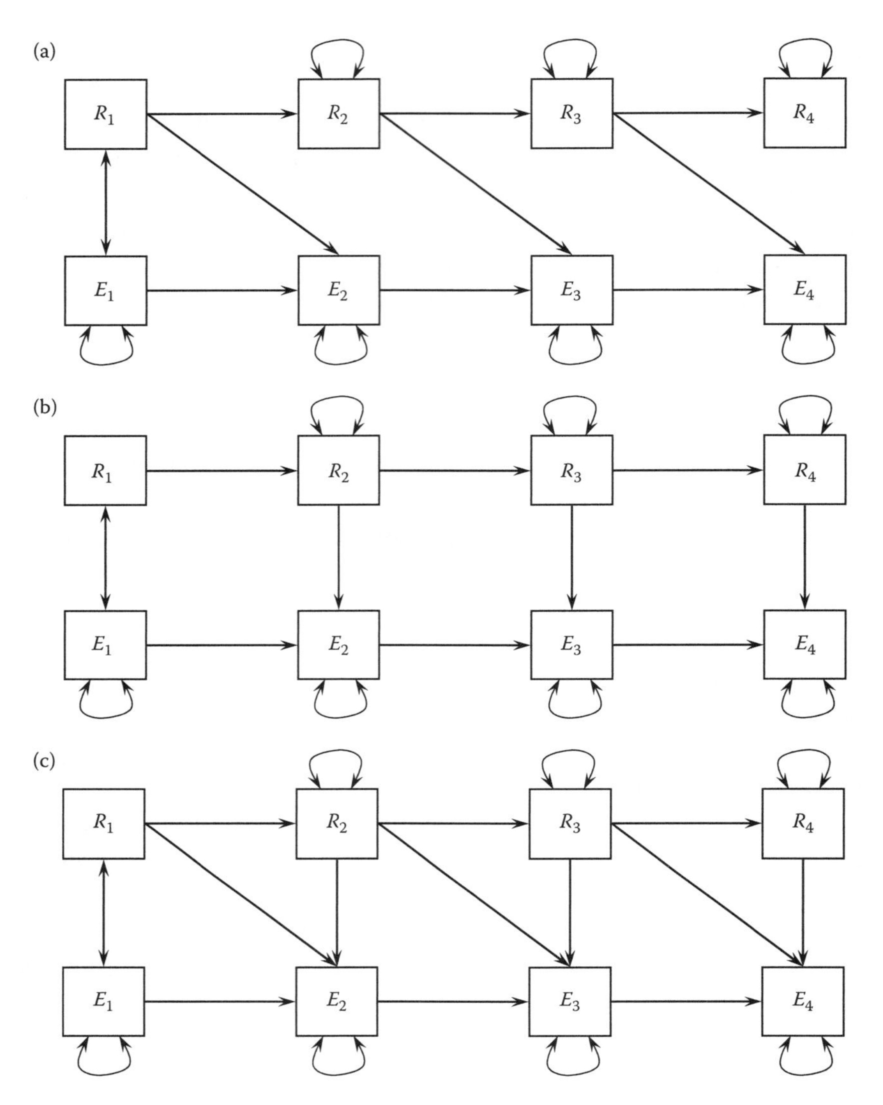

FIGURE 14.8 Possible models for the analysis of ACTIVE data (R_t and E_t represent the reasoning ability and everyday problem test score at occasion t); (a) Model 1, (b) Model 2, and (c) Model 3.

on the everyday problem-solving ability. This model implies that an improvement in reasoning ability may not convert to an improvement in everyday problem-solving ability all at once or just in a short time. The whole conversion process may spread over multiple measurement occasions.

TABLE 14.2

Model Fit Statistics for the Models in Figure 14.8

	Chi-Square/df	AIC	BIC	RMSEA
Model 1	110/36	8958	9298	0.085
Model 2	84/36	8932	9272	0.069
Model 3	71/27	8938	9320	0.077

Note: df: degrees of freedom; AIC: Akaike information criterion; BIC: Bayesian information criterion; RMSEA: root mean square error of approximation.

To determine which model fits the data best, each model was fitted to the ACTIVE data. Goodness of fit indexes such as chi-square value, AIC, and BIC were used to compare the model fit. The three fit statistics are provided in Table 14.2. Based on the fit statistics, we can see that Model 2 fits the current data better than the other proposed models. This could indicate that an improvement in reasoning ability can immediately convert to an improvement in everyday problem-solving ability or the conversion time from improvement in reasoning ability to improvement in everyday problem-solving ability, is much shorter than the one year time interval between occasions.

Note that although the regression path from reasoning to everyday problem solving links two concurrent variables, an inherent time lag has been built into the design of the ACTIVE study; for example, the participants were trained before the test was administered. Thus, Model 2 in Figure 14.8 still reflects the main ideas of longitudinal mediation shown in Model 1. In the following data analysis, Model 2 is used.

14.4.7 Mediation Analysis

After determining that Model 2 in Figure 14.8b represents the data relatively better, we further investigate how training improves the everyday problem-solving ability. The mediation model for the ACTIVE data is portrayed in Figure 14.9. In this model, initial training has a direct influence on everyday problem-solving ability at the second occasion. It also has an indirect influence through the mediation of R_2. The initial training effects on E_3 and E_4 are both indirect. Both the direct and indirect effects can be tested to check whether they are significant or not. For evaluating the booster training effects, we can use similar procedures.

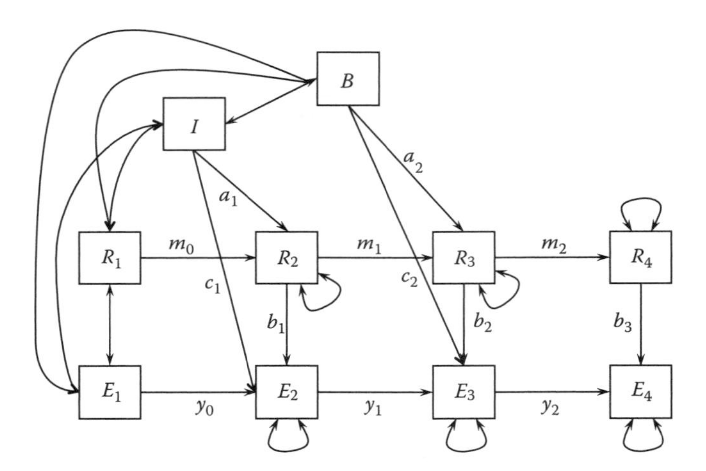

FIGURE 14.9 The mediation model for the ACTIVE data (R_t and E_t represent the reasoning ability and everyday problem test score at occasion t).

The estimated direct and indirect effects of initial training on E_2 and of booster training on E_3 are given in Table 14.3. Based on the confidence intervals, the direct effects of both initial c_1 and booster c_2 training were not significantly different from 0. However, the indirect effects were both significantly positive. Thus, the training effects on everyday problem-solving ability were totally mediated by reasoning ability. In the upcoming analysis, we fixed $c_1 = c_2 = 0$.

Based on the model with constraints ($c_1 = c_2 = 0$), the initial and booster training effects at different observed occasions were estimated and summarized in Table 14.4. It can be seen that training showed increased effects over time within the observed occasions. The initial training effect on

TABLE 14.3

Estimated Direct and Indirect Training Effects

		Estimate	Lower	Upper
		Initial		
Direct	c_1	−0.058	−0.167	0.038
Indirect	a_1b_1	0.103	0.055	0.157
		Booster		
Direct	c_2	−0.016	−0.137	0.081
Indirect	a_2b_2	0.049	0.025	0.082

Note: Lower and upper denotes the lower and upper bounds of confidence intervals.

TABLE 14.4

Estimated Training Effects at Different Observed Occasions and Confidence Intervals

	Initial Training Effect Only			Booster Training Effects Only			Overall		
	Estimate	Lower	Upper	Estimate	Lower	Upper	Estimate	Lower	Upper
E2	0.103	0.055	0.157				0.103	0.055	0.157
E3	0.155	0.097	0.216	0.049	0.025	0.082	0.204	0.139	0.274
E4	0.182	0.128	0.241	0.093	0.054	0.143	0.275	0.206	0.358

Note: Lower and upper denotes the lower and upper bounds of confidence intervals.

E_4 was larger than that on E_3, which, in turn, was larger than that on E_2. Furthermore, the booster training effect on E_4 was also larger than that on E_3.

14.4.8 Stationarity and Prediction

In the previous section, we have discussed that one can calculate or predict training effects beyond observed occasions if a model is stationary. From Table 14.4, we found that training effects actually increased with time. Thus, it will be interesting to investigate how the training effects change over time after the fourth measurement occasion. To predict the training effects, we first test the stationarity of the model in Figure 14.9 for each group.

14.4.8.1 Stationarity of the Control Group

For the control group, here, testing stationarity is to test H_0: $m_1 = m_2$, $b_1 = b_2 = b_3$, and $y_1 = y_2$. Note that we did not test whether $m_0 = m_1$ because the time interval between the first and second occasions was not the same as the later time intervals. To implement the test, we first fitted the model in Figure 14.9 without any constraints and obtained the $\chi^2 =$ 409.13 with degrees of freedom df $= 18$. Then, we fitted the model again with the constraints $m_1 = m_2, b_1 = b_2 = b_3$, and $y_1 = y_2$ and obtained the $\chi^2 = 416.04$ with df $= 22$. The difference between the models is $\Delta\chi^2 =$ 6.91 with Δdf $= 4$.The p-value is 0.14. The possible individual tests, such as $m_1 = m_2$, $b_1 = b_2 = b_3, y_1 = y_2$ versus $m_1 \neq m_2$, $b_1 = b_2 = b_3, y_1 =$ y_2, were also conducted and found no significant results. Thus, we can conclude that the model for the control group is stationary given the current data. The estimated path coefficients are given in Table 14.5.

TABLE 14.5

Estimated Path Coefficients for the Three Groups

	Control		Initial		Booster	
	Estimate	s.e.	Estimate	s.e.	Estimate	s.e.
$R_1 \rightarrow E_1$	0.773	0.043	0.799	0.069	0.909	0.054
$R_1 \rightarrow R_2$	0.952	0.021	0.995	0.039	0.959	0.034
$R_2 \rightarrow R_3$	0.916	0.014	0.913	0.022	0.914	0.025
$R_3 \rightarrow R_4$	0.916	0.014	0.913	0.022	0.937	0.025
$E_1 \rightarrow E_2$	0.701	0.026	0.731	0.042	0.716	0.040
$E_2 \rightarrow E_3$	0.731	0.021	0.741	0.031	0.677	0.036
$E_3 \rightarrow E_4$	0.731	0.021	0.741	0.031	0.733	0.040
$R_2 \rightarrow E_2$	0.228	0.020	0.211	0.029	0.216	0.046
$R_3 \rightarrow E_3$	0.228	0.020	0.211	0.029	0.290	0.033
$R_4 \rightarrow E_4$	0.228	0.020	0.211	0.029	0.290	0.033

Note: s.e.: standard error. $X \rightarrow Y$ represents the path from X to Y. R_t and E_t represent the reasoning ability and everyday problem test score at occasion t.

14.4.8.2 Stationarity of the Initial Training Group

For the initial training group, testing stationarity is also to test H_0: $m_1 = m_2$, $b_1 = b_2 = b_3$, and $y_1 = y_2$. We first fitted the model without any constraints and obtained $\chi^2 = 117.99$ with degrees of freedom df $= 18$. Then, we fitted the model again with the constraints $m_1 = m_2$, $b_1 = b_2 = b_3$, and $y_1 = y_2$ and obtained $\chi^2 = 123.07$ with df $= 22$. The difference between the models is $\Delta\chi^2 = 5.08$ with Δdf $= 4$. The p-value is 0.28. Individual tests were also conducted and no significant results were found. Thus, we can also conclude that the model for the initial group is stationary. The estimated path coefficients are given in Table 14.5.

14.4.8.3 Stationarity of the Booster Training Group

For the booster training group, there is no reason to test $m_1 = m_2$ and $y_1 = y_2$ because the coefficients before and after the booster training can vary. Here we can only test H_0: $b_2 = b_3$. We obtained $\Delta\chi^2 = 0.98$ with Δdf $= 1$. The p-value is 0.32. The estimated path coefficients are also given in Table 14.5.

14.4.9 Predicting Training Effects over Time

Given the current observed data in the ACTIVE study, there is no way to test whether $m_2 = m_t, t \geq 3$, $b_3 = b_t, t \geq 4$, and $y_2 = y_t, t \geq 3$. Thus, we have to assume that the model was stationary beyond the fourth occasion, if we want to extrapolate beyond the observed occasions. With this assumption, we can calculate or predict the training effects beyond the observed data occasions.

Let $I(t)$ and $B(t)$ represent the initial and booster training effects on everyday problem-solving ability at occasion t. Clearly, $I(1) = 0$ and $B(1) = B(2) = 0$. With the parameter estimates in Table 14.5, we have

$$I(2) = a_1 b_1^{(1)} = 0.091,$$

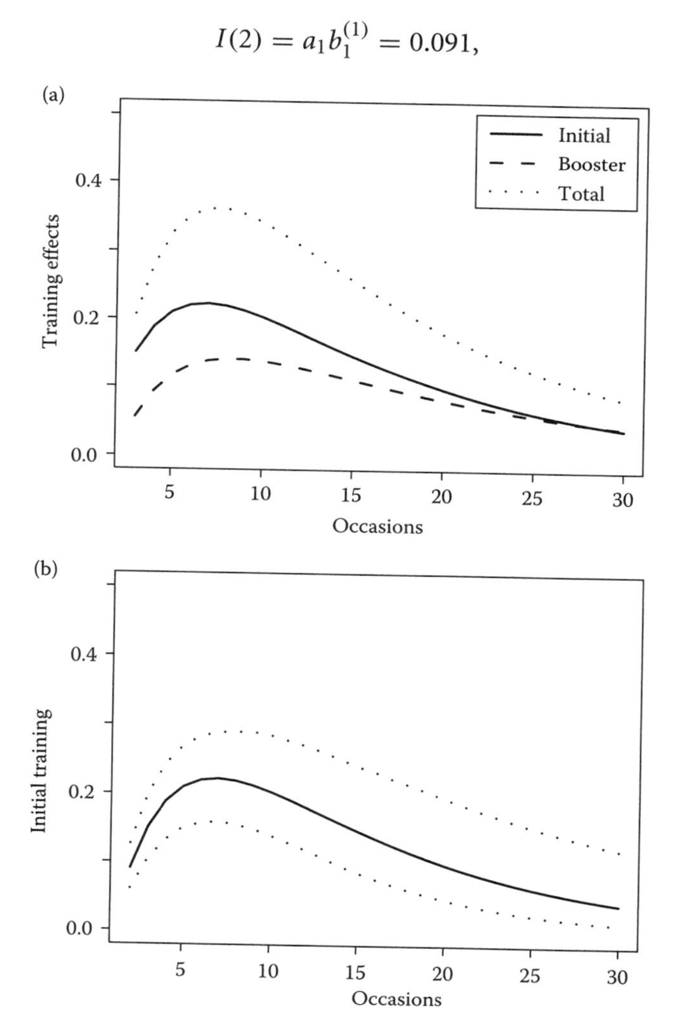

FIGURE 14.10 Plot of estimated training effects and 95% confidence intervals; (a) training effects, (b) CI for initial training, (c) CI for booster training, and (d) CI for total training.

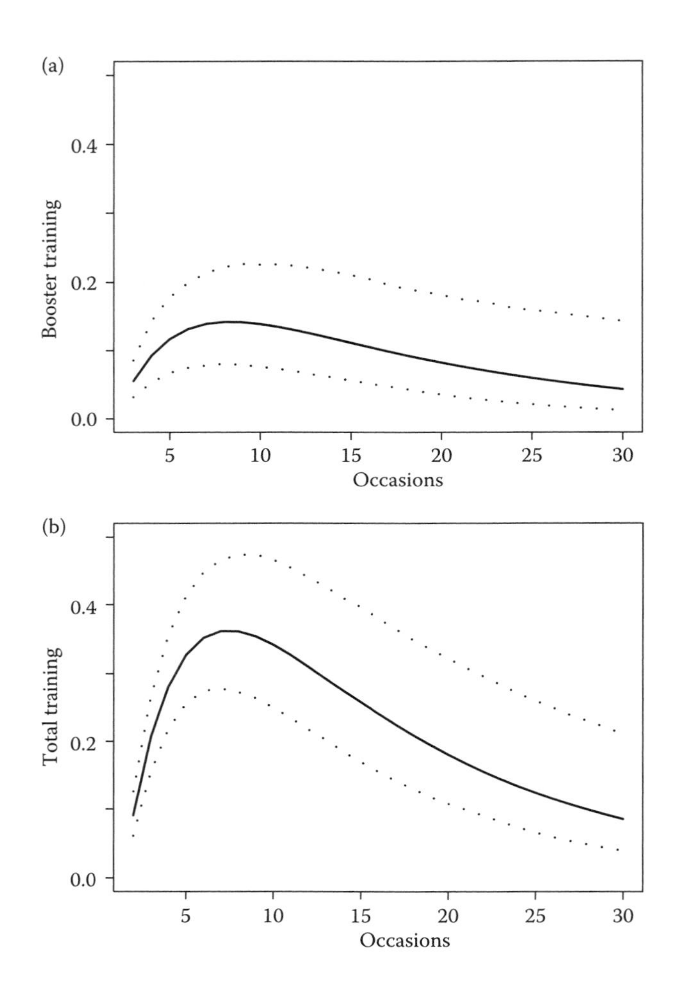

FIGURE 14.10 continued

and

$$I(3) = I(2)y_1^{(1)} + a_1 m_1^{(1)} b_1^{(1)} = 0.151,$$

where $^{(1)}$ denotes that the parameters were from the initial training group. In general, we have

$$\begin{aligned} I(t) &= I(t-1)y_1^{(1)} + a_1[m_1^{(1)}]^{t-2} b_1^{(1)}, \\ &= 0.741 I(t-1) + 0.091(0.913)^{t-2}, \end{aligned} \qquad t \geq 3.$$

Similarly, we can calculate the booster training effects as

$$B(3) = a_2 b_2^{(2)} = 0.056$$

and

$$\begin{aligned} B(t) &= B(t-1)y_2^{(2)} + a_2[m_2^{(2)}]^{t-2} b_2^{(2)}, \\ &= 0.733B(t-1) + 0.056(0.937)^{t-2}, \end{aligned} \qquad t \geq 4,$$

where $^{(2)}$ denotes that the parameters were from the booster training group. Note that the training effects here are slightly different from those in Table 14.4 because the estimated parameters used here were under equality constraints. The overall training effects $O(t)$ can be calculated as

$$O(t) = I(t) + B(t).$$

The predicted initial, booster, and total training effects from time $t = 5$ to $t = 30$ are plotted in Figure 14.10a. The maximum initial training effect will be demonstrated at time $t = 7, I(7) = 0.222(0.033)$, about 6 years after the initial training. The maximum booster training effect will be demonstrated at time $t = 8, B(8) = 0.141(0.037)$, also about 6 years after the booster training. The total training effect peaked at time $t = 7, O(7) = 0.361(0.049)$.

Figure 14.10 also plots the 95% confidence intervals for the initial (Figure 14.10b), booster (Figure 14.10c), and total training effects (Figure 14.10d). The R codes for obtaining the confidence intervals can be found in the CD that comes with the book. Based on the confidence intervals, we can see that the initial training improved the everyday problem-solving ability and the booster training had significant effect above and beyond the initial training.

14.5 CONCLUSION AND DISCUSSION

We have outlined a variation on the longitudinal mediation model (Cole & Maxwell, 2003) adapted for application to intervention research. This model allows for the evaluation of not only the direct effects of an intervention, but also evaluation of mediation and changes to path coefficients themselves. The model was then applied to data from the ACTIVE study, to test the effects and longevity of the effects of reasoning training on everyday tasks. The results showed that the training effects on everyday problem-solving ability were totally mediated by reasoning ability and an improvement in reasoning ability can immediately convert to an improvement in everyday problem-solving ability. Based on the assumption that the model was stationary, the training effects over time were predicted and investigated through difference equations. The prediction showed that total training effects reached a peak after 6 years of the initial training or 5 years of the booster training.

While evaluating training, interventions may be studied more simply by adding group information into the model directly as covariates, and there could be practical difficulties in implementing this. Training may not only influence the level of the mediation variable and the output variable, but also the longitudinal relationship between the mediation variable and the output variable and the longitudinal structure of the mediation variable and the output variable. To simultaneously estimate the change in the level of the mediation variable and the longitudinal structure in one model, many interaction terms must be added to the model. Of course, when the intervention variable only influences the level of the mediation variable, the interaction method can be implemented with greater ease in commonly used SEM software. In this study, a multiple group method was discussed and applied to analyze the data.

Among the features of the proposed approach is its ability to predict training effects over time. Once stationarity is established or assumed, researchers can extrapolate what the process would look like beyond collected data. There are of course many concerns with such a process. In the analysis presented here, this assumption of stationarity may not be true in reality due to the nature of the ACTIVE sample. The average age of participants is 73.30, and the current model makes no adjustments to longitudinal prediction based on age. Participants may face sudden decline or terminal decline in the cognitive ability (Wilson, Beckett, Bienias, Evans, & Bennett, 2003; Wilson, Beck, Bienias, & Bennett, 2007). Thus, the predicted training effects can only be viewed as the maximum effects in ideal conditions.

The analysis of training intervention effects in the current study can also be interpreted from a dynamic systems analysis perspective. One may view the phenomenon to be investigated as a system developing in a certain way before training or intervention; for instance, the system may be in its stationary status. The training can be viewed as a shock to an element (e.g., the mediator variable) of the system at a time-point. And the training or intervention may not only result in a change in the element (the mediator) on which the training directly influences, but also a change in the structure of the whole system. Using the ACTIVE study as an example, training not only increased the level of reasoning ability, but also changed the relationship between reasoning ability and everyday problem-solving ability. To study the training effects over time is equivalent to investigating how the effect of the shock evolves over time. With the methods we proposed, one can separate the training effects (shock) from the other confounding variables and study how the pure training effects change over time. Thus, even when the observed trajectories of the outcome variables decline or remain flat over time, the training effects, by themselves, may still be increasing over time. The reason why people observe declining trajectories of the outcome variable may be that the positive training effects cannot balance off the overall decline in the outcome variables.

While the longitudinal mediation model in this study was developed with psychological and medical intervention research in mind, it is applicable to many types of longitudinal studies with similar research designs. The intervention variables presented here can be replaced by a grouping variable at any number of time-points, provided the intervention variables are nominal (i.e., dummy coded). For instance, this model could be used in lifespan developmental research, where the intervention variables are replaced by a set of variables indicating presence or absence of dementia at some time-point. This model would closely resemble Cole & Maxwell's original model as shown in Figure 14.2 (Cole & Maxwell, 2003), with the added benefit that the relationships between the mediator and output variables could take any of the forms shown in Figure 14.8. The longitudinal mediation model is not inherently limited to a set number of intervention variables (or alternatively, a set number of groups), and thus can be applied to a number of situations that mirror these research designs.

Several perspectives of the current study can be improved in the future. First, longitudinal mediation analysis is useful for studying lag relationship in the data. It will be useful to investigate how to design a longitudinal mediation study that can best utilize the merits of longitudinal mediation analysis. Second, longitudinal mediation models (e.g., Collins et al.,

1998; Cole & Maxwell, 2003) and their ancestor (Baron & Kenny, 1986) seem to be able to analyze the intrinsic temporal relationship, or causal relationship, among input, mediator, and output variables. However, how to scientifically relate these models with causal inference still needs much investigation. Third, a very weak definition of stationarity—the invariance of autoregressive coefficients—was adopted in this chapter. Even so, because of the limitation of only four measurement occasions, weak stationarity cannot be fully tested in the long-term prediction. Additional research is desired on how the stationarity influences the longitudinal mediation model performance.

REFERENCES

Baron, R.M., & Kenny, D.A. (1986). The moderator-mediator variable distinction in social psychological research: Conceptual, strategic, and statistical considerations. *Journal of Personality and Social Psychology, 51*, 1173–1182.

Bauer, D.J., Preacher, K.J., & Gil, K.M. (2006). Conceptualizing and testing random indirect effects and moderated mediation in multilevel models: New procedures and recommendations. *Psychological Methods, 11*(2), 142–163.

Bollen, K.A., & Stine, R.A. (1990). Direct and indirect effects: Classical and bootstrap estimates of variability. *Sociological Methodology, 20*, 115–140.

Cheong, J., MacKinnon, D.P., & Khoo, S.T. (2003). Investigation of mediational processes using parallel process latent growth curve modeling. *Structural Equation Modeling, 10*, 238–262.

Cheung, M.W.-L. (2007). Comparison of approaches to constructing confidence intervals for mediating effects using structural equation models. *Structural Equation Modeling, 14*(2), 227–246.

Cole, D.A., & Maxwell, S.E. (2003). Testing mediational models with longitudinal data: Questions and tips in the use of structural equation modeling. *Journal of Abnormal Psychology, 112*, 558–577.

Collins, L.M., Graham, J.W., & Flaherty, B.P. (1998). An alternative framework for defining mediation. *Multivariate Behavioral Research, 33*, 295–312.

Diehl, M., Willis, S.L., & Schaie, K.W. (1995). Everyday problem solving in older adults: Observational assessment and cognitive correlates. *Psychological Aging, 10*, 478–491.

Efron, B., (1979). Bootstrap methods: Another look at the jackknife. *The Annals of Statistics, 7*(1), 1–26.

Efron, B. (1987). Better bootstrap confidence intervals. *Journal of the American Statistical Association, 82*(397), 171–185.

Efron, B., & Tibshirani, R. (1993). *An introduction to the bootstrap*. New York: CRC Press.

Ekstrom, R.B., French, J.W., Harman, H.H., & Derman, D. (1976). *Manual for the kit of factor–referenced cognitive tests*. Princeton, NJ: Educational Testing Service.

Gollob, H., & Reichardt, C. (1991). Interpreting and estimating indirect effects assuming time lags really matter. In L. Collins & J. Horn (Eds.), *Best methods for the analysis of change: Recent advances, unanswered questions, future directions* (pp. 243–259). Washington, DC: American Psychological Association.

Gonda, J., & Schaie, K.W. (1985). *Schaie–Thurstone mental abilities test: Word series test.* Palo Alto, CA: Consulting Psychologists Press.

Jobe, J.B., Smith, D.M., Ball, K., Tennstedt, S.L., Marsiske, M., Willis, S.L., et al. (2001). Active: A cognitive intervention trial to promote independence in older adults. *Controlled Clinical Trials, 22*(4), 453–479.

Judd, C.M., & Kenny, D.A. (1981a). *Estimating the effects of social interventions.* New York: Cambridge University Press.

Judd, C.M., & Kenny, D.A. (1981b). Process analysis: Estimating mediation in treatment evaluations. *Evaluation Review, 5*, 602–619.

Kenny, D. A. (1979). *Correlation and causality*. New York: Wiley.

Kenny, D.A., Bolger, N., & Korchmaros, J. (2003). Lower-level mediation in multilevel models. *Psychological Methods, 8*, 115–128.

Krull, J.L., & MacKinnon, D.P. (1999). Multilevel mediation modeling in group-based intervention studies. *Evaluation Review, 23*, 418–444.

Krull, J.L., & MacKinnon, D.P. (2001). Multilevel modeling of individual and group level mediated effects. *Multivariate Behavioral Research, 36*(2), 249–277.

MacKinnon, D.P. (1994). Analysis of mediating variables in prevention intervention studies. In A. Cázares & L.A. Beatty (Eds.), *Scientific methods for prevention intervention research: NIDA research monograph 139* (pp. 127–153). Washington, DC: U.S. Department of Health and Human Services.

MacKinnon, D.P. (2000). Contrasts in multiple mediator models. In J. Rose, L. Chassin, C.C. Presson, & S.J. Sherman (Eds.), *Multivariate applications in substance use research: New methods for new questions* (pp. 141–160). Mahwah, NJ: Erlbaum.

MacKinnon, D.P., & Dwyer, J.H. (1993). Estimating mediated effects in prevention studies. *Evaluation Review, 17*, 144–158.

MacKinnon, D.P., Fairchild, A.J., & Fritz, M.S. (2007). Mediation analysis. *Annual Review of Psychology, 58*, 593–614.

MacKinnon, D.P., Lockwood, C.M., Hoffman, J.M., West, S.G., & Sheets, V. (2002). A comparison of methods to test mediation and other intervening variable effects. *Psychological Methods, 7*, 83–104.

Muthén, L.K., & Muthén, B.O. (1998–2007). *Mplus user's guide* (5th ed.). Los Angeles, CA: Muthén and Muthén. (http://www.statmodel.com)

Preacher, K.J., & Hayes, A.F. (2004). Spss and sas procedures for estimating indirect effects in simple mediation models. *Behavior Research Methods, Instruments, & Computers, 36*, 717–731.

R Development Core Team. (2005). R: A language and environment for statistical computing [Computer software manual]. Vienna, Austria. Available from http://www.R-project.org (ISBN 3-900051-07-0).

Rutter, A., & Hine, D. W. (2005). Sex differences in workplace aggression: An investigation of moderation and mediation effects. *Aggressive Behavior, 31*, 254–270.

Salthouse, T.A. (1991). Mediation of adult age differences in cognition by reductions in working memory and speed of processsing. *Psychological science, 2*(3), 179–183.

Salthouse, T.A. (1993). Speed mediation of adult age differences in cognition. *Developmental Psychology, 29*(3), 722–738.

Salthouse, T.A. (1996). The processing-speed theory of adult age differences in cognition. *Psychological Review, 103*(3), 403–428.

Schlaug, G., Norton, A., Overy, K., & Winner, E. (2005). Effects of music training on the child's brain and cognitive development. *Annals of the New York Academy of Sciences, 1060*(1), 219–230.

Shrout, P.E., & Bolger, N. (2002). Mediation in experimental and nonexperimental studies: New procedures and recommendations. *Psychological Methods, 7*, 422–445.

Sobel, M.E. (1982). Asymptotic confidence intervals for indirect effects in structural equation models. In S. Leinhardt (Ed.), *Sociological methodology* (pp. 290–312). San Francisco: Jossey-Bass.

Sobel, M.E. (1986). Some new results on indirect effects and their standard errors in covariance structure models. In N. Tuma (Ed.), *Sociological methodology* (pp. 159–186). Washington, D.C.: American Sociological Association.

Tennstedt, S. (2001). *ACTIVE (advanced cognitive training for independent and vital elderly), 1999–2001 [UNITED STATES] [Computer file]. ICPSR04248-v1. Watertown, MA: New England Research Institute [producer], 2001. Ann Arbor, MI: Inter-university Consortium for Political and Social Research [distributor], 2005-10-11.*

Thurstone, L.L., & Thurstone, T.G. (1949). *Examiner manual for the sra primary mental abilities test (form 10–14)*. Chicago: Science Research Associates.

Willis, S.L. (1987). Cognitive training and everyday competence. In K.W. Schaie (Ed.), *Annual review of gerontology and geriatrics* (Vol. 7). New York: Springer.

Willis, S.L. (1996). Everyday cognitive competence in elderly persons: Conceptual issues and empirical findings. *Gerontologist, 36*, 595–601.

Willis, S.L., Jay, G.M., Diehl, M., & Marsiske, M. (1992). Longitudinal change and prediction of everyday task performance in the elderly. *Research on Aging, 14*, 68–91.

Willis, S.L., & Marsiske, M. (1993). *Manual for the everyday problems test.* University Park, PA: Pennsylvania State University.

Willis, S.L., & Nesselroade, C.S. (1990). Long-term effects of fluid ability training in old-old age. *Developmental Psychology, 26*(6), 905–910.

Willis, S.L., Tennstedt, S.L., Marsiske, M., Ball, K., Elias, J., Koepke, K.M., et al. (2006). Long-term effects of cognitive training on everyday functional outcomes in older adults. *JAMA, 296*(23), 2805–2814. Available from http://jama.ama-assn.org/cgi/content/abstract/296/23/2805

Wilson, R.S., Beck, T.L., Bienias, J.L., & Bennett, D. A. (2007). Terminal cognitive decline: Accelerated loss of cognition in the last years of life. *Psychosomatic Med, 69*(2), 131–137.

Wilson, R.S., Beckett, L.A., Bienias, J.L., Evans, D.A., & Bennett, D.A. (2003). Terminal decline in cognitive function. *Neurology, 60*(11), 1782–1787.

Zhang, Z., & Wang, L. (2008). Methods for evaluating mediation effects: Rationale and comparison. In K. Shigemasu, A. Okada, T. Imaizumi, & T. Hoshino (Eds.), *New trends in psychometrics* (pp. 595–604). Tokyo: Universal Academy Press.

15

Exploring Intraindividual, Interindividual, and Intervariable Dynamics in Dyadic Interactions

Emilio Ferrer, Shu-Chun Chen, Sy-Miin Chow, and Fushing Hsieh

15.1 INTRODUCTION: DYADIC INTERACTIONS

A fundamental goal in the study of dyadic interactions is to understand the dynamics underlying the interrelations between two units in a dyad. In psychological research, most of the work on dyadic interactions concerns interactions between two individuals (i.e., parent–child, husband–wife, teacher–student). Psychological theories pertaining to dyadic interactions postulate such interactions in dynamic terms (e.g., attachment theory; Bowlby, 1982; Mikulincer & Shaver, 2007). In spite of this theoretical description, there is not much empirical work showing evidence for such dyadic interactions in dynamic terms, with attention to processes over time. One possibility for this mismatch between theory and empirical work is the lack of adequate methodology for uncovering the dynamics between two individuals from multiple time series. In this chapter, we propose a set of exploratory techniques designed to extract patterns of dynamics from dyadic interactions.

The chapter is organized as follows. We first describe common techniques used to analyze dyadic interactions and identify some limitations. We then introduce the basics of our proposed approach and elaborate on each of the steps using empirical data in a different section. We conclude the chapter by summarizing the results and discussing possible methodological and theoretical implications.

15.1.1 Modeling Dyadic Interactions

To capture the dynamics underlying dyadic interactions, several features are necessary. First, measures need to be collected with enough frequency to reflect the dyad's fluctuations over time as well as the time dependency of such fluctuations. Second, the postulated models need to be able to accurately and reliably capture such dynamics. Various approaches have been used to examine dyadic interactions in the past, yielding different types of information about interrelations between the two individuals in the dyad. Examples of these models are dynamic factor analysis, dynamic systems of differential equation models, multilevel models, sequential analysis models, and state-space models, to mention a few.

Dynamic factor analysis models, for example, have been used to examine affective processes in dyadic interactions (Ferrer, 2006; Ferrer & Nesselroade, 2003; Ferrer & Widaman, 2007). Multilevel models, another common set of techniques for the analysis of dyadic interactions, have also been used to distinguish among actor, partner, and interaction effects (Campbell & Kashy, 2002; Kenny, Kashy, Cook, & Simpson, 2006), to examine change within married couples (Raudenbush, Brennan, & Barnett, 1995), to model affect corregulation between romantic partners (Butner, Diamond, & Hicks, 2007), daily intimacy and disclosure in married couples (Laurenceau, Troy, & Carver, 2005), and to identify emotional contagion in couples under stress (Thomson & Bolger, 1999).

Differential equation models, as a continuous-time alternative to difference equation-based approaches such as the dynamic factor analysis models, have been used as a theoretical representation of different types of interactions in dyads (Felmlee, 2006; Felmlee & Greenberg, 1999). They have also been applied to various types of dyadic interaction data, including turn-taking in conversations (Buder, 1991; Newtson, 1993), the development of various types of social relationships and marriages (Baron, Amazeen, & Beek, 1994), the emotional interaction between spouses with implications for break-up (Gottman, Murray, Swanson, Tyson, & Swanson, 2002), and daily intimacy and disclosure in married couples (Boker & Laurenceau, 2006). Finally, another popular technique for analyzing single- or low-dimensional time series of dyadic interactions is the state-space models. This technique has been employed, for example, to investigate the dynamics of emotional experiences between individuals in close relationships (Chow, Ferrer, & Nesselroade, 2007; Song & Ferrer, in press).

15.1.2 Limitations and Current Approach

Many contemporary dynamic models used to represent human dynamics are based on the notion of a stationary system; that is, they do not account for the possibly changing dynamics of a system, which may occur due to a combination of different intrinsic and extrinsic factors. Furthermore, when modeling empirical data on, say, dyadic interactions, several key issues arise with respect to the choice of the factors regulating the dynamics of the system. First, the structural assumptions underlying such factors can dictate the methodology and interpretation of the results. The validity of these functions can often be greatly bolstered by evaluating evidence from exploratory information prior to confirmatory model fitting. Second, detecting dynamics in high-dimensional time-series data is often a formidable task. The number of parameters typically grows exponentially as the dimensions in the series increase. Utilizing exploratory information prior to model fitting provides helpful insights into (a) possible ways of reducing the dimensionality of the data, (b) critical recurrence patterns in the data, and (c) cues for determining the choice for the factors underlying the dynamics.

In the present chapter, we introduce three exploratory techniques for examining patterns of dyadic interactions. The first two techniques are nonparametric in nature and they assume no prior knowledge about possible coupling relationships—or any other form of dynamics—between both units of the system. The first technique utilizes the Lempell–Ziv (L–Z) measure, a measure of algorithmic complexity from information theory (Cover & Thomas, 1991), to describe change features embedded in different time series. The second technique, termed hierarchical segmentation (HS), was originally proposed by Hsieh, Hwang, Lee, Lan, and Horng (2006) for representing nonstationary dynamics in animal behavior. The third technique proposed in the present chapter is based on stochastic transition networks. This is a graphical approach for summarizing dynamic information coded in nonparametric terms. We show how these techniques can be used to extract systematic patterns of change in high-dimensional data from dyadic interactions and, together with exploratory techniques

TABLE 15.1

Positive and Negative Affect Items

Positive	Negative
Interested	Irritable
Alert	Distressed
Excited	Ashamed
Inspired	Upset
Strong	Nervous
Determined	Scared
Attentive	Hostile
Enthusiastic	Jittery
Active	Afraid
Proud	Guilty

such as clustering analysis, to identify intraindividual, interindividual, and intervariable patterns of information.

15.2 ILLUSTRATIVE DATA: DAILY FLUCTUATIONS IN AFFECT

The empirical data used to illustrate our proposed approach consist of daily measurements of affect from a married couple. Details of data collection, participants, and measures are reported elsewhere (Ferrer & Nesselroade, 2003). The variables from the data represent self-reports of emotional experiences using the Positive and Negative Affective Scale (PANAS; Watson, Clark, & Tellegen, 1988) reported by both individuals daily for 182 days. The PANAS scale contains 20 items describing positive and negative affective states. Participants are asked to mark the extent to which they experienced each of the items on a 5-point Likert-type scale ranging from 1 (*very slightly* or *not at all*) to 5 (*extremely*). Table 15.1 lists all the positive and negative items of the PANAS scale.

15.3 LEMPELL–ZIV (L–Z) COMPLEXITY

In the first set of analyses, we explored characteristics of the 20 PANAS items over time to summarize key differences between the variables. That is, rather than attempting to create composite or theoretically guided factor scores based on the valence of the items (i.e., positive affect and negative affect items), as is routinely done in the literature, we first evaluated the parallels and differences among the items using a measure of algorithmic complexity, the L–Z complexity measure.

The idea behind algorithmic complexity is to identify the "shortest" length of a computer program needed to regenerate a given time series. The L–Z measure is an estimate of this uncomputable complexity (Cover & Thomas, 1991; see Kaspar & Schuster, 1987, for details). For example, inspecting the wife's responses on the "afraid" variable in our illustrative data reveals no variability over time (i.e., the data consist of a constant value "1"). Thus, the program needed to regenerate this time series would be very simple. In contrast, such a program would be much longer when trying to regenerate the time series for the husband's variable "enthusiastic," which is associated with frequent fluctuations between high and low values. Hence, the time series of these two affect variables can be described as having very low and high L–Z complexity, respectively. Heuristically, the L–Z complexity is a way of measuring the amount of repeated patterns embedded within a digital string. Thus, a digital string with more unique patterns would yield higher complexity than a digital string with more repeated patterns.

Computationally, the L–Z algorithm involves two operations: "copy" and "insert." The complexity measure of a digital string is the number of digital patterns separated by the "insert" operation in the process of regenerating the string. An illustration of this algorithm is as follows (see Kaspar & Schuster, 1987, for a detailed description)

Consider the following data string of base-3 and length 12: $A = 122010112200$. For the first and second digits, 1 and 2, we need to execute the "insert" operation twice because these digits are new in the string. We mark the construction up to this point by $1 \cdot 2 \cdot$. The third digit is 2, which is repeated. Thus, we only need to execute the "copy" operation. But the fourth digit, 0, is new, so we need to "insert" again and the reconstructed string becomes $1 \cdot 2 \cdot 20 \cdot$. The fifth digit, 1, is repeated so we need to "copy" only. Before making this "copy" operation, however, we ask whether the fifth and sixth digits, 10, can be copied from $1 \cdot 2 \cdot 20 \cdot 1$. The answer is negative, so we need one more "insert" and then the reconstructed string becomes $1 \cdot 2 \cdot 20 \cdot 10 \cdot \cdots$. Likewise, for the seventh and eigth digits, 11, we need one more "insert" to accommodate the new pattern with the reconstructed string as $1 \cdot 2 \cdot 20 \cdot 10 \cdot 11 \cdot$. The next three-digit pattern 220 has appeared in $1 \cdot 2 \cdot 20 \cdot 10 \cdot 11 \cdot$, but not the pattern 2200 in $1 \cdot 2 \cdot 20 \cdot 10 \cdot 11 \cdot 220$. Hence, we need one more "insert" and then we regenerate the string $S = 1 \cdot 2 \cdot 20 \cdot 10 \cdot 11 \cdot 2200 \cdot$ with six digital patterns. Thus, the L–Z measure of complexity for the string A is 6, and is denoted as $H(A) = 6$.

In sum, the L–Z complexity—a tool from information theory—is a way of measuring the amount of repeated patterns embedded within a digital string. The example above illustrates the fact that the algorithmic complexity characterizes the number of unique patterns of information in a given time series. Thus, a string with more unique patterns would result in higher complexity, whereas a string with more repeated patterns would have less complexity.* Consider now a new data string that is constructed by augmenting itself, denoted by $A \oplus A$. The complexity of this new series would only increase by one; that is, $H(A \oplus A) = H(A) + 1$. This points to the fact that if a new string B consists of many digital patterns contained in string A, then the algorithmic complexity of the augmented string $A \oplus B$ will only increase by a small amount relative to $H(B)$. On the other hand, if B is very different from A, the increment $H(A \oplus B)$ could be comparable to $H(B)$. Hence, we define the mutual L–Z measure of complexity as

$$H(A : B) = H(A \oplus B) - H(B) + H(B \oplus A) - H(A). \tag{15.1}$$

Heuristically, the idea behind mutual L–Z complexity is to compute the amount of unknown patterns that are not in common between two digital strings.

Without assuming a particular model for each string, there is no information regarding possible patterns on which both strings could differ. Thus, the mutual L–Z complexity is particularly suited for situations without parametric assumptions imposed on the digital strings, especially those

* One reviewer pointed out that a time series with greater within-person over-time variance may be characterized by greater L–Z complexity, thereby complicating the use of this measure as a "strict" measure of complexity in cases involving arbitrary scaling differences. We acknowledge this potential complication but note that the L–Z complexity is simply one way to summarize and extract the regularity contained in a data string. Thus, information such as variance as well as other essential characteristics of a variable as expressed through the digital string would collectively define the magnitude of the complexity measure. A researcher has to decide whether differences in variance—either within person over time, or across individuals—are simply an artifact that needs to be removed prior to data analysis or something that is of theoretical interest within the context of a data analytic problem.

derived from potentially nonstationary time series. Here, we emphasize that greater complexity does not always imply the existence of nonstationarities in the data, nor do nonstationary data always yield greater algorithmic complexity than stationary data. For instance, the sequence 000111222 is nonstationary (linearly increasing), but its L–Z complexity is smaller than 211020120 (which could be stationary). The L–Z complexity measures can be used to characterize stationary as well as nonstationary processes; however, nonstationary processes may show critical changes in their statistical properties in ways that are not clearly understood by contemporary researchers. In these cases, fitting a misspecified stationary (or nonstationary) model to the corresponding data can lead to misleading conclusions. In contrast, because the mutual L–Z complexity measure simply quantifies the amount of unknown patterns that are not in common between two digital strings without making prior postulates on possible patterns on which both strings could differ, this kind of exploratory index is especially useful for revealing the patterns embedded in more complex processes, of which nonstationary processes are just one possible example. The univariate L–Z complexity measure is useful in a similar way.

Finally, we propose an index of relative increment as

$$DH(A:B) = \frac{H(A \oplus B) - H(B)}{H(B)} + \frac{H(B \oplus A) - H(A)}{H(A)}. \tag{15.2}$$

This index of relative increment of mutual L–Z complexity, $DH(A:B)$, captures a weighted average of the additional complexity contained in each time series that is not shared with the other time series. It can also be thought of as the "quasi-distance" between two time series or two sets of variables.

15.3.1 Clustering between-Variable Dynamics Based on the Mutual L–Z Complexity

To summarize the differences (or similarities) among the different PANAS items, we use the mutual L–Z complexity, $H(A:B)$, in a hierarchical clustering analysis. Our goal here is to identify a clustering tree for the 20 time series of PANAS items based on their complexity over time.

Figure 15.1 presents the clustering trees for all the times series of both individuals (panels a and b). The y-axis in this figure represents the mutual L–Z complexity between each pair of variables. The husband's tree (panel a)

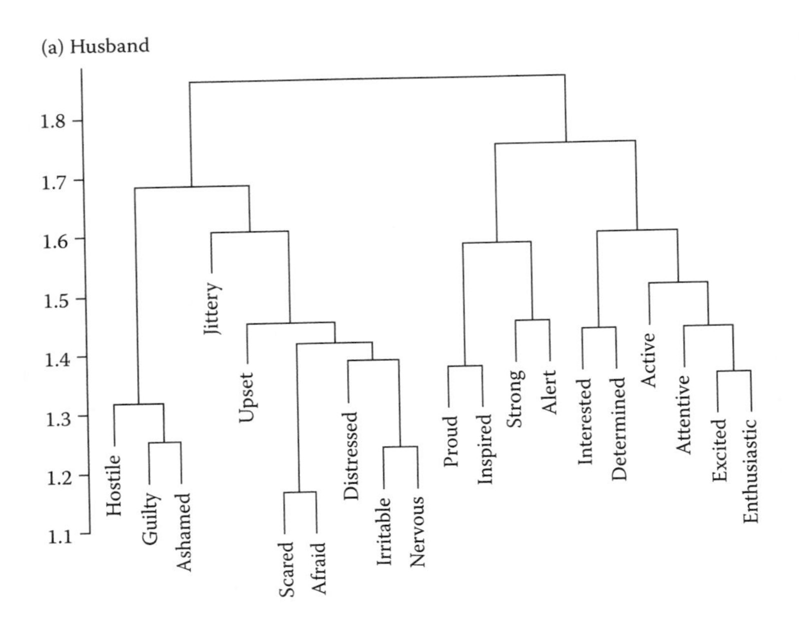

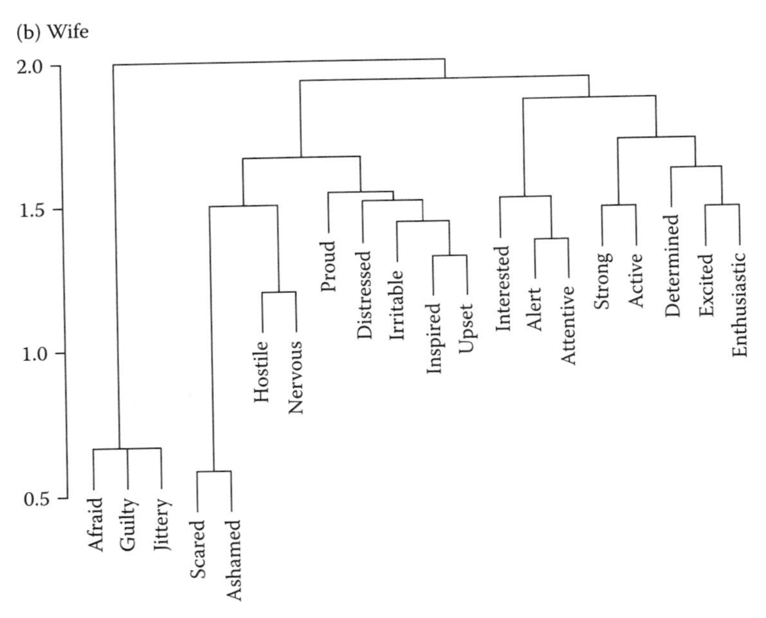

FIGURE 15.1 Clustering trees based on mutual complexity for all the times series of both individuals.

has two main branches: one that includes all positive affect variables and another with all negative emotions. The clustering tree for the wife's affect, however, has three main branches. The first branch contains three variables with very low complexity, including "afraid," "guilty," and "jittery." The second branch consists of mainly negative emotions and two positive variables ("inspired" and "proud"). The last branch includes all the remaining positive affect variables.

The arrangement of branches in these trees indicates similarity (or dissimilarity) among the time series of all the variables. For example, variables that are located in the same subbranches are similar in complexity, and the lower the location of the subbranch, the more similar the variables. Thus, a major subbranch would likely stand for a group of "similar" emotions. Hence, these hierarchical clustering trees offer insights into the complexity of this dyad's affect. In particular, they suggest a hierarchical structure in the wife's affective dynamics, namely, there exist subgroups of emotions with varying degrees of complexity. Conversely, a more uniform pattern of complexity was evident across the husband's emotions.

The clustering results revealed information about the structure underlying the couple's affects. Specifically, the husband's affect items seem to be organized based on the valence of the emotion items: positive emotion items were classified with other positive items and negative items were classified with other negative items. In the wife's clustering tree, however, two positive items, "proud" and "inspired," were actually grouped with other negative items such as "distressed" and "irritable." This is because these two items, just as other items in the same branch, were only endorsed very sparingly. This shows that valence may not be the only dimension along which the PANAS items can be organized. We now turn to our second approach to extract dynamic information from the data.

15.4 HIERARCHICAL SEGMENTATION

Hierarchical segmentation (HS) is a nonparametric technique for grouping multivariate time series into segments with similar discrete-state recurrence patterns. The HS algorithm was originally developed for pattern recognition in animal behavior data (Hsieh et al., 2006) and has also been applied to affect data (Hsieh, Ferrer, Chen, & Chow, 2008a). In principle, this algorithm is applicable to any time series data, especially high-dimensional time series. Before describing the steps of the HS algorithm, we discuss some basics and rationales for performing nonparametric decoding, a necessary step for HS.

15.4.1 Background on Nonparametric Decoding

One of the goals in the empirical analysis of time-series data is to identify potential changes in the dynamics of a system. Some of the parametric approaches for identifying the possible point(s) at which a system deviates from a stationary trajectory include change-point models (Carlin, Gelfand, & Smith, 1992) and regime switching models (Kim & Nelson, 1999). Alternatively, this task can be accomplished via nonparametric decoding procedures. Such procedures should provide a means of aggregating patterns of a defined event and, in doing so, help differentiate "regimes" that are characterized by similar patterns or dynamics of the event of interest.

In the context of our empirical data on dyadic interactions of affect, one important focus is the possible changes between persistently high and persistently low affective states. Then, a reasonable choice of an "event" of interest is extreme values in positive or negative affect. Frequent recurrence of such an extreme event constitutes a persistently high regime of unusual dynamics, which can, in turn, help reveal the driving force leading to the emergence of such a regime. The question then becomes how to identify such a period of persistently high regime from other regimes.

To illustrate the goal of nonparametric decoding more concretely, consider the following scenario. Let a discrete time series $\mathcal{X}_n = \{X(t): t = 1, 2, \ldots, n\}$ of length n be the observable trajectory generated from the nonautonomous dynamics of interest. Now let an n-dimensional state-space vector $\mathcal{S}_n = \{S(t): t = 1, 2, \ldots, n\}$ be postulated as the unobserved driving force that dictates the dynamics of the system. For simplicity, we can assume that $S(t)$ takes only two possible values, 0 or 1, for each time t. Hence, the task of estimation of $\mathcal{S}_n$ is to find the "most likely" unobserved state of the system (i.e., $\mathcal{S}_n$) based on the manifest $\mathcal{X}_n$. This task, termed "decoding," can be interpreted as a change-point analysis but without knowledge about the number of change-points in the data.

Decoding is a signal processing technique used, for example, to estimate the discrete state-space vector in hidden Markov models (HMM). Within the HMM approach, the Viterbi—or Baum–Welch—algorithm is typically used to estimate such discrete state-space vectors (see pp. 339–340, Rabiner & Juang, 1993; Viterbi, 1967). Similarly, in state-space models with linear and Gaussian noise structures, the Kalman filtering algorithm (Kalman, 1960) is used for the same purpose. Although common in their application, both algorithms involve different but related notions: the former is based on conditional probabilities, whereas the latter is based on condition expectations. The data in our analyses are discrete and, thus, we use decoding. Furthermore, we make no assumptions about the state-space structures of our data. We simply use the HS algorithm as a decoding tool to map out where a system changes from one possible subset of patterns to another. Portions of the data that show similar patterns constitute a "regime" that may represent some meaningful psychological states. By grouping portions of the data that show similar characteristics into different regimes, exploratory results from our decoding algorithm can be used as a starting point for constructing other change-point or regime-switching models.

Unlike decoding in the HMM setting, the decoding task described here is highly computationally demanding. In some cases, it can be infeasible without any parametric assumptions about the mechanisms governing the dynamics of $S(t)$. In our analyses, for instance, we make no assumptions about state-space structures. Thus, the Viterbi algorithm, which can be derived as a discrete version of the EM algorithm, the so-called Baum–Welch algorithm, is not the appropriate technique. Furthermore, we make no structural assumptions nor use mathematical programming techniques. In these cases, the Viterbi algorithm is not applicable and an exhaustive search for an optimal solution involves 2^n procedural computations or, in other words, the number of all possible configurations 2^n. From this perspective, we can see how much we have imposed on the state-space model assumption in general. This exponential growth rate of computation with n is called the *NP* problem in the mathematical computation literature. In our empirical data, for example, the computational loading based on each of the 40 time series $\mathcal{X}_{182}$ would translate into the need to discover one sequence $\mathcal{S}_{182}$ out of 2^{182} candidates in a 182-dimensional state-space vector.

15.4.2 Steps for HS

The goal of HS is to decode the underlying "states" in a multivariate time series. The term "states" is used broadly in the present context to denote latent regimes or discrete categories for grouping portions of the data that show similar dynamics. Similar "dynamics" can refer to similarities in the level or intensity of an event (in our case, affect), the scarcity of extreme events (i.e., extreme affects), or the rapid recurrence of extreme events (affects) within the context of HS. Specifically, given an observable event in the time series $\mathcal{X}_n$, the HS algorithm follows the following steps:

Step 1: Based on a defined event, the time series $\mathcal{X}_n$ is transformed into a 0–1–2 digital string of base-3 following the scheme: code 0 for $X(t)$ when an extremely high value of an event is observed at time t, code 2 for an unusually low extreme, and code 1 for a nonextreme event. This first level 0–1–2 string is denoted by the code sequence C_1.

Step 2: A histogram is constructed based on the 0-event recurrent time distribution from C_1. The sequence of recurrence time (inter-event-spacing) is denoted as $\mathcal{R}_2$.

Step 3: Upper and lower percentile values are chosen to transform the sequence of recurrence time in $\mathcal{R}_2$ into another 0–1–2 digital string. We describe this procedure as the second-level coding scheme. A recurrent time (i.e., the time interval between two "0" events) smaller than the lower percentile is coded as 2_2. A recurrent time greater than the upper percentile is coded as 0_2, and a recurrence time falling in between the two percentiles is coded as 1_2. The resulting digital string of base-3 is denoted by the code sequence C_2.

Step 4: Based on the new code sequence C_2, code 0_2 is taken as another "new" event and its corresponding recurrent time histogram is constructed. Similarly, a sequence of inter-0_2-event recurrence time is computed and labeled as $\mathcal{R}_3$.

Step 5: A second set of upper and lower percentile values is chosen based on the histogram of inter-0_2-event recurrence time. The sequence of recurrence time in $\mathcal{R}_3$ is then recoded into another 0–1–2 digital string. This is the third (and top) level coding scheme. An inter-0_2-event interval that is smaller than the lower percentile value is coded as 2_3. An inter-0_2-event interval greater than the upper percentile value is coded as 0_3, and the recurrence time falling between the two percentiles is coded as 1_3. The third sequence of digital strings of base-3 is denoted as C_3.

Step 6: The resulting code sequence C_3 is mapped onto the original time series to create m partitions of elements in $\mathcal{R}_3$ on the time span $[1, n]$. We denote this partition as $\mathcal{N}$.

The code sequence C_3 serves as the top level of the HS hierarchy because it effectively summarizes information contained in the first two levels, namely, the sequences C_1 and C_2. For example, a given segment, say corresponding to the 0_3-code, is a period of time points falling between two widely separated 0_2-codes. The wide separation of two successive 0_2-codes implies that there are many 0-codes on the particular segment of code sequence C_1 and, equivalently, many extreme events (e.g., a very high positive affect or a negative affect) being observed on the segment of $\mathcal{X}_n$. This is denoted as a segment of rapid recurrence of high affect intensity. In contrast, a segment corresponding to 1_3 or 2_3 would present an extended period of many 1- and 2-codes, but very sparse 0-codes. This is denoted as a segment of moderate to slow recurrence of extreme affect.

In sum, the partition $\mathcal{N}(\mathcal{X}_n)$ serves to separate segments with distinct patterns of dynamics. The three flags, 0_1, 0_2, and 0_3, each serve different functions. Each 0-code marks an instance of extremely high affect (e.g., an especially good day). Each 0_2-code marks a segment with extreme scarcity of high affect (e.g., a prolonged absence of good days). Finally, each 0_3-code indicates a segment with unusually frequent recurrence of high affect (e.g., a string of consecutive good days).

The number of levels in the HS algorithm depends on the segmentation of interest. The three-level segmentation that we use in our analyses allows us to discriminate between the aggregation versus sparsity of event of interest. If patterns of aggregation of segments are the main interest, a fourth—or above—level may be selected. If the time series is not long enough, however, any level above three might be questionable. In this regard, the number of levels is not arbitrary, but depends on the question of interest as well as the characteristics of the data.

15.4.3 Empirical Illustration

A schematic illustration of the HS algorithm as applied to a segment of the empirical data is given in Figure 15.2. In this figure, the data represent a

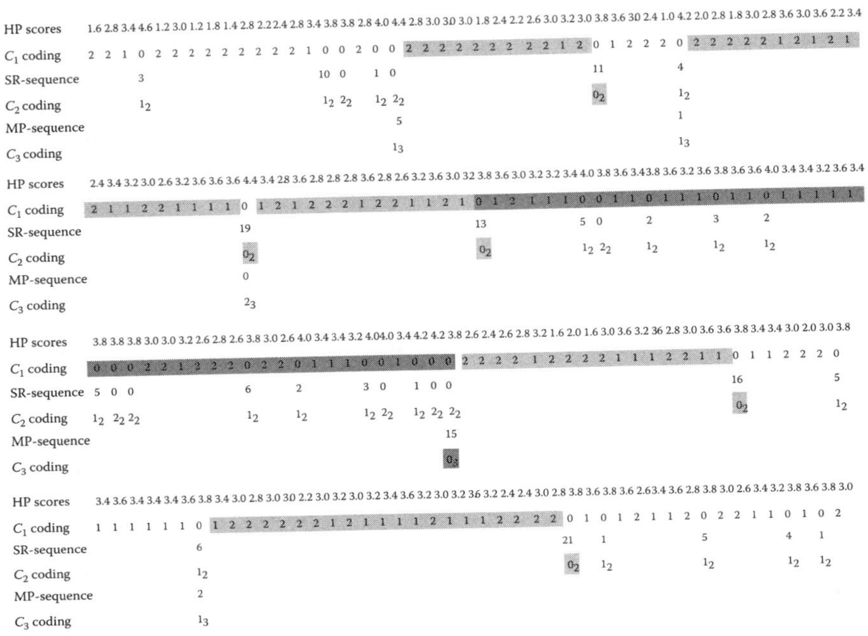

HP scores 1.6 2.8 3.4 4.6 1.2 3.0 1.2 1.8 1.4 2.8 2.2 2.4 2.8 3.4 3.8 3.8 2.8 4.0 4.4 2.8 3.0 30 3.0 1.8 2.4 2.2 2.6 3.0 3.2 3.0 3.8 3.6 30 2.4 1.0 4.2 2.0 2.8 1.8 3.0 2.8 3.6 3.0 3.6 2.2 3.4
C_1 coding 2 2 1 0 2 2 2 2 2 2 2 2 2 1 0 0 2 0 0 2 2 2 2 2 2 2 2 2 1 2 0 1 2 2 2 0 2 2 2 2 2 1 2 1 2 1
SR-sequence 3 10 0 1 0 11 4
C_2 coding 1_2 1_2 2_2 1_2 2_2 0_2 1_2
MP-sequence 5 1
C_3 coding 1_3 1_3

HP scores 2.4 3.4 3.2 3.0 2.6 3.2 3.6 3.6 3.6 4.4 3.4 28 3.6 2.8 2.8 2.8 3.6 2.8 2.6 3.2 3.6 3.0 32 3.8 3.6 3.0 3.2 3.2 3.4 4.0 3.8 3.6 3.43.8 3.6 3.2 3.6 3.8 3.6 3.6 4.0 3.4 3.4 3.2 3.6 3.4
C_1 coding 2 1 1 2 2 1 1 1 1 0 1 2 1 2 2 2 1 2 2 1 1 2 1 0 1 2 1 1 1 0 0 1 1 0 1 1 1 0 1 1 0 1 1 1 1 1
SR-sequence 19 13 5 0 2 3 2
C_2 coding 0_2 0_2 1_2 2_2 1_2 1_2 1_2
MP-sequence 0
C_3 coding 2_3

HP scores 3.8 3.8 3.8 3.0 3.0 3.2 2.6 2.8 2.6 3.8 3.0 2.6 4.0 3.4 3.4 3.2 4.04.0 3.4 4.2 4.2 3.8 2.6 2.4 2.6 2.8 3.2 1.6 2.0 1.6 3.0 3.6 3.2 36 2.8 3.0 3.6 3.6 3.8 3.4 3.4 3.0 2.0 3.0 3.8
C_1 coding 0 0 0 2 2 1 2 2 2 0 2 2 0 1 1 1 0 0 1 0 0 0 2 2 2 2 1 2 2 2 2 1 1 1 2 2 1 1 0 1 1 2 2 2 0
SR-sequence 5 0 0 6 2 3 0 1 0 0 16 5
C_2 coding 1_2 2_2 2_2 1_2 1_2 1_2 2_2 1_2 2_2 2_2 0_2 1_2
MP-sequence 15
C_3 coding 0_3

HP scores 3.4 3.6 3.4 3.4 3.4 3.6 3.8 3.4 3.0 2.8 3.0 30 2.2 3.0 3.2 3.0 3.2 3.4 3.6 3.2 3.0 3.2 36 3.2 2.4 2.4 3.0 2.8 3.8 3.6 3.8 3.6 2.63.4 3.6 2.8 3.8 3.0 2.6 3.4 3.2 3.8 3.6 3.8 3.0
C_1 coding 1 1 1 1 1 1 0 1 2 2 2 2 2 2 1 2 1 1 1 1 2 1 1 1 2 2 2 2 0 1 0 1 2 1 1 2 0 2 2 1 1 0 1 0 2
SR-sequence 6 21 1 5 4 1
C_2 coding 1_2 0_2 1_2 1_2 1_2 1_2
MP-sequence 2
C_3 coding 1_3

FIGURE 15.2 Full sequential coding for a selected composite data segment.

composite (husband's positive affect) based on the 10 positive items.* This figure depicts the full sequence coding from the HS algorithm, from the raw data to the top level of the sequence hierarchy. The first line in each section shows a segment of the raw data. The second line represents the C_1 code sequence, resulting from the first transformation of the raw data. The codes 0, 1, and 2 indicate large, medium, and low expression of positive affect, respectively.

To recode the raw data in level 1 of the HS, we chose cut-off points separately for each of the time series. Because of the positive skewness of the negative items, we used each individual's 75th and 85th percentiles as the cut-off points for defining low, medium, and high expression. Such skewness is typical in affect data, with a high frequency of small values and rare occurrences of high values. For the positive items, in contrast, we used each individual's 50th and 85th percentiles as the cut-off points.

* Note that the composite score for positive affect is calculated based on the theoretically posited valence of the PANAS items, not their algorithmic complexity as in our earlier L–Z complexity analysis.

It is worth noting that the 0, 1, and 2 codes are created based on the percentiles of the observed variables and are invariant to changes in variances. Of course, any *ad hoc* categorization of responses requires a researcher to determine the cut-off points that are used to separate the different categories. Occasions marked as extreme events using one set of cut-off points may not be identified as extreme events using another set of cut-off points. Using our current coding scheme, the same percentage of cases would be classified as low, medium, and extreme events across individuals, but the actual values of the data that form the cut-off points differ by individual. Doing so helps create some consistency across participants and reduces potential artifacts due to interindividual differences in response variability and intervariable differences in measurement scales.

Figure 15.3a and b depict actograms for all time series (i.e., individual variables) of both individuals in the dyad. Actograms are a type of graph commonly used in circadian research in which activity is plotted against time (Winfree, 1987). Here, these figures summarize information extracted from the HS. For these data, we stack the sequence coding of all the husband's (panel a) and wife's (panel b) time series, separately, and arrange them in line with the hierarchical clustering tree from Figure 15.1. We used the flags 0_{3+} and 0_{3-} to indicate occurrences of positive and negative value, respectively. To identify these values, we first considered the number of extreme events, irrespective of the valence. At the third level of HS, when a segment was coded as 0_3, we counted the number of positive and negative events for that segment. If the number of positive events was greater than the number of negative events, the segment was coded as 0_{3+} and vice versa (see Hsieh et al., 2008a).

These actograms show several sequences of regime changes with synchrony among the variables within each individual. These patterns are indicative of intraindividual dynamics, with relationships among the affective time series. For the husband's time series (panel a), items that were clustered together earlier based on their mutual L–Z complexity scores tended to show periods of rapid recurrence (marked with 0_3) and periods with prolonged scarcity of extreme intensities (marked with 0_2) in synchrony throughout the 182 days. In other words, items of similar algorithmic complexity tended to change together for the husband.

The wife's data (panel b), in contrast, showed less of such interitem coherence. Examining results from the HS reveals that some of the items were clustered together earlier based on their mutual L–Z complexity because

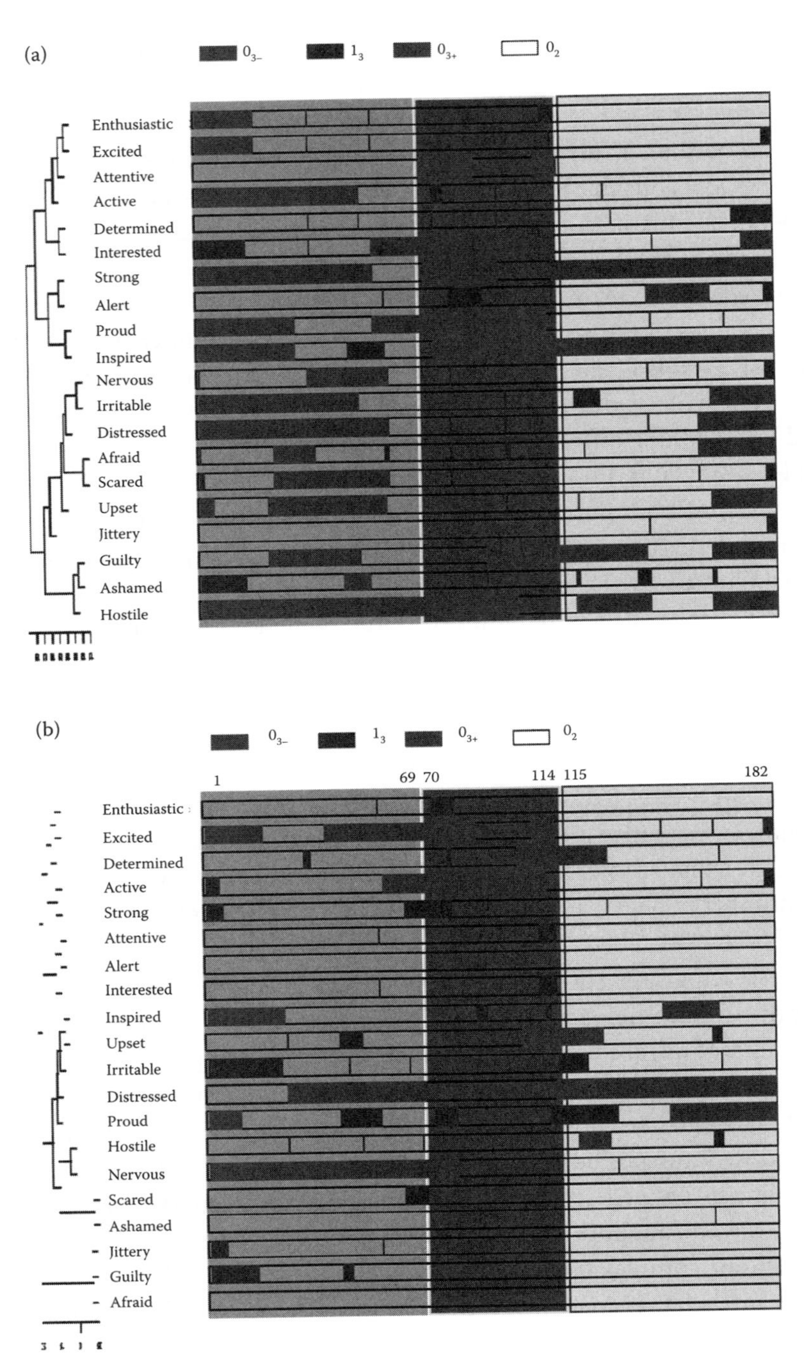

FIGURE 15.3 Actograms for all the time series of both individuals (panels a and b, respectively).

these items were generally endorsed with low frequencies by the wife. Between 70 and 114 days, the wife started to show frequent recurrence of several positive emotions (e.g., "excited," "enthusiastic," "determined," "active," and "alert") and this period also coincided with frequent recurrence of several positive emotions in the husband (e.g., "determined," "interested," "inspired," and "proud").

Slight discrepancies also arose between the HS results and the results from our earlier clustering analysis. Specifically, judging from the wive's mutual L–Z complexity, the item "inspired" was classified as more similar to items such as upset, irritable, and distressed than items such as nervous, hostile, and ashamed. According to results from the HS, however, the item "inspired," just as "nervous" and "hostile," did not show any extreme occurrence. This shows that the HS algorithm and the L–Z complexity are two separate techniques that are looking at very different aspects of change. The HS identifies *relatively extreme* events and marks their *temporal location* when these events occur in sequential segments. In contrast, the mutual L–Z complexity of two time series, A and B, quantifies the number of patterns of A that cannot be found in B, as well as the number of patterns in B that are not in A. The precise temporal ordering of these patterns contributes to the overall complexity but is not the only determinant.

Inspecting both panels of Figure 15.3 further suggests the existence of three periods with different affective dynamics. The first period consists of data points 1–69. In this period, the husband's data present a pattern of persistent high negative affect while the wife's data show relatively low positive and negative affect. In the second period (i.e., data points 70–114), both individuals show aggregation of positive affective extremes. In the final period (i.e., points 115–182), both individuals have few aggregations of affect extremes. We do not have further information from the current data set to deduce whether these three periods coincided with any major external event. However, these three periods can be used as the basis for constructing other confirmatory models of change.

Thus, combining results from the HS with the graphical summary information from the actograms helped uncover informative coupling relationships between the two dyad members. For example, the affect of both individuals shows synchrony during the second period, with aggregate extreme positive affect. Moreover, the wife's affect in the first period reveals consistently mild negative affect, which aligns with the husband's aggregate extreme negative affect. Finally, they share low-positive and low-negative affective regimes throughout the entire third period, with just a few sparse affect extremes.

15.5 STOCHASTIC TRANSITION NETWORKS

15.5.1 Stochastic Transition Networks

As a way of depicting daily transitions in the data, we use stochastic transition networks (STNs). These STNs are derived from the vast literature on small-world networks, a method first proposed by Milgram (1967) for describing human friendship networks and acquaintance connection. The notion of small-word networks was later popularized by Watts and Strogatz (1998; Watts, 1999). In particular, Watts and Strogatz (1998, 1999) defined two key features in small-world networks, path length and neighboring cluster size. They then used these features to classify all networks into three major categories, namely (1) regular networks, (2) random networks, and (3) small-world networks. Path length represents the average steps needed to go from one node to another. Cluster size indicates the average connectedness of the nodes with their neighbors (i.e., the average number of edges connecting a node to its neighbors). These two aspects of the wiring pattern are correlated, but are not identical. For example, given a network with all nodes k being wired to each other, the path length would be one and cluster size $k - 1$.

Small-world networks have short characteristic path lengths just as random networks, but they are highly clustered just as regular networks. They have been used to characterize social networks (Amaral, DiazGuilera, Moreira, Goldberger, & Lipsitz, 2004), the collaboration graph of film actors, the power grid of the western United States (*cf.*, Watts & Strogatz, 1998), the world wide web (Albert, Jeong, & Barabási, 1999), and traffic patterns (Chowell, Hyman, Eubank, & Castillo-Chavez, 2003). Our development of STNs was inspired largely by features of small-world networks, but our focus resides primarily in how network-based approaches can be used to summarize the shared dynamics between two time series over time. The key features of small-world networks, namely, average path length and cluster size, are still an integral part of our approach but classifying networks into one of the three major types of networks, in terms of path length and cluster size, is not the main focus here. Rather, our STNs reflect several key adaptations designed specifically to extract co-varying dynamics in dyadic interaction data.

First, the "nodes" in our application are nonparametric, ordinal states thought to represent important affective states based on information from the data. In our empirical illustration, the ordinal states are taken to be the raw ratings on the PANAS items, or C_1 codes from the HS. Second, the wiring between nodes is constituted by the transition from one affective state to another, and the resultant network is thus more a *transition network*, as opposed to a static network. Third, our proposed networks have path lengths and cluster sizes that are stochastic across nodes and over time. Thus, they are stochastic networks (see Hsieh et al., 2008a, for more details).

15.5.2 Steps for Constructing STNs

We construct STNs as a way to represent the transition of the dyad between different affective states. Say, for instance, that the C_1 codes 0, 1, and 2 obtained from HS are used to define the states. Each STN is constructed as follows. Consider two variables P_H and Q_W representing the affect of two individuals in a dyad. Let the combination (p,q) of the C_1 codes for both people be the nine nodes of the network. For instance, the node (0,0) represents a state where both the husband and wife show extremely high levels on the particular affect of interest. By taking the node of the combination (p,q) on the first day as the starting point, we then draw a connecting line to the node of the corresponding combination on the second day, and so on until completing the entire sequence. A repeated transition would increase the width of the connecting line by a fixed amount. Thus, the width of the line between two nodes indicates the frequency of a specific transition. A transition from a given state to itself can be represented by a circle attaching to the node.

15.5.3 Empirical Illustration

Following the steps detailed earlier, Figure 15.4 presents STNs of the time series of each of the PANAS items for the husband and wife. All the items were rated on a scale of 1 to 5 so, in this particular case, each node in the STNs represents a possible rating on this five-point scale. Wirings—or edges—in these STNs reflect the transition in affect from one value to another and the thickness of the wiring depicts the frequency of such transition along the entire time series. Thus, a STN not only depicts the frequencies of endorsing the different intensity levels on the PANAS but also the transition probabilities of moving from one affect intensity level to another.

The plots in Figure 15.4a and d show that some affect variables have very similar transition patterns and other variables are very different from each other. Moreover, some networks display a relatively complex wiring, whereas others seem rather simple. In addition, most positive affect items have patterns of transition that spread across all nodes (i.e., data values) although with more frequency for higher nodes, but with the exception of the variables "inspired" and "proud" for the wife. In contrast, the negative affect variables show very similar patterns of transition. Such transitions cluster around very low values and, in many cases, without ever leaving the lowest node.

Based on results from our earlier HS analysis, we partition the entire 182-day series into three periods: (i.e., 1–69, 70–114, and 115–182). Within each of these periods, we expect the covariations between the dyad members to show a higher degree of stationarity than was found earlier by applying HS to the entire 182-day study span. The four STNs representing the husband and wife's positive affect's are reported in Figure 15.5, while those representing negative affect's are displayed in Figure 15.6. An inspection of these STNs reveals that they are not structurally regular, nor do they appear to be completely random. This is reasonable given that dyadic interactions can follow organized patterns but can also be easily perturbed by many internal and external factors.

Inspection of the STNs for positive affect for each of the three periods (panels b, c, and d in Figure 15.5) reveals distinct wiring patterns across periods. The network of the first period is tilted to the right side, in nodes that represent low PA for both individuals. The network of the second period, in contrast, features nodes of high and medium PA, showing frequent transitions to nodes with discrepant affect between the two individuals (e.g., nodes [0,1] and [0,2]). Finally, the network of the third period shows activity in nodes of low and middle PA for both individuals.

The STNs for negative affect (Figure 15.6) reveal a different type of synchrony between the transition of both individuals' affect. The wiring structure in the STN for the first period (panel b) is spread out, with

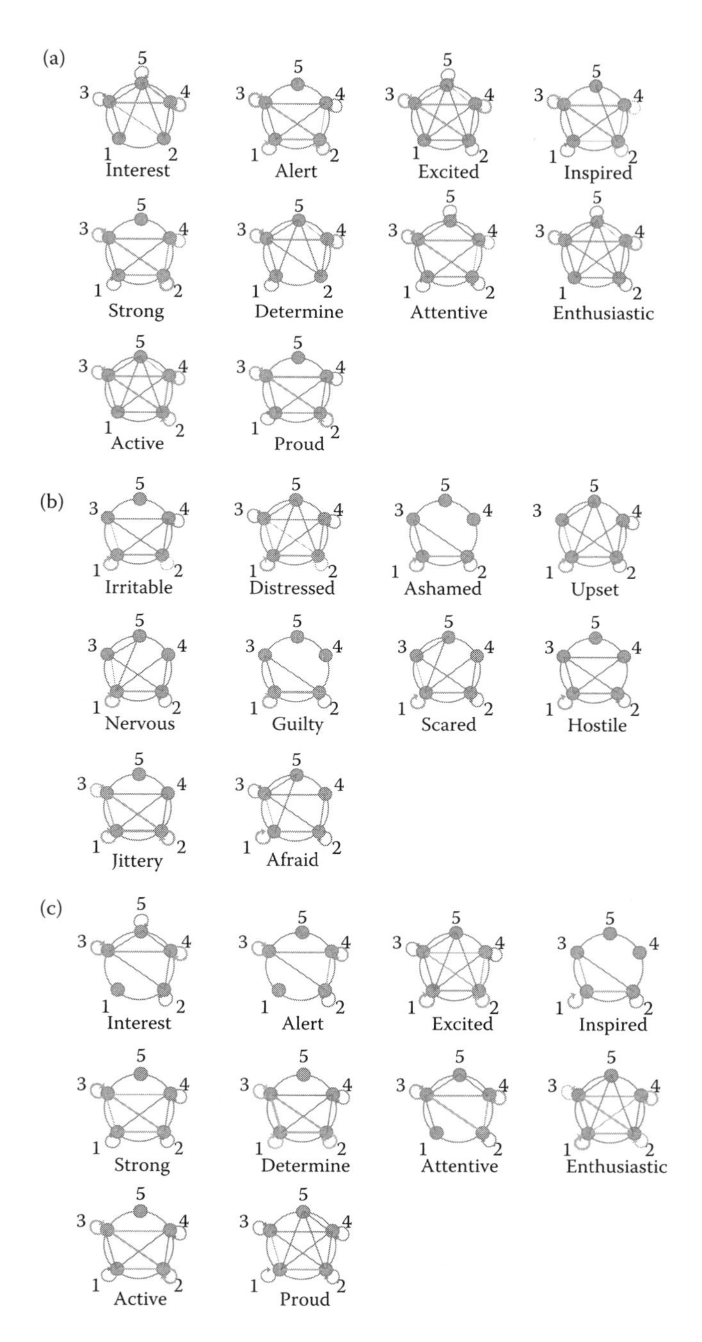

FIGURE 15.4 Stochastic transition networks (STNs) of self-reports of the husband (panels a and b) and wife (panels c and d) on the positive and negative affect items.

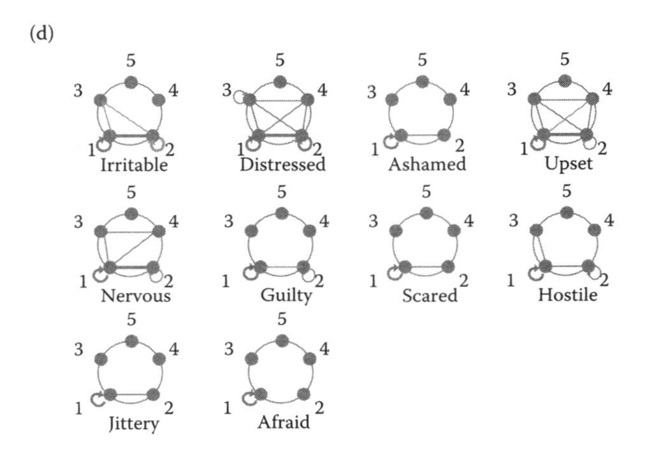

FIGURE 15.4 Continued.

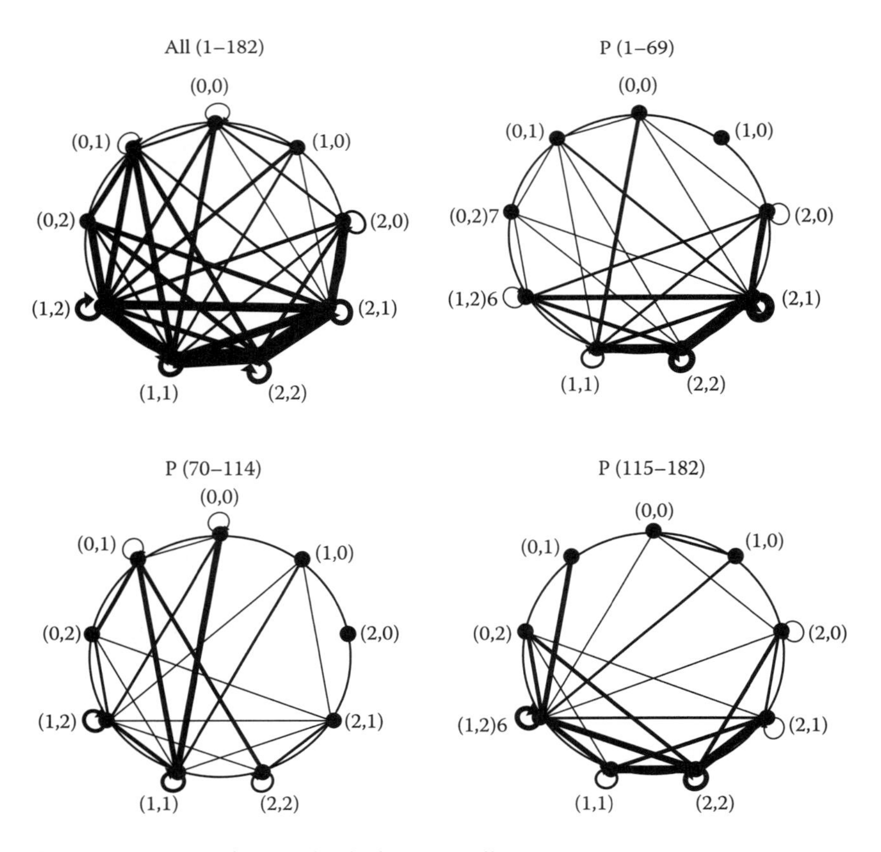

FIGURE 15.5 STN of interindividual positive affect.

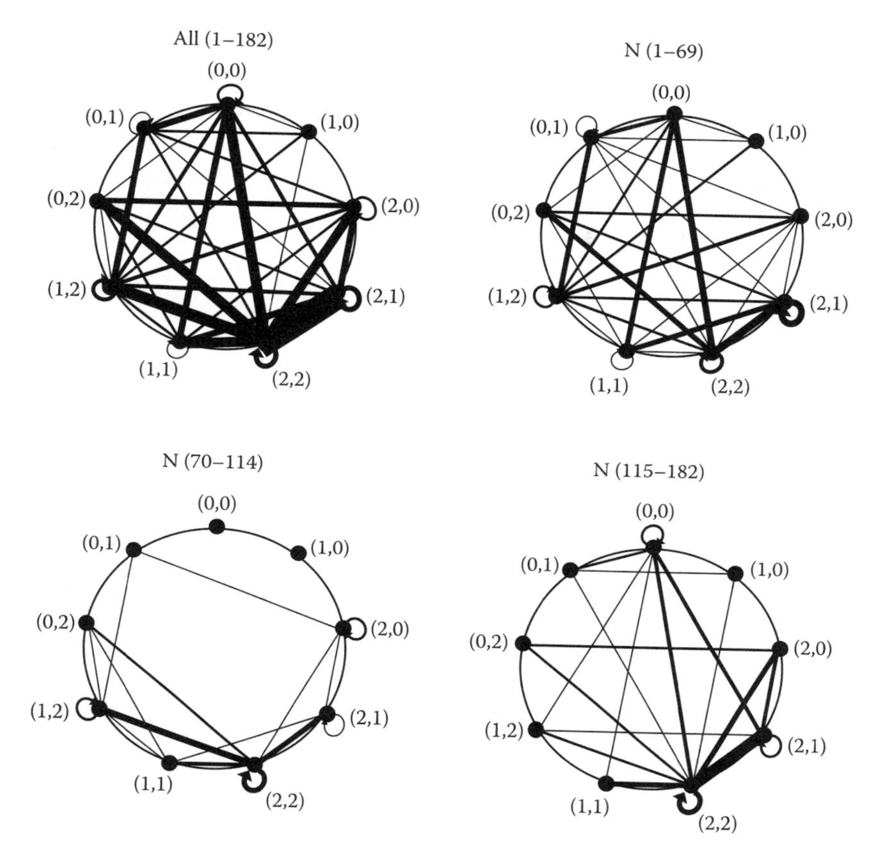

FIGURE 15.6 STN of interindividual negative affect.

multiple expressions of high NA and frequent transitions between opposite extreme states (e.g., between nodes [0,0] and [2,2]). This feature indicates that, during this period, the couple expresses high NA very often (i.e., nodes with code 0 are visited frequently), also showing some transitions between nodes of opposite emotional valence. The STNs of the second and third periods, however, show transitions clustered around lower levels of NA (e.g., nodes with code 2) and with a strong synchrony between both individuals (e.g., [2,2] node). However, whereas the transitions in the second period cluster around nodes of low negative affect with very few wirings between nonadjacent nodes, the STN of the third period is connected across all nodes.

In sum, Figures 15.5 and 15.6 reveal clear differences in the structure of the STNs corresponding to the three periods. These differences suggest distinct coupling patterns between both individuals' affect across these three periods. In our present formulation, only the first-order transition probabilities are used to construct the STNs. Higher-order lagged dependencies can, in principle, be incorporated if needed. However, appropriate graphical adaptations will have to be made (e.g., by using three-dimensional plots) to effectively convey such higher-order dependencies.

15.5.4 Simulation to Determine the Time-Varying Properties of STNs

We emphasize in our STNs differences in the frequency of wiring among the three networks. This is the reason why these networks are based on conditional transition probabilities as well as marginal probabilities, which are expressed in the thickness of the wiring between any two connected nodes. Thus an STN is simply a visual representation of the empirical transition probability matrix of the bivariate discrete time series over a period of time. One important restriction remains in the portrayal of the STNs, however. That is, an STN provides a snapshot of the probabilities of transitioning between different affective states/nodes for a pre-specified period. In cases where nonstationary dynamics are expected to emerge, and one transition probability matrix can no longer characterize the dynamics of all portions of the data, the information may not be immediately apparent from visual inspection of an STN.

To formally evaluate whether or not there are time-varying changes in the probabilities of transitioning between different affective nodes, we conducted a simulation study. The logic behind the simulation is as follows. We first computed one empirical transition probability matrix from each STN across the entire 182 days. For illustrative purposes, our simulation consists of two STNs: one involving the covariations between the husband's and the wife's positive affect, and the other involving the covariations with regard to negative affect. We then constructed an STN with wiring patterns determined by the transition probability matrix. This process was then repeated over a large number of Monte Carlo runs to yield multiple replications of time series whose values are simply the different affective nodes of the STNs (e.g., 0, 1, and 2 in our application). All of these simulated time series conformed to the same transition probability matrix. We then computed the L–Z complexity for each of these time series and their associated summary statistics. These summary statistics can then be compared with the

L–Z complexity of the observed empirical time series to see if the algorithmic complexity of the latter statistically exceeds the complexity contained in the simulated time series. To summarize, the simulation was conducted according to the following steps:

Step 1: A node of an STN is randomly selected based on the marginal distribution of nine nodes from a corresponding transition matrix of interest (i.e., the transition matrix for the dyad's covariations in positive affect or covariations in negative affect).
Step 2: From the starting node, a simulated trajectory of the same length as the empirical time series under comparison (e.g., 182 steps in this specific application) is simulated and its L–Z complexity is computed.
Step 3: The simulated trajectory is partitioned into three segments based on the results from HS (i.e., segments for days 1–69, 70–114, and 115–182), with L–Z complexity computed on each of them.
Step 4: Steps 1–3 are repeated a sufficiently large number of times (e.g., 1000 in our experiment).

The end product that arises from this sequence of steps is generically called a surrogate digital string. The simulated time series retains the second-order (i.e., second HS level) transition property of the original digital string through STN. These simulated digital strings are stationary and the resultant 99% confidence interval of the L–Z complexity of the simulated series captures the potential variability in L–Z complexity one may expect to get across different samples even though all of them conform to the same population transition probability matrix. If the transition probability matrix alone can sufficiently reproduce the patterns (or specifically, complexity) embedded within the observed digital string, then we should have the observed L–Z complexity measurement falling within the 99% simulated confidence regions. Consequently if the observed L–Z complexity measurement is beyond the simulated confidence regions, we see that there are patterns which could not be described through the STN. From this sense, the observed digital string is not stationary (with respect to the transition probability matrix used to generate the STN), or the lag-one transition probabilities alone cannot adequately capture the dynamics embedded in the data. Thus, this specific simulation is not a test of the stationarity of the data *per se*, but rather a test of the discrepancy

TABLE 15.2

Comparison between Observed and Simulated L–Z Complexity

	HP versus WP		HN versus WN	
	Observed	Simulated (99%)	Observed	Simulated (99%)
Overall	65	62/(55, 66)	59	56/(48, 62)
Period I	30	29/(24, 32)	31	26/(20, 31)
Period II	25	21/(17, 24)	15	19/(14, 23)
Period III	27	28/(24, 32)	22	27/(20, 31)

between the complexity of an actual set data and the complexity implied by a stationary lag-one transition probability matrix.

From this simulation we obtained four histograms of the L–Z complexity (i.e., entire series and each of the three segments) for positive affect and four histograms for negative affect. The results from this simulation are reported in Table 15.2. The values represent the observed estimates and the mode (and 99% range) of L–Z complexity. With regard to the overall time series, these results indicate that the observed trajectories of the dyad's dynamics are within the 99% range of complexities of the simulated trajectories generated from one overall transition probability matrix. When considering the different periods, only one of the six observed L–Z complexities of the segments fall outside the 99% simulated regions, and one falls on the region boundary. This result indicates that only the STNs of Period II on positive affect and of Period I on negative affect do not capture important features of the corresponding bivariate time series. This suggests that the transition probability matrix used for simulation purposes to a great extent captures an aggregate of the transition dynamics across the 182 days. Only some local changes and more complex patterns (e.g., regime changes) are overlooked. It is worth noting that the reliability of these inferences depends heavily upon the stability of L–Z complexity performed on finite length digital strings of base 9 (corresponding to the nine "nodes" of the STN).

The same simulation procedure can, in principle, be applied to transition matrices covering smaller windows of time (e.g., for each of the three periods identified by the HS). Our goal here is to illustrate a simple method for examining possible nonstationarity in the transition patterns across different categorical states over time. Although the procedure is relatively simple and straightforward, it is flexible enough for use with any time series data (nominal, ordinal, and interval). Our empirical illustration shows that the dynamics contained in the empirical time series were largely captured by one aggregate transition probability matrix, with the exception of the second period. The changes during this specific period were more complex than those predicted from a stationary lag-one transition matrix.

15.6 DISCUSSION

15.6.1 Summary Results and Application to Dyadic Interactions

In this paper, we introduced a set of nonparametric techniques for examining dyadic interactions with multivariate data. We illustrated some possibilities of using these techniques with empirical data on daily emotional experiences from two individuals in a couple. Our analyses yielded a number of results not immediately apparent in the observed data. First, hierarchical clustering based on L–Z mutual complexity revealed different clustering patterns of affect for the two individuals in the dyad. Whereas the husband's variables clustered in positive and negative affect separately, the wife's were mixed showing a less uniform complexity.

The L–Z mutual complexity can be used as an alternative distance measure for hierarchical clustering purposes. We have successfully applied this technique to data with multiple couples and found its performance to be more reliable than other clustering algorithms that use Kulback distance of spectrum densities derived from Walsh–Fourier transformations (Hsieh, Ferrer, Chen, & Chow, 2008b). Furthermore, the current findings from hierarchical clustering are quite similar to those obtained from dynamic factor analysis (Ferrer, 2006).

The second main result from our application concerns the segmentation of data at the factor level. Based on the different individual variables, we constructed "factors" or, rather, "segments" representing regions of the data with similar dynamics. Our HS analyses indicated the existence of three periods in the time series, each with different patterns of dynamics in the affective interrelations between the two individuals. Such differences were not immediately apparent in the observed data and would be difficult to detect with other existing methods. These results, showing nonstationarity of dynamics in the various segments, could then be used in further analyses investigating regime switching in more detail, such as using confirmatory techniques.

15.6.2 Methodological Implications and Future Extensions

The computational procedure introduced in this chapter is the HS algorithm. This is a decoding technique for mapping out possible regime changes underlying time-series data. In our analyses, we combined the results of HS with hierarchical clustering and actograms to examine similarity and differences in complexity among all the time series in the data. This information can also be used to identify groups of variables that exhibit synchrony—or coherence—on the unobservable trajectory of state-space and regime processes.

HS is a nonparametric bottom-up approach for exploring and discovering coupling relationships in dyadic dynamics. This technique involves simple yet informative computations that are applicable to other dyadic or more complex systems. More generally, this approach can be used to examine questions about dynamics in psychology and other social and behavioral sciences in which (a) knowledge about the driving forces underlying the data is rarely available, (b) statistical assumptions are not testable or justifiable, and (c) the time-series data available are relatively short. Under these conditions the HS can be used to decode the state-space vector and yield information about the possible regime changes on a relatively short time series under no parametric assumptions.

In our analyses, we demonstrated the use of the HS algorithm together with other aiding methods. Again, this is a new approach with promising possibilities for modeling dyadic interactions, but more research is needed to further examine its full potential. In particular, some possibilities to be examined in more detail include the minimum number of data points required to reliably detect information from random noise or the maximum number of variables that can be simultaneously included in the analyses.

In sum, we propose in this chapter a set of nonparametric methodologies for examining dyadic interactions. These exploratory techniques can handle multiple time-series data and capture complex dynamics based on multivariate relationships. We believe these techniques can facilitate the extraction of hidden dynamics in empirical data and serve as a basis for more confirmatory, model-based analysis.

ACKNOWLEDGMENT

This study was supported in part by grants from the National Science Foundation (BCS-05-27766, BCS-08-27021, and BCS-08-26844) and NIH-NINDS (R01 NS057146-01). All computer programs are available on the book's website.

REFERENCES

Amaral, L. A. N., DiazGuilera, A., Moreira, A. A., Goldberger, A. L., & Lipsitz, L. A. (2004). Emergence of complex dynamics in a simple model of signaling network. *Proceedings of the National Academy of Sciences, 101*, 155551–155555.

Albert, R., Jeong, H., & Barabási, A.-L. (1999). Diameter of the worldwide web. *Nature, 401*, 130–131.

Baron, R. M., Amazeen, P. G., & Beek, P. J. (1994). Local and global dynamics of social relations. In R. R. Vallacher & A. Nowak (Eds.), *Dynamical systems in social psychology* (pp. 111–138). San Diego, CA: Academic Press.

Boker, S. M., & Laurenceau, J.-P. (2006). Dynamical systems Modeling: An application to the regulation of intimacy and disclosure in marriage. In T.A. Walls & J.L. Schafer (Eds.), *Models for intensive longitudinal data* (pp. 195–218). New York: Oxford University Press.

Browne, M. W., & Nesselroade, J. R. (2005). Representing psychological processes with dynamic factor models: Some promising uses and extensions of ARMA time series models. In A. Maydeu-Olivares & J. J. McArdle (Eds.), *Advances in psychometrics: A festschrift to Roderick P. McDonald* (pp. 415–451). Mahwah, NJ: Erlbaum.

Bowlby, J. (1982). *Attachment and loss: Vol. 1. Attachment* (2nd ed.). New York: Basic Books. (Original work published 1969).

Butner, J., Diamond, L.M., & Hicks, A.M. (2007). Attachment style and two forms of affect corregulation between romantic partners. *Personal Relationships, 14*, 431–455.

Buder, E. (1991). A nonlinear dynamic model of social interaction. *Communications Research 18*(2), 174–198.

Campbell, L., & Kashy, D.A. (2002). Estimating actor, partner, and interaction effects for dyadic data using PROC MIXED and HLM: A guided tour. *Personal Relationships, 9*, 327–342.

Carlin, B.P., Gelfand, A.E., & Smith, A.F.M. (1992). Hierarchical Bayesian analysis of changepoints problems. *Applied Statistics, 41*, 389–405.

Chowell, G., Hyman, J. M., Eubank, S., & Castillo-Chavez, C. (2003). Scaling laws for the movement of people between locations in a large city. *Physical Review, 68*, 066102–066109.

Chow, S-M., Ferrer, E., & Nesselroade, J.R. (2007). An unscented Kalman filter approach to the estimation of nonlinear dynamical systems models. *Multivariate Behavioral Research, 42*, 283–321.

Cover, T.M., & Thomas, J.A. (1991). *Elements of information theory*. New York: John Wiley & Sons.

Felmlee, D. H. (2006). Application of dynamic systems analysis to dyadic interactions. In A.D. Ong & M. van Dulmen (Eds.), *Handbook of methods in positive psychology* (pp. 409–422). New York: Oxford University Press.

Felmlee, D. H., & Greenberg, D.F. (1999). A dynamic systems model of dyadic interaction. *Journal of Mathematical Sociology, 23*, 155–180.

Ferrer, E. (2006). Application of dynamic factor analysis to affective processes in dyads. In A.D. Ong & M. van Dulmen (Eds.), *Handbook of methods in positive psychology* (pp. 41–58). New York: Oxford University Press.

Ferrer, E., & Nesselroade, J.R. (2003). Modeling affective processes in dyadic relations via dynamic factor analysis. *Emotion, 3*, 344–360.

Ferrer, E., & Widaman, K. F. (2007). Dynamic factor analysis of dyadic affective processes with inter-group differences. In N. A. Card, J. Selig, & T. D. Little (Eds.), *Modeling dyadic and interdependent data in the development and behavioral sciences* (pp. 107–137). Hillsdale, NJ: Psychology Press.

Ferrer, E., Chen, S., Chow, S.-M., & Hsieh, F. (in press). Exploring nonstationary dynamics in dyadic interactions via hierarchical segmentation. *Psychometrika*.

Gottman, J. M., Murray, J. D., Swanson, C. C., Tyson, R., & Swanson, K. R. (2002). *The mathematics of marriage: Dynamic nonlinear models*. Cambridge, MA: MIT Press.

Hsieh, F., Hwang, C-R., Lee, H-C., Lan, Y-C., & Horng, S-B. (2006). Testing and mapping non-stationarity in animal behavioral processes: A case study on an individual female bean weevil. *Journal of Theoretical Biology, 238*, 805–816.

Hsieh, F., Ferrer, E., Wang, Y.-F., & Chen, S.-C.(2008b). *Hierarchical clustering affective time series with mutual algorithmic complexity as pseudo-distance*. Technical Report. Department of Statistics, University of California, Davis.

Kalman, R. E. (1960). A new approach to linear filtering and prediction problems. *Transactions of the ASME–Journal of Basic Engineering, Series D, 82*, 35–45.

Kaspar, F., & Schuster, H. G. (1987). Easily calculable measure of the complexity of spatiotemporal patterns. *Physical, Review. A. 36*, 842–848.

Kenny, D.A., Kashy, D.A., Cook, W.L., & Simpson, J.A. (2006). *Dyadic data analysis*. New York: Guilford Press.

Kim, C.-J., & Nelson, C. R. (1999). *State-space models with regime switching: Classical and Gibbs-sampling approaches with applications*. Cambridge, MA: MIT Press.

Laurenceau, J.-P., Troy, A.B., & Carver, C.S. (2005). Two distinct emotional experiences in romantic relationships: Effects of perceptions regarding approach of intimacy and avoidance of conflict. *Personality and Social Psychology Bulletin, 31*, 1123–1133.

Lotka, A. J. (1925). *Elements of physical biology*. Baltimore, MD: Williams and Wilkins.

Manuca, R., & Savit, R. (1996). Stationarity and nonstationarity in time series analysis. *Physica D. 99*, 134–161.

Mikulincer, M., & Shaver, P.R. (2007). *Attachment in adulthood: Structure, dynamics, and change*. New York: Guilford Press.

Milgram, S. (1967). The small-world problem. *Psychology Today, 1*(1), 60–67.

Newtson, D. (1993). The dynamics of action and interaction. In L. B. Smith & E. Thelen (Eds.), *A dynamic systems approach to development: Applications* (pp. 241–264). Cambridge, MA: MIT Press.

Rabiner, L. R. (1989). A tutorial on Hidden markov models and selected applications in speech recognition. *Proceedings of the IEEE, 77*, 257–286.

Rabiner, L., & Juang, B.-H (1993) Fundamentals of Speech Recognition. Prentice Hall, New Jersey.

Raudenbush, S.W., Brennan, R.T., & Barnett, R.C. (1995). A multivariate hierarchical model for studying psychological change within married couples. *Journal of Family Psychology, 9*, 161–174.

Song, H., & Ferrer, E. (2009). State-space modeling of dynamic psychological processes via the Kalman smoother algorithm: Rationale, finite sample properties, and applications. *Structural Equation Modeling, 16*, 338–363.

Thomson, A., & Bolger, N. (1999). Emotional transmission in couples under stress. *Journal of Marriage & the Family, 61*, 38–48.

Viterbi, A. J. (1967). Error bounds for convolutional codes and an asymptotically optimal decoding algorithm. *IEEE Transactions on Information Theory, IT-13*, 260–269.

Volterra, V. (1926). Fluctuations in the abundance of a species considered mathematically. *Nature, 118*, 558–560.

Watson, D., Clark, L. A., & Tellegen, A. (1988). Development and validation of brief measures of positive and negative affect: The PANAS scales. *Journal of Personality and Social Psychology, 54*, 1063–1070.

Watts, D.J. (1999). *Small Worlds: The dynamics of networks between order and randomness.* Princeton, NJ: Princeton University Press.

Watts, D.J., & Strogatz, S.H. (1998). Collective dynamics of 'small-world' networks. *Nature, 393*, 440–442.

Weigend, A. S., Mangeas, M., & Srivastava, A. N. (1995). Nonlinear gated experts for time series: Discovering regimes and avoiding overfitting. *International J. of Neural Systems, 6*, 373–399.

West, M., & Harrison, J. (1997). *Bayesian Forecasting and dynamic models.* (2nd ed.). New York: Springer.

Winfree, A. T. (1987) *The Timing of Biological Clocks.* New York: Scientific American Library.

Author Index

C

D

E

F

G

H

I

J

K

L

M

N

O

P

Q

R

S

T

U

V

W

X

Y

Z

Subject Index

C

D

I

K

L